Knee Osteoarthritis: Assessment, Diagnosis and Treatment

Knee Osteoarthritis: Assessment, Diagnosis and Treatment

Edited by Joyce Kennedy

hayle medical

New York

Hayle Medic Floor,
750 Third Av USA
New York, N

Visit us World Wide Web at:
www.h edical.com

ISBN: 978-1-64647-101-0

Cataloging-in-Publication Data

Knee osteoarthritis : assessment, diagnosis and treatment / edited by Joyce Kennedy.
p. cm.
Includes bibliographical references and index.
ISBN 978-1-64647-101-0
1. Osteoarthritis. 2. Knee--Diseases. 3. Knee--Diseases--Diagnosis.
4. Knee--Diseases--Treatment. I. Kennedy, Joyce.
RC931.O67 K64 2022
616.722 3--dc23

Table of Contents

Preface

Over the recent decade, advancements and applications have progressed exponentially. This has led to the increased interest in this field and projects are being conducted to enhance knowledge. The main objective of this book is to present some of the critical challenges and provide insights into possible solutions. This book will answer the varied questions that arise in the field and also provide an increased scope for furthering studies.

Osteoarthritis is a condition in which the cartilage between joints wears away. Osteoarthritis can occur in specific joints only, such as knee osteoarthritis which only affects the knee joints. The symptoms of knee arthritis include pain, feeling of warmth in the joint, swelling, decreased mobility of the knee, stiffness in the knee, etc. The diagnosis of knee osteoarthritis requires a physical examination of the symptoms experienced, X-ray and MRI scans. Blood tests can ensure that other conditions such as rheumatoid arthritis are ruled out. The goals of the treatment of knee osteoarthritis are to return mobility and relieve the pain. The chief strategies employed to manage the condition include weight loss, stretching exercises, using braces to support the knee and relieve pressure, prescription of anti-inflammatory and pain relieving drugs, injection of corticosteroids into the knees, etc. This book includes some of the vital pieces of work being conducted across the world, on various topics related to the assessment, diagnosis and treatment of knee osteoarthritis. It provides significant information on osteoarthritis to help develop a good understanding. The book is appropriate for students seeking detailed information of this medical condition as well as for experts.

I hope that this book, with its visionary approach, will be a valuable addition and will promote interest among readers. Each of the authors has provided their extraordinary competence in their specific fields by providing different perspectives as they come from diverse nations and regions. I thank them for their contributions.

Editor

1

Dose-response relationship between lower serum magnesium level and higher prevalence of knee chondrocalcinosis

Chao Zeng[1], Jie Wei[2,7], Robert Terkeltaub[3,4], Tuo Yang[1], Hyon K. Choi[5], Yi-lun Wang[1], Dong-xing Xie[1], David J. Hunter[6], Yuqing Zhang[5], Hui Li[1], Yang Cui[8], Liang-jun Li[1,9] and Guang-hua Lei[1*]

Abstract

Background: The aim was to assess serum magnesium levels in relation to prevalence of knee chondrocalcinosis in two population-based Chinese studies.

Methods: Data included in this analysis consisted of two population-based cross-sectional studies, i.e., the Xiangya Hospital Health Management Center Study and the Xiangya Osteoarthritis (XO) Study I. A bilateral knee anteroposterior radiograph was obtained from each subject. Radiographic knee chondrocalcinosis was present if there was definite linear cartilage calcification. Serum magnesium concentration was measured using the chemiluminescence method. We examined the relation of serum magnesium levels to prevalence of knee chondrocalcinosis using generalized estimating equations.

Results: The prevalence of knee chondrocalcinosis was 1.4% in the Xiangya Hospital Health Management Center Study (n = 12,631). Compared with the lowest tertile, the age, sex and body mass index (BMI)-adjusted odds ratios (ORs) of chondrocalcinosis were 0.59 (95% CI 0.40–0.87) and 0.49 (95% CI 0.33–0.72) in the second and the third tertiles of serum magnesium, respectively (P for trend <0.001). The prevalence of knee chondrocalcinosis in the XO Study I (n = 1316) was 4.1%. The age, sex and BMI-adjusted ORs of chondrocalcinosis were 0.67 (95% CI 0.34–1.30) in the second and 0.45 (95% CI 0.21–0.94) in the third tertile of serum magnesium when compared with the lowest tertile (P for trend = 0.030). Similar results were observed in men and women in both studies. Adjusting for additional potential confounders did not change the results materially.

Conclusions: Subjects with lower levels of serum magnesium, even within the normal range, had higher prevalence of knee chondrocalcinosis in a dose-response relationship manner, suggesting that magnesium may have a preventive or therapeutic potential for knee chondrocalcinosis.

Keywords: Chondrocalcinosis, Magnesium, Knee

Background

Calcium pyrophosphate deposition (CPPD) in articular fibrocartilage and hyaline cartilage, termed chondrocalcinosis, has been considered to be associated with both aging and osteoarthritis [1]. CPPD, together with basic calcium phosphate (BCP), are the two main components of calcium-containing crystals in cartilage in osteoarthritis [2, 3]. While most subjects with chondrocalcinosis have no clinical symptoms (asymptomatic CPPD) [4], CPPD may promote articular degeneration (osteoarthritis with CPPD) and traffic of the crystals from articular cartilage into the joint space; and thus can stimulate acute episodic crystal arthritis and can also lead to chronic inflammatory arthritis.

To date, only a few risk factors have been identified for the occurrence of chondrocalcinosis. Studies have shown that prevalence of chondrocalcinosis varied in different ethnic groups. For example, prevalence of chondrocalcinosis was much lower in Beijing Osteoarthritis Study participants (1.8% in men, 2.7% in women) than that in white

* Correspondence: lei_guanghua@csu.edu.cn
[1]Department of Orthopaedics, Xiangya Hospital, Central South University, #87 Xiangya Road, Changsha, Hunan Province 410008, China
Full list of author information is available at the end of the article

subjects among the predominantly white participants in the Framingham Study (6.2% in men, 7.7% in women) [5]. Several studies also found that knee chondrocalcinosis is associated with low levels of serum magnesium [6–11]. For instance, patients with hypomagnesemia (e.g., poor parenteral nutrition, short bowel syndrome, Gitelman syndrome or familial heredity) had a much higher prevalence of chondrocalcinosis (up to 23.1%) [6–11]. However, these findings were often based on subjects with extremely low serum magnesium, and it remains unclear whether more modest variations of magnesium levels observed in the general population are associated with the prevalence of chondrocalcinosis. Such potential associations and their quantification would have an implication in public health and clinical practices.

To fill in this knowledge gap, we used data collected from two large population-based studies (i.e., Xiangya Hospital Health Management Center Study and Xiangya Osteoarthritis (XO) Study I) and examined the relation of serum magnesium levels with the prevalence of knee chondrocalcinosis and to determine the shape of the dose-response relationship between serum magnesium levels and the prevalence of knee chondrocalcinosis.

Methods

Study population

Xiangya Hospital Health Management Center Study

Subjects included in this study were residents living in Hunan, China, who were undergoing routine health examination at Xiangya Hospital, Central South University, China. The study design has been published elsewhere [12–14]. In brief, routine health checkup included anthropometric (e.g., height, weight, etc.), basic clinical examination (e.g., blood pressure, heart rate, etc.), and biochemical (e.g., blood routine examination, hepatic function, renal function, trace elements test, etc.) and imaging tests (e.g., chest radiography, weight-bearing bilateral anteroposterior knee radiography, etc.). Subjects included in the current analysis were those who: (1) had health checkup between October 2013 and December 2015; (2) were age ≥40 years; (3) underwent a serum magnesium test; and (4) had bilateral weight-bearing anteroposterior radiographs. All interviewers, clinical examiners and x-ray technicians were trained by the principal investigators (CZ and GL) before the study began.

Of 14,715 participants who underwent routine health examination, 2081 (14.1%) were excluded from the analysis for the following reasons: (1) age <40 years old (n = 1408); (2) low quality of weight-bearing anteroposterior knee radiographs (n = 63); (3) the Kellgren-Lawrence (K-L) [15] grades of both knees were 4 (n = 8); and (4) repeated health examinations in the same person during the study period (n = 604). Finally, 12,631 participants were included in the analysis.

Xiangya Osteoarthritis Study I (XO Study I)

Subjects included in this study were a randomly selected sample of residents, age ≥50 years, from eight rural mountainous communities of Longshan County [16], Hunan Province, for a study of osteoarthritis. All of the villages in the selected communities were listed in a random order. Beginning with the first village in the first community, all residents age ≥50 years were invited to participate in our study. The village-to-village recruitment continued until the number of subjects in that community met the predetermined quota according to the Sixth National Census Data of Longshan County (2010). Subjects were recruited at the site near their home and were transported to the hospital for interview and clinical examination between November 2015 and January 2016. Trained health professional interviewers administered a standardized questionnaire that focused on sociodemographic factors, lifestyle habits, joint symptoms, joint functions, quality of life, dietary intake, medication use and other potential risk factors for osteoarthritis. Clinical examination, laboratory testing and radiography were also conducted at the time of interview. All interviewers, clinical examiners and x-ray technicians were trained under the supervision of the study principal investigators (CZ and GL).

Of 1739 age-eligible (i.e., age ≥50 years) residents randomly selected in Longshan County, 270 (15.5%) subjects declined to participate the study. There was no significant difference in sex and age distribution between subjects who consented to participate and who declined ($P = 0.42$ and 0.47, respectively). Among 1469 participants in the XO Study I, 153 were excluded from the analysis because of: (1) history of lower limb surgery (n = 37); (2) history of pelvic surgery (n = 1); (3) lower extremity disability due to cerebrovascular diseases (n = 2) or spinal diseases (n = 2); (4) rheumatoid arthritis (n = 61); (5) unavailability of knee radiographs (n = 3); (6) low quality of weight-bearing anteroposterior radiographs of the knees (n = 1); (7) K-L grades of 4 (n = 5) in both knees; and (8) unavailability of a serum magnesium test (n = 41). Finally, 1316 participants were included in the analysis.

Blood biochemical analysis

All blood samples were drawn after a 12-hour overnight fast and were stored at 4 °C until analysis. The serum magnesium concentration was measured using the chemiluminescence method by Beckman Coulter AU 5800 (Beckman Coulter Inc., Brea, CA, USA). The inter-assay and intra-assay coefficients of variation were tested by low concentrations (0.60 mmol/L of serum magnesium) and high concentrations (1.00 mmol/L of serum magnesium) of standard human samples. The intra-assay coefficients of variation were 1.86% (0.60 mmol/L) and 1.65% (1.00 mmol/L) for serum magnesium, and the inter-assay coefficients of variation were 1.87% (0.60 mmol/L) and 1.70% (1.00 mmol/L) for serum magnesium. Measuring methods and reliability data of potential confounders (e.g., serum parathyroid hormone, iron, ferritin, total iron binding capacity, calcium, copper, zinc, phosphorus and vitamin D) are shown in Additional file 1.

Assessment of radiographic knee chondrocalcinosis

All radiographs were assessed by two orthopedic surgeons (TY and YLW) who were blinded to subjects' clinical symptoms and biochemical test results. Radiographic chondrocalcinosis was defined as present when there was evidence of definite linear cartilage calcification in the knee [17]. Specifically, prior to starting the assessment, these two orthopedists re-read 200 radiographs from the Osteoarthritis Initiative (OAI) to calibrate their reading. Formal readings of batches of randomly selected radiographs did not start until the readers reached a high level of agreement with previous readings from OAI (the specific cutoff of simple kappa for inter-rater reliability was 0.70). During the formal reading, one batch of knee radiographs (100 radiographs) consisting of 10 previously read radiographs selected at random and 90 unread radiographs were mingled and read. For each batch, 90 unread radiographs were used to test inter-rater reliability and 10 previously read radiographs were used to test intra-rater reliability, respectively. Two readers both assessed all radiographs and inconsistencies were resolved through discussion. The kappa value for reliability readings of radiographs from Xiangya Hospital Health Management Center Study was 0.72 (95% CI 0.67 – 0.77) for inter-rater reliability and 0.76 (95% CI 0.67–0.85) for intra-rater reliability. The kappa value for reliability readings of radiographs from XO Study I was 0.75 (95% CI 0.68–0.83) for inter-rater reliability and 0.80 (95% CI 0.65–0.94) for intra-rater reliability.

Statistical analysis

Continuous data were expressed as the mean ± standard deviation, and categorical data were expressed as proportion (percentage). The serum magnesium concentration was classified into three categories based on the tertiles distribution in each study population (i.e., ≤ 0.86, 0.87–0.91 and ≥ 0.92 mmol/L in the Xiangya Hospital Health Management Center Study and ≤ 0.89, 0.90–0.95 and ≥ 0.96 mmol/L in the XO Study I). We calculated the sex-specific prevalence of chondrocalcinosis for each category of serum magnesium. We examined the association of serum magnesium categories and prevalence of chondrocalcinosis using generalized estimating equations (GEE) [18], adjusting for the potential confounders (knee specific analysis). Odds ratios (OR) and related 95% confidence intervals (95% CI) of chondrocalcinosis among different categories of serum magnesium were calculated using the PROC GENMOD procedure in SAS with binomial distribution and logit links, and the lowest tertile of serum magnesium was considered as the reference. We also calculated the OR and the related 95% CI by using the category ≤0.70 mmol/L (dividing the lowest category of serum magnesium into two categories: ≤0.70 mmol/L and 0.71–0.86 in the Xiangya Hospital Health Management Center Study, and the category ≤0.70 mmol/L and 0.71–0.89 in the XO Study I) as the reference group. Specifically, in the Xiangya Hospital Health Management Center Study we first adjusted for age (40–49, 50–59, 60–69, ≥70 years), body mass index (BMI) (<25, ≥25 kg/m^2) and sex (male, female). Then we added each of the following covariates separately: serum iron (tertiles), serum ferritin (tertiles), serum calcium, serum zinc (tertiles), serum copper (tertiles), serum phosphorus (tertiles), education (high school or above, lower than high school) and occupation (manual labor, non-manual labor) in the regression model adjusted for age, sex and BMI. In the XO Study I, we first adjusted for age (50–59, 60–69, ≥70 years), BMI (<25, ≥25 kg/m^2) and sex (male, female), and then added each of the following covariates separately in the regression models. These covariates included knee injury, serum parathyroid (tertiles), serum iron (tertiles), serum total iron binding

Table 1 Basic characteristics of the population in the Xiangya Hospital Health Management Center Study (n = 12,631)

	Tertiles of serum Mg (mmol/L)		
	1 (≤0.86)	2 (0.87–0.91)	3 (≥0.92)
Number	4633	3720	4278
Median Mg level (mmol/L)	0.83	0.89	0.95
Sex (female, %)	45.3	42.5	40.9
Age (years)	52.1 ± 8.1	52.4 ± 8.1	52.5 ± 7.9
40–49 (%)	43.5	41.1	39.5
50–59 (%)	37.5	39.5	40.4
60–69 (%)	15.2	15.9	17.2
≥70 (%)	3.8	3.5	2.9
BMI (kg/m^2)	24.5 ± 3.4	24.4 ± 3.3	24.4 ± 3.2
<25 (%)	57.6	59.2	58.6
≥25 (%)	42.4	40.8	41.4
Serum iron (μmol/L)	18.1 ± 6.5	18.4 ± 6.3	18.9 ± 6.5
Serum ferritin (μg/L)	78.4 ± 67.3	78.3 ± 68.2	81.5 ± 62.8
Serum calcium (mmol/L)	2.4 ± 0.1	2.4 ± 0.1	2.4 ± 0.1
Serum zinc (μmol/L)	13.1 ± 2.5	13.5 ± 2.6	13.7 ± 3.1
Serum copper (μmol/L)	16.1 ± 3.6	16.2 ± 3.4	16.8 ± 3.8
Serum phosphorus (mmol/L)	1.2 ± 0.2	1.2 ± 0.2	1.2 ± 0.2
Education (high school or above, %)	42.3	49.8	49.0
Occupation (manual labor, %)	20.1	17.2	17.5

Mg magnesium, *BMI* body mass index

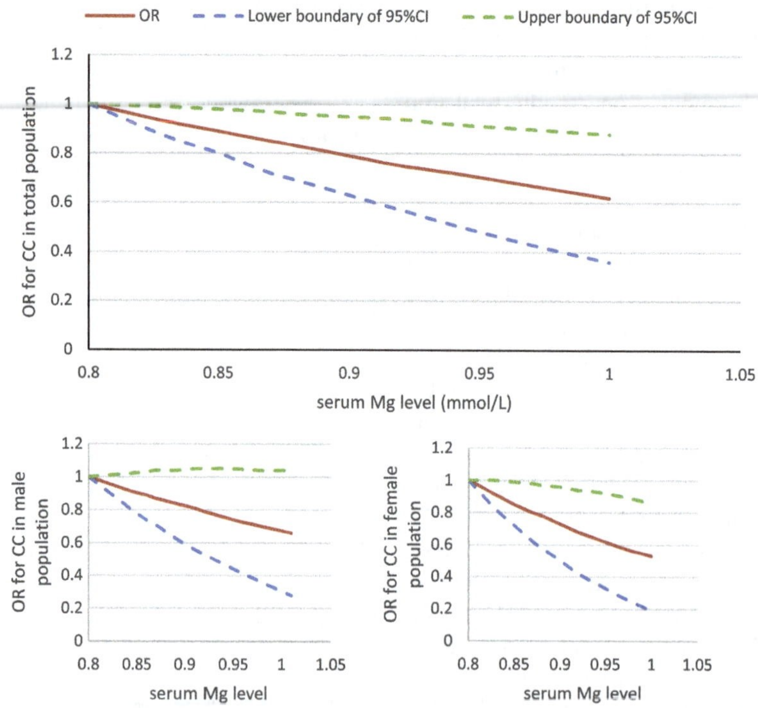

Fig. 1 Dose-response relationship between serum magnesium (Mg) level and the odds ratio (OR) for knee chondrocalcinosis (CC) in the Xiangya Hospital Health Management Center Study. CI, confidence interval

capacity (tertiles), serum unsaturated iron binding capacity (tertiles), serum calcium (tertiles), serum 25(OH)D (tertiles), serum zinc (tertiles), serum copper (tertiles), serum phosphorus (tertiles), education (educated, non-educated) and occupation (farmer, non-farmer).

In addition, we performed sex-specific analysis to examine the levels of serum magnesium and prevalence of chondrocalcinosis. The dose-response relationship between levels of serum magnesium and the prevalence of knee chondrocalcinosis was evaluated by restricted cubic splines regression with two knots defined by the tertile distribution of serum magnesium [19, 20]. We also used the value 0.7 mmol/L as an additional knot, to evaluate the dose-response association between serum magnesium and the prevalence of knee chondrocalcinosis.

Results

Xiangya Hospital Health Management Center Study

Of the remaining 12631 participants from the initially included 14,715 participants, 43.0% (n = 5428) were

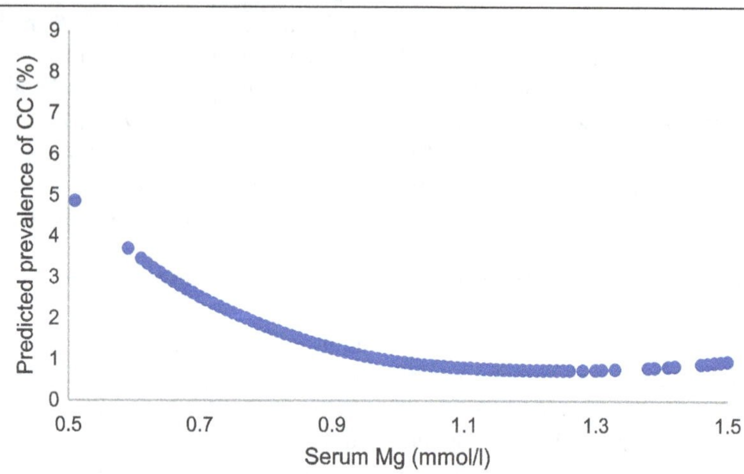

Fig. 2 Association between serum magnesium (Mg) and predicted prevalence of chondrocalcinosis (CC) analyzed by spline regression in the Xiangya Hospital Health Management Center Study

Table 2 Association between serum Mg and knee chondrocalcinosis in the Xiangya Hospital Health Management Center Study (n = 12,631)

	Tertiles of serum Mg (mmol/L)			*P* for trend
	1 (≤0.86)	2 (0.87–0.91)	3 (≥0.92)	
Total				
N for knee*	9263	7438	8497	-
Knee chondrocalcinosis (%)	1.3	0.8	0.6	-
Model 1 (95% CI)	1.00 (reference)	0.59 (0.40, 0.87)	0.49 (0.33, 0.72)	<0.001
Model 2 (95% CI)	1.00 (reference)	0.59 (0.39, 0.89)	0.53 (0.36, 0.78)	0.001
Model 3 (95% CI)	1.00 (reference)	0.69 (0.36, 1.32)	0.38 (0.20, 0.71)	0.002
Model 4 (95% CI)	1.00 (reference)	0.60 (0.41, 0.89)	0.48 (0.33, 0.71)	<0.001
Model 5 (95% CI)	1.00 (reference)	0.58 (0.39, 0.88)	0.52 (0.35, 0.78)	0.001
Model 6 (95% CI)	1.00 (reference)	0.57 (0.38, 0.86)	0.49 (0.33, 0.73)	<0.001
Model 7 (95% CI)	1.00 (reference)	0.60 (0.41, 0.89)	0.48 (0.33, 0.72)	<0.001
Model 8 (95% CI)	1.00 (reference)	0.83 (0.43, 1.58)	0.46 (0.23, 0.90)	0.021
Male				
N for knee*	5065	4279	5058	-
Knee chondrocalcinosis (%)	1.4	0.7	0.5	-
Model 1 (95% CI)	1.00 (reference)	0.56 (0.33, 0.95)	0.43 (0.25, 0.74)	0.002
Model 2 (95% CI)	1.00 (reference)	0.54 (0.31, 0.96)	0.45 (0.26, 0.78)	0.003
Model 3 (95% CI)	1.00 (reference)	0.65 (0.27, 1.56)	0.37 (0.16, 0.84)	0.017
Model 4 (95% CI)	1.00 (reference)	0.57 (0.34, 0.98)	0.42 (0.24, 0.73)	0.002
Model 5 (95% CI)	1.00 (reference)	0.54 (0.30, 0.94)	0.45 (0.26, 0.78)	0.003
Model 6 (95% CI)	1.00 (reference)	0.54 (0.31, 0.94)	0.41 (0.24, 0.72)	0.001
Model 7 (95% CI)	1.00 (reference)	0.57 (0.33, 0.98)	0.42 (0.24, 0.73)	0.002
Model 8 (95% CI)	1.00 (reference)	0.92 (0.40, 2.11)	0.51 (0.21, 1.24)	0.134
Female				
N for knee*	4198	3159	3494	-
Knee chondrocalcinosis (%)	1.2	0.9	0.8	-
Model 1 (95% CI)	1.00 (reference)	0.64 (0.36, 1.13)	0.54 (0.30, 0.96)	0.034
Model 2 (95% CI)	1.00 (reference)	0.65 (0.36, 1.19)	0.60 (0.33, 1.09)	0.094
Model 3 (95% CI)	1.00 (reference)	0.78 (0.29, 2.13)	0.41 (0.14, 1.21)	0.091
Model 4 (95% CI)	1.00 (reference)	0.65 (0.37, 1.15)	0.54 (0.31, 0.96)	0.035
Model 5 (95% CI)	1.00 (reference)	0.65 (0.36, 1.18)	0.59 (0.33, 1.07)	0.081
Model 6 (95% CI)	1.00 (reference)	0.65 (0.35, 1.19)	0.60 (0.33, 1.10)	0.096
Model 7 (95% CI)	1.00 (reference)	0.65 (0.36, 1.14)	0.54 (0.30, 0.96)	0.034
Model 8 (95% CI)	1.00 (reference)	0.67 (0.24, 1.88)	0.37 (0.13, 1.12)	0.073

Model 1 included age (40–49, 50–59, 60–69, ≥70 years), body mass index (BMI) (<25, ≥25 kg/m^2) and sex (age and BMI for the sex subgroup) (n = 12,631)
Model 2 added serum iron (tertiles) on the basis of model 1 (n = 12,149)
Model 3 added serum ferritin (tertiles) on the basis of model 1 (n = 5113)
Model 4 added serum calcium (tertiles) on the basis of model 1 (n = 12,479)
Model 5 added serum zinc (tertiles) on the basis of model 1 (n = 12,154)
Model 6 added serum copper (tertiles) on the basis of model 1 (n = 12,153)
Model 7 added serum phosphorus (tertiles) on the basis of model 1 (n = 12490)
Model 8 added education (high school or above, lower than high school) and occupation (manual labor, non-manual labor) on the basis of model 1 (n = 5844)
*Five right knees and four left knees with Kellgren-Lawrence grade 4were excluded from analysis (data from the contralateral knees were retained)
Mg magnesium, *N* number, *CI* confidence interval

Table 3 Basic characteristics of the study population in XO Study I (n = 1316)

	Tertiles of serum Mg (mmol/L)		
	1 (≤0.89)	2 (0.90-0.95)	3 (≥0.96)
Number	490	400	426
Median Mg level (mmol/L)	0.85	0.92	1.00
Sex (female, %)	48.6	50.3	55.2
Age (years)	63.6 ± 8.9	63.3 ± 8.4	61.6 ± 8.5
50–59 (%)	37.1	36.3	46.4
60–69 (%)	36.3	40.0	34.9
≥70 (%)	26.7	23.8	18.7
BMI (kg/m^2)	24.1 ± 3.5	24.3 ± 3.9	24.3 ± 3.4
< 25 (%)	67.6	61.0	59.9
≥25 (%)	32.4	39.0	40.1
Knee injury (yes, %)	5.5	3.8	5.2
Serum PTH (μmol/L)	52.5 ± 38.0	54.8 ± 23.1	51.3 ± 20.2
Serum iron (μmol/L)	20.2 ± 8.6	19.8 ± 7.2	20.3 ± 7.8
Serum TIBC (μmol/L)	58.3 ± 11.3	59.1 ± 11.6	60.2 ± 11.4
Serum UIBC (μmol/L)	38.2 ± 13.5	39.5 ± 13.2	40.0 ± 13.1
Serum calcium (mmol/L)	2.3 ± 0.1	2.3 ± 0.1	2.3 ± 0.1
Serum 25(OH)D (μg/L)	25.8 ± 11.3	24.9 ± 9.9	25.9 ± 10.9
Serum zinc (μmol/L)	17.3 ± 3.5	18.5 ± 3.7	19.9 ± 6.1
Serum copper (μmol/L)	16.3 ± 3.2	16.4 ± 3.7	16.8 ± 3.5
Serum phosphorus (mmol/L)	1.2 ± 0.2	1.2 ± 0.2	1.2 ± 0.2
Education (educated, %)	70.2	66.5	67.8
Occupation (farmer, %)	85.5	87.3	85.7

Mg magnesium, *BMI* body mass index, *PTH* parathyroid hormone, *TIBC*, total iron binding capacity, *UIBC* unsaturated iron-binding capacity

women, the average age was 52.3 ± 8.0 years, and the mean BMI was 24.5 kg/m^2 (SD = 3.3 kg/m^2). The prevalence of knee chondrocalcinosis was 1.3% in men and 1.5% in women (Table 1).

As shown in Fig. 1, serum magnesium, even within the normal range, was inversely associated with the OR for knee chondrocalcinosis in a dose-response-relationship manner (test for trend $P = 0.03$ for total population; $P = 0.16$ for the male population; $P = 0.05$ for the female population). The prevalence of knee chondrocalcinosis (knee-specific analysis) decreased from 1.3% in the lowest tertile of serum magnesium to 0.8% in the second, and 0.6% in the highest tertile of serum magnesium. Figure 2 showed the linear association between the serum magnesium and predicted prevalence of chondrocalcinosis. After adjusting for age, sex and BMI, the ORs for knee chondrocalcinosis were 0.59 (95% CI 0.40–0.87) in the middle and 0.49 (95% CI 0.33–0.72) in the highest tertile of serum magnesium, respectively, compared with the lowest tertile (*P* value for trend <0.001). Adding each of the potential confounders (e.g., serum iron, ferritin, calcium, zinc, copper and phosphorus) into the age, sex and BMI-adjusted model, or sensitivity analysis with exclusion of participants with chronic renal failure, also did not change the results materially. The association was also consistent in men and women (Table 2). When 0.70 mmol/L was used as an additional knot for spline regression, and the category ≤0.70 was used as reference group for GEE analysis, the results did not change significantly (see Additional file 2).

XO Study I

Of 1469 participants in the XO Study I, 1316 were included in the current analysis. About half (51.2%, n = 674) were women, average age was 62.9 ± 8.7 years and mean BMI was 24.2 kg/m^2 (SD = 3.6). The prevalence of knee chondrocalcinosis was 3.1% in men and 5.0% in women (Table 3).

Serum magnesium, even within the normal range, was inversely associated with the OR for prevalence of knee chondrocalcinosis in a dose-response-relationship manner (Fig. 3, test for trend $P = 0.06$ for the total population; $P = 0.25$ for the male population; $P = 0.14$ for the female population). As shown in Table 4, the prevalence of knee chondrocalcinosis (knee-specific analysis) decreased from 4.8% in the lowest tertile of serum magnesium to 3.2% in the second, and 2.0% in the highest tertile of serum magnesium. Figure 4 shows the linear association between the serum magnesium and predicted prevalence of chondrocalcinosis. After adjusting for age, sex and BMI, compared with the lowest tertile, ORs for knee chondrocalcinosis were 0.67 (95% CI 0.34–1.30) in the middle and 0.45 (95% CI 0.21–0.94) in the highest tertile of serum magnesium, respectively (*P* value for trend = 0.030). Adding each of the potential confounders (e.g., knee injury, serum parathyroid hormone, iron, total iron binding capacity, unsaturated iron binding capacity, calcium, 25(OH)D, zinc, copper and phosphorus) into the age, sex and BMI-adjusted model, or sensitivity analysis with exclusion of participants with chronic renal failure or who used diuretics, also did not change the results materially. The association was consistent in men and women (Table 4). When 0.70 mmol/L was used as an additional knot for spline regression, and the category ≤0.70 was used as the reference group for GEE analysis, the results did no change significantly (see Additional file 2).

Discussion

In two population-based cross-sectional studies, we found that serum magnesium, even within the normal range, was inversely associated with the prevalence of knee chondrocalcinosis in a dose-response-relationship manner. In both studies, prevalence of knee chondrocalcinosis among subjects in the highest tertile of serum

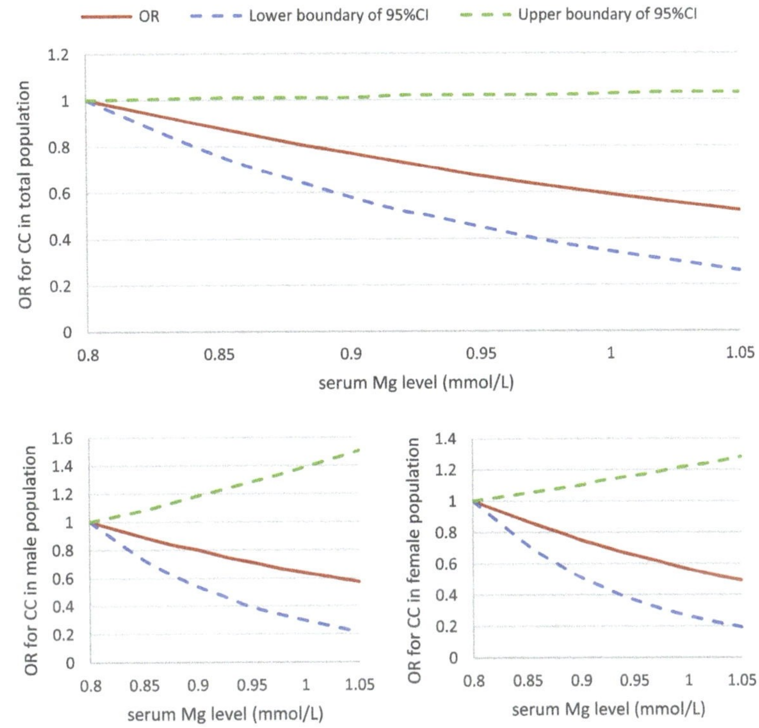

Fig. 3 Dose-response relationship between serum magnesium (Mg) and the odds ratio (OR) for knee chondrocalcinosis (CC) in the XO Study I. CI, confidence interval

magnesium was approximately 50% lower than those in the lowest tertile of serum magnesium. Such an association was consistent in men and women.

A few case-reports and case-series studies have shown that chondrocalcinosis often co-occurs with hypomagnesemia or with hypomagnesemia owing to bowel syndrome and Gitelmen syndrome [7–11]. For example, in 2007 Richette et al. compared serum magnesium and the prevalence of chondrocalcinosis in 72 patients with intestinal failure and 72 age-matched and sex-matched patients with back pain [6]. They found that serum magnesium was significantly lower ($P < 0.001$) among patients with intestinal failure (0.75 mmol/L) than those with back pain (0.81 mmol/L). On the other hand, the prevalence of chondrocalcinosis was sevenfold higher ($P = 0.006$) among patients with intestinal failure (16.6%) than among patients with back pain (2.7%). Furthermore, serum magnesium, globular magnesium and 24-hour urinary magnesium were significantly lower in patients with intestinal failure than those with back pain.

Several in vivo studies have demonstrated that decreasing magnesium intake induces calcification formation in different animal models [21–24]. However, few in vivo studies, if any, have examined the effect of magnesium supplementation or intake on the inhibition of cartilage calcification. In a double-blind randomized clinical trial assessing the effect of a magnesium carbonate supplement among patients with chronic pyrophosphate arthropathy, there was no significant difference in the radiographic appearance of chondrocalcinosis between the treatment and placebo groups; however, the treatment group had a uniform trend towards improvement in pain, stiffness, effusion, tenderness and overall subjective and objective assessment compared with the placebo group over a 6-month period [25]. This finding could be explained by the physiologic N-methyl-D-aspartate (NMDA) receptor antagonist property of magnesium, and consequently, increasing serum magnesium level may reduce the incidence of symptomatic calcium-deposition-related diseases [26]. Furthermore, in a large population-based study, Zhang et al. reported that the prevalence of knee chondrocalcinosis was much lower among participants in the Beijing Osteoarthritis Study than in their counterparts in the Framingham Study (age-standardized prevalence ratios = 0.34 in men and 0.43 in women); however, no difference in the levels of magnesium in the tap drinking water was found between the two cities [5].

Several mechanisms linking magnesium and chondrocalcinosis have been postulated [27]. These include that high serum magnesium may inhibit the formation of calcium phosphate apatite and of calcium-acidic phospholipid-phosphate complexes [28, 29], may increase the expression of calcification inhibitors (e.g., matrix gla protein, osteopontin, and bone morphogenetic protein 7), may decrease the

Table 4 Association between serum Mg and knee chondrocalcinosis of study population in the XO Study I (n = 1316)

	Tertiles of serum Mg (mmol/L)			*P* for trend
	1 (≤0.89)	2 (0.90–0.95)	3 (≥0.96)	
Total				
N for knee*	977	793	848	-
Knee chondrocalcinosis (%)	4.8	3.2	2.0	-
Model 1 (95% CI)	1.00 (reference)	0.67 (0.34, 1.30)	0.45 (0.21, 0.94)	0.030
Model 2 (95% CI)	1.00 (reference)	0.68 (0.35, 1.32)	0.45 (0.22, 0.94)	0.046
Model 3 (95% CI)	1.00 (reference)	0.73 (0.37, 1.47)	0.41 (0.18, 0.93)	0.028
Model 4 (95% CI)	1.00 (reference)	0.71 (0.35, 1.41)	0.41 (0.18, 0.91)	0.025
Model 5 (95% CI)	1.00 (reference)	0.73 (0.37, 1.46)	0.42 (0.19, 0.94)	0.032
Model 6 (95% CI)	1.00 (reference)	0.71 (0.36, 1.41)	0.40 (0.18, 0.91)	0.024
Model 7 (95% CI)	1.00 (reference)	0.67 (0.34, 1.30)	0.45 (0.21, 0.94)	0.030
Model 8 (95% CI)	1.00 (reference)	0.69 (0.35, 1.34)	0.45 (0.21, 0.95)	0.032
Model 9 (95% CI)	1.00 (reference)	0.71 (0.36, 1.42)	0.43 (0.20, 0.95)	0.020
Model 10 (95% CI)	1.00 (reference)	0.68 (0.35, 1.33)	0.41 (0.19, 0.88)	0.034
Model 11 (95% CI)	1.00 (reference)	0.68 (0.35, 1.32)	0.45 (0.21, 0.95)	0.033
Model 12 (95% CI)	1.00 (reference)	0.65 (0.33, 1.28)	0.46 (0.21, 0.96)	0.036
Male				
N for knee*	502	397	380	-
Knee chondrocalcinosis (%)	3.8	2.5	1.1	-
Model 1 (95% CI)	1.00 (reference)	0.72 (0.26, 2.01)	0.34 (0.08, 1.37)	0.115
Model 2 (95% CI)	1.00 (reference)	0.75 (0.28, 2.05)	0.34 (0.08, 1.38)	0.114
Model 3 (95% CI)	1.00 (reference)	0.81 (0.29, 2.30)	0.39 (0.09, 1.66)	0.195
Model 4 (95% CI)	1.00 (reference)	0.78 (0.28, 2.21)	0.39 (0.09, 1.62)	0.184
Model 5 (95% CI)	1.00 (reference)	0.87 (0.31, 2.48)	0.40 (0.10, 1.64)	0.198
Model 6 (95% CI)	1.00 (reference)	0.84 (0.30, 2.35)	0.39 (0.09, 1.60)	0.183
Model 7 (95% CI)	1.00 (reference)	0.72 (0.26, 2.00)	0.34 (0.09, 1.37)	0.117
Model 8 (95% CI)	1.00 (reference)	0.65 (0.19, 2.25)	0.47 (0.11, 1.88)	0.254
Model 9 (95% CI)	1.00 (reference)	0.81 (0.27, 2.42)	0.21 (0.04, 1.08)	0.077
Model 10 (95% CI)	1.00 (reference)	0.72 (0.26, 2.00)	0.17 (0.04, 0.83)	0.024
Model 11 (95% CI)	1.00 (reference)	0.63 (0.23, 1.74)	0.32 (0.08, 1.32)	0.094
Model 12 (95% CI)	1.00 (reference)	0.67 (0.24, 1.93)	0.34 (0.08, 1.38)	0.116
Female				
N for knee*	475	396	468	-
Knee chondrocalcinosis (%)	5.9	3.8	2.8	-
Model 1 (95% CI)	1.00 (reference)	0.64 (0.27, 1.52)	0.50 (0.20, 1.23)	0.128
Model 2 (95% CI)	1.00 (reference)	0.65 (0.27, 1.55)	0.50 (0.20, 1.24)	0.130
Model 3 (95% CI)	1.00 (reference)	0.66 (0.27, 1.65)	0.40 (0.15, 1.10)	0.069
Model 4 (95% CI)	1.00 (reference)	0.62 (0.25, 1.54)	0.40 (0.14, 1.09)	0.067
Model 5 (95% CI)	1.00 (reference)	0.66 (0.26, 1.63)	0.42 (0.15, 1.17)	0.090
Model 6 (95% CI)	1.00 (reference)	0.63 (0.25, 1.58)	0.41 (0.15, 1.10)	0.071
Model 7 (95% CI)	1.00 (reference)	0.64 (0.27, 1.53)	0.50 (0.20, 1.23)	0.126
Model 8 (95% CI)	1.00 (reference)	0.66 (0.27, 1.59)	0.50 (0.20, 1.23)	0.129
Model 9 (95% CI)	1.00 (reference)	0.66 (0.27, 1.59)	0.53 (0.21, 1.33)	0.174
Model 10 (95% CI)	1.00 (reference)	0.66 (0.27, 1.60)	0.53 (0.21, 1.32)	0.171

Table 4 Association between serum Mg and knee chondrocalcinosis of study population in the XO Study I (n = 1316) *(Continued)*

	Tertiles of serum Mg (mmol/L)			*P* for trend
	1 (≤0.89)	2 (0.90–0.95)	3 (≥0.96)	
Model 11 (95% CI)	1.00 (reference)	0.68 (0.29, 1.64)	0.52 (0.21, 1.28)	0.149
Model 12 (95% CI)	1.00 (reference)	0.63 (0.26, 1.50)	0.48 (0.19, 1.21)	0.116

Model 1 included age (50–59, 60–69, ≥70 years), body mass index (BMI) (<25, ≥25 kg/m^2) and sex (age and BMI for the sex subgroup) (n = 1316)
Model 2 added knee injury on the basis of model 1 (n = 1316)
Model 3 added serum parathyroid hormone (tertiles) on the basis of model 1 (n = 1250)
Model 4 added serum iron (tertiles) on the basis of model 1 (n = 1250)
Model 5 added serum total iron binding capacity (tertiles) on the basis of model 1 (n = 1241)
Model 6 added serum unsaturated iron binding capacity (tertiles) on the basis of model 1 (n = 1241)
Model 7 added serum calcium (tertiles) on the basis of model 1 (n = 1316)
Model 8 added serum 25(OH)D (tertiles) on the basis of model 1 (n = 1306)
Model 9 added serum zinc (tertiles) on the basis of model 1 (n = 1292)
Model 10 added serum copper (tertiles) on the basis of model 1 (n = 1292)
Model 11 added serum phosphorus (tertiles) on the basis of model 1 (n = 1316)
Model 12 added education (educated, non-educated) and occupation (farmer, non-farmer) on the basis of model 1 (n = 1316)
*Six right knees and eight left knees with Kellgren-Lawrence grade 4 were excluded from analysis (data from the contralateral knees were retained)
Mg magnesium, *CI* confidence interval

expression of calcification promoters (e.g., alkaline phosphatase, bone morphogenetic protein 2 and runt-related transcription factor 2) and apoptosis [30–33], may activate calcium-sensing receptors [34–36], modulate vitamin D receptor, fibroblast growth factor-1 receptor and its co-receptor klotho [36], or may block various calcium channels to impair excessive calcium uptake [37, 38].

Several characteristics of our study are noteworthy. First, compared with other studies, the sample size of the current two studies was relatively large, and the prevalence of knee chondrocalcinosis found in these two studies (1.4% in the Xiangya Hospital Health Management Center Study and 4.1% in the XO Study I) was similar to another population-based study (i.e., the Beijing Osteoarthritis Study) conducted among residents in Beijing (1.8% in men and 2.7% in women) [5]. These findings suggest that the prevalence of knee chondracalcinosis is lower than in the predominantly white participants in the Framingham Study [5]. In addition, we also showed that prevalence of hypomagnesemia appeared to be lower among the participants in the current two studies than that among subjects in the Rotterdam Study [39]. Second, an inverse association between serum magnesium levels and prevalence of knee chondrocalcinosis was found in our two study populations and across the sex categories, and the magnitude of association was also quite similar when several potential confounders (e.g., knee injury, serum parathyroid hormone, iron, ferritin, total iron binding capacity, unsaturated iron binding capacity, calcium, copper, zinc, phosphorus and 25(OH)D) was added into the age, sex and BMI adjusted model, respectively, indicating the robustness of our findings. Third, we also showed that even within the normal range of serum magnesium, the levels of magnesium were still inversely associated with the prevalence of knee chondrocalcinosis in a dose-response-relationship manner. This finding suggests that increased serum magnesium not only among subjects with hypomagnesium but also among subjects who were within the normal range of magnesium may help to reduce the risk of chondrocalcinosis.

The prevalence of radiographic chondrocalcinosis in the XO Study I was two to three times higher than that in the Xiangya Hospital Health Management Center Study. Such a difference may be due to the age difference between the two study populations in that the average age in the XO Study I (62.9 ± 8.7 years) was almost 10 years older than that in the Xiangya Hospital Health Management Center Study (52.3 ± 8.0 years). While the age distribution is similar in the XO Study I, and the Beijing Osteoarthritis Study restricted participants to 60 years and older, the prevalence in the XO Study I was higher than in the Beijing Osteoarthritis study. This may because of the heavy physical labor (82.4% of men and 91.6% of women were farmers) and frequent climbing (mountain area) of participants in the XO Study I, which of course warrants further study for confirmation.

Our study has some limitations. First, this is a cross-sectional study, thus, we cannot be certain that the causal relationship between serum levels of magnesium and prevalence of knee chondrocalcinosis. Second, we did not assess the dietary intake of magnesium in relation to the prevalence of knee chondrocalcinosis in the present study. While previous studies have shown that dietary intake of magnesium is strongly associated with the serum levels of magnesium [40, 41], studies of dietary intake of magnesium and risk of knee chondrocalcinosis are warranted. Third, we did not use other views of the knee (e.g., lateral or skyline) to ascertain radiographic choncrocalcinosis; thus, it may have resulted in underestimation of the prevalence of radiographic CPPD. However, we postulate that such misclassification of the prevalence of knee CPPD is likely to be non-differential; thus the association between serum

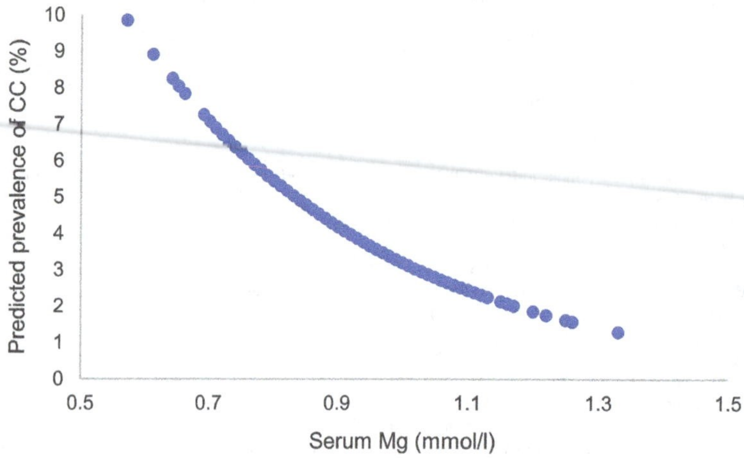

Fig. 4 Association between serum magnesium (Mg) and predicted prevalence of chondrocalcinosis (CC) analyzed by spline regression in the XO Study I

magnesium levels and prevalence of knee radiographic CPPD may be even stronger than we have observed. In addition, as almost half of cases of wrist, hip, symphysis pubis, and metacarpophalangeal joint chondrocalcinosis occur without knee chondrocalcinosis [42], the examination of the association of magnesium levels with a predisposition to form CPPD crystals would ideally include radiographs from other joint sites. Fourth, a synovial fluid test taken from the joint should be more sensitive and specific to detect crystals than radiographs, and some of the articular CPPD deposition (alone or mixed with BCP [2, 3]) may be too small to be detected on radiographs; thus, our estimate of the prevalence of knee chondrocalcinosis is likely to be underestimated. However, as we stated previously, that prevalence estimate of knee chondrocalcinosis was similar to another study [5] conducted in Chinese subjects that used the same protocol to assess the presence of knee chondrocalcinosis. The proportion of persons with chondrocalcinosis identified on radiographs who develop clinical symptoms related to this is small. Fifth, data on some other potential confounders (e.g., osteoporosis and use of bisphosphonates) were not collected in either study and could impact the results. We performed sensitivity analysis to assess to what extent the residual confounding could explain the association, using the E-value proposed by VanderWeele and Ding [43]. The observed OR of 0.49 for prevalence with the highest levels of magnesium in Xiangya Hospital Health Management Center Study could be explained if an OR of an unmeasured confounder with either high serum magnesium or with the prevalence of chondrocalcinosis is at least 3.50, which is above and beyond the measured confounders. There should be a similar magnitude of residual confounders to explain the findings in the XO Study I. To our best knowledge we are unaware that there is such a strong confounder between magnesium and the prevalence of chondrocalcinosis.

Our study findings have potential clinical implications. The existing in vivo and in vitro studies showed that magnesium supplementation may have a protective effect on cartilage or chondrocytes [44]. Two large epidemiological studies conducted in twins and in the general population reported an inverse association between serum magnesium levels and radiographic knee osteoarthritis [12, 45]. Furthermore, several studies have reported that chondrocalcinosis may be a potential risk factor for osteoarthritis [46–52]. Thus, it is not unreasonable to speculate that increasing serum magnesium may be beneficial in decreasing the risk of osteoarthritis through reducing the incidence of chondrocalcinosis. Future studies are warranted to test this hypothesis.

Conclusions

We found that low serum magnesium, even within the normal range, was associated with higher prevalence of knee chondrocalcinosis in a dose-response-relationship manner. Future studies of dietary intake, including magnesium supplementary intake, on the risk of chondrocalcinosis are warranted.

Additional files

Additional file 1: Measuring methods and reliability data of potential confounders. (DOCX 15 kb)

Additional file 2: Table S1. Association between serum Mg and knee chondrocalcinosis in the Xiangya Hospital Health Management Center Study (n = 12,631). **Table S2.** Association between serum Mg and knee chondrocalcinosis in the XO Study I (n = 1316). **Figure S1.** Association between serum Mg and OR of CC analyzed by spline regression (3 knots, 0,7 as reference) in the Xiangya Hospital Health Management Center Study ($P = 0.049$). Mg, magnesium; CC, chondrocalcinosis; OR, odds ratio; CI, confidence interval. **Figure S2.** Association between serum Mg and OR of CC analyzed by spline regression (3 knots, 0,7 as reference) in the XO Study I ($P = 0.060$). Mg, magnesium; CC, chondrocalcinosis; OR, odds ratio; CI, confidence interval. (DOCX 1720 kb)

Abbreviations

BCP: Basic calcium phosphate; BMI: Body mass index; CPPD: Calcium pyrophosphate deposition; K-L: Kellgren-Lawrence; NMDA: N-methyl-D-aspartate; OAI: Osteoarthritis Initiative; ORs: Odds ratios; XO Study I: Xiangya Osteoarthritis Study I

Acknowledgements

The authors appreciate the support of Orthopedics Research Institute of Xiangya Hospital.

Funding

This work was supported by the National Natural Science Foundation of China (No. 81472130, 81672225, 81601941, 81501923, 81772413, 81702207, 81702206), the VA Research Service and National Institutes of Health (NIH) (P0AG07996), the Postdoctoral Science Foundation of Central South University (182130), the Young Investigator Grant of Xiangya Hospital, Central South University (2016Q03, 2016Q06), the Scientific Research Project of the Development and Reform Commission of Hunan Province ([2013]1199), the Scientific Research Project of Science and Technology Office of Hunan Province (2013SK2018), the Key Research and Development Program of Hunan Province (2016JC2038), the Xiangya Clinical Big Data System Construction Project of Central South University (No. 45), the Clinical Scientific Research Foundation of Xiangya Hospital, Central South University (2015 L03), the Fundamental Research Funds for the Central Universities of Central South University (2015zzts112), the Postdoctoral Science Foundation of Central South University (182130), the Young Investigator Grant of Xiangya Hospital, Central South University (2016Q03, 2016Q06) and the Natural Science Foundation of Hunan Province (2017JJ3491, 2017JJ3492).

Authors' contributions

GHL, CZ and JW had full access to the data in the study and take responsibility for the integrity of the data and the accuracy of the data analysis. GHL, CZ and JW conceived the study. GHL, CZ and JW were responsible for conception and design of the study and drafted the manuscript. CZ, JW, TY, YLW, DXX, HL, YC and LJL contributed to data collection. CZ, TY, YLW, DXX, LJL and GHL contributed to assessment of radiographs. JW contributed to preparation and data analysis. RT, HKC, DJH, YQZ and GHL contributed to revision of the manuscript. All the authors contributed to the interpretation of the data and critically reviewed the manuscript for publication. All authors read and approved the final manuscript.

Authors' information

Not applicable.

Competing interests

The authors declare that they have no competing interests.

Author details

[1]Department of Orthopaedics, Xiangya Hospital, Central South University, #87 Xiangya Road, Changsha, Hunan Province 410008, China. [2]Health Management Center, Xiangya Hospital, Central South University, Changsha, Hunan Province 410008, China. [3]VA San Diego Medical Center, San Diego, CA 92161, USA. [4]Department of Medicine, UCSD, San Diego, CA 92161, USA. [5]Division of Rheumatology, Allergy, and Immunology, Department of Medicine, Massachusetts General Hospital, Boston, MA 02114, USA. [6]Rheumatology Department, Royal North Shore Hospital and Institute of Bone and Joint Research, Kolling Institute, University of Sydney, Sydney, NSW 2065, Australia. [7]Department of Epidemiology and Health Statistics, Xiangya School of Public Health, Central South University, Changsha, Hunan Province 410008, China. [8]International Medical Center, Xiangya Hospital, Central South University, Changsha, Hunan Province 410008, China. [9]Department of Orthopaedics, Changsha Central Hospital, Changsha, Hunan 410000, China.

References

1. Zhang W, Doherty M, Bardin T, Barskova V, Guerne PA, Jansen TL, Leeb BF, Perez-Ruiz F, Pimentao J, Punzi L, et al. European League Against Rheumatism recommendations for calcium pyrophosphate deposition. Part I: terminology and diagnosis. Ann Rheum Dis. 2011;70(4):563–70.
2. Fuerst M, Bertrand J, Lammers L, Dreier R, Echtermeyer F, Nitschke Y, Rutsch F, Schafer FK, Niggemeyer O, Steinhagen J, et al. Calcification of articular cartilage in human osteoarthritis. Arthritis Rheum. 2009;60(9):2694–703.
3. Nguyen C, Bazin D, Daudon M, Chatron-Colliet A, Hannouche D, Bianchi A, Come D, So A, Busso N, Busso N, et al. Revisiting spatial distribution and biochemical composition of calcium-containing crystals in human osteoarthritic articular cartilage. Arthritis Res Ther. 2013;15(5):R103.
4. Rosenthal AK, Ryan LM. Calcium pyrophosphate deposition disease. N Engl J Med. 2016;374(26):2575–84.
5. Zhang Y, Terkeltaub R, Nevitt M, Xu L, Neogi T, Aliabadi P, Niu J, Felson DT. Lower prevalence of chondrocalcinosis in Chinese subjects in Beijing than in white subjects in the United States: The Beijing Osteoarthritis Study. Arthritis Rheum. 2006;54(11):3508–12.
6. Richette P, Ayoub G, Lahalle S, Vicaut E, Badran A, Joly F, Messing B, Bardin T. Hypomagnesemia associated with chondrocalcinosis: a cross-sectional study. Arthritis Rheum. 2007;57(8):1496–501.
7. Ellman MH. Images in clinical medicine. Chondrocalcinosis and hypomagnesemia. N Engl J Med. 2009;360(1):71.
8. Milazzo SC, Ahern MJ, Cleland LG, Henderson DR. Calcium pyrophosphate dihydrate deposition disease and familial hypomagnesemia. J Rheumatol. 1981;8(5):767–71.
9. Smilde TJ, Haverman JF, Schipper P, Hermus AR, van Liebergen FJ, Jansen JL, Kloppenborg PW, Koolen MI. Familial hypokalemia/hypomagnesemia and chondrocalcinosis. J Rheumatol. 1994;21(8):1515–9.
10. Richette P, Ayoub G, Bardin T, Bouvet S, Orcel P, Badran AM. Hypomagnesemia and chondrocalcinosis in short bowel syndrome. J Rheumatol. 2005;32(12):2434–6.
11. Ea HK, Blanchard A, Dougados M, Roux C. Chondrocalcinosis secondary to hypomagnesemia in Gitelman's syndrome. J Rheumatol. 2005;32(9):1840–2.
12. Zeng C, Wei J, Li H, Yang T, Zhang FJ, Pan D, Xiao YB, Yang TB, Lei GH. Relationship between serum magnesium concentration and radiographic knee osteoarthritis. J Rheumatol. 2015;42(7):1231–6.
13. Li H, Zeng C, Wei J, Yang T, Gao SG, Luo W, Li YS, Xiong YL, Xiao WF, Lei GH. Associations of dietary and serum magnesium with serum high-sensitivity C-reactive protein in early radiographic knee osteoarthritis patients. Mod Rheumatol. 2017;27(4):669–74.
14. Zeng C, Wang YL, Wei J, Yang T, Li H, Xie DX, Li YS, Lei GH. Association between low serum magnesium concentration and hyperuricemia. Magnes Res. 2015;28(2):56–63.
15. Kellgren JH, Lawrence JS. Radiological assessment of osteo-arthrosis. Ann Rheum Dis. 1957;16(4):494–502.
16. The gate-way website of the Longshan County People Government. http://www.xxls.gov.cn. Accessed 1 May 2015.
17. Abhishek A, Doherty S, Maciewicz R, Muir K, Zhang W, Doherty M. Chondrocalcinosis is common in the absence of knee involvement. Arthritis Res Ther. 2012;14(5):R205.
18. Zhang Y, Glynn RJ, Felson DT. Musculoskeletal disease research: should we analyze the joint or the person? J Rheumatol. 1996;23(7):1130.
19. Rothman KJ, Moore LL, Singer MR, Nguyen US, Mannino S, Milunsky A. Teratogenicity of high vitamin A intake. N Engl J Med. 1995;333(21):1369–73.
20. Schöttker B, Herder C, Rothenbacher D, Perna L, Müller H, Brenner H. Serum 25-hydroxyvitamin D levels and incident diabetes mellitus type 2: a competing risk analysis in a large population-based cohort of older adults. Eur J Epidemiol. 2013;28(3):267–75.
21. Britton WM, Stokstad EL. Aorta and other soft tissue calcification in the magnesium-deficient rat. J Nutr. 1970;100(12):1501–5.
22. Planells E, Llopis J, Peran F, Aranda P. Changes in tissue calcium and phosphorus content and plasma concentrations of parathyroid hormone and calcitonin after long-term magnesium deficiency in rats. J Am Coll Nutr. 1995;14(3):292–8.
23. Altura BT, Brust M, Bloom S, Barbour RL, Stempak JG, Altura BM. Magnesium dietary intake modulates blood lipid levels and atherogenesis. Proc Natl Acad Sci U S A. 1990;87(5):1840–4.
24. King JL, Miller RJ, Blue JP, O'Brien WD, Erdman JW. Inadequate dietary magnesium intake increases atherosclerotic plaque development in rabbits. Nutr Res. 2009;29(5):343–9.

25. Doherty M, Dieppe P. Double blind, placebo controlled trial of magnesium carbonate in chronic pyrophosphate arthropathy. Ann Rheum Dis. 1983;42 Suppl 1:106.
26. Tramer MR, Schneider J, Marti RA, Rifat K. Role of magnesium sulfate in postoperative analgesia. Anesthesiology. 1996;84(2):340–7.
27. Massy ZA, Drueke TB. Magnesium and cardiovascular complications of chronic kidney disease. Nat Rev Nephrol. 2015;11(7):432–42.
28. Cheng PT, Grabher JJ, LeGeros RZ. Effects of magnesium on calcium phosphate formation. Magnesium. 1988;7(3):123–32.
29. Lagier R, Baud CA. Magnesium whitlockite, a calcium phosphate crystal of special interest in pathology. Pathol Res Pract. 2003;199(5):329–35.
30. Louvet L, Buchel J, Steppan S, Passlick-Deetjen J, Massy ZA. Magnesium prevents phosphate-induced calcification in human aortic vascular smooth muscle cells. Nephrol Dial Transplant. 2013;28(4):869–78.
31. Kircelli F, Peter ME, Sevinc Ok E, Celenk FG, Yilmaz M, Steppan S, Asci G, Ok E, Passlick-Deetjen J. Magnesium reduces calcification in bovine vascular smooth muscle cells in a dose-dependent manner. Nephrol Dial Transplant. 2012;27(2):514–21.
32. Montezano AC, Zimmerman D, Yusuf H, Burger D, Chignalia AZ, Wadhera V, van Leeuwen FN, Touyz RM. Vascular smooth muscle cell differentiation to an osteogenic phenotype involves TRPM7 modulation by magnesium. Hypertension. 2010;56(3):453–62.
33. De Schutter TM, Behets GJ, Geryl H, Peter ME, Steppan S, Gundlach K, Passlick-Deetjen J, D'Haese PC, Neven E. Effect of a magnesium-based phosphate binder on medial calcification in a rat model of uremia. Kidney Int. 2013;83(6):1109–17.
34. Henaut L, Boudot C, Massy ZA, Lopez-Fernandez I, Dupont S, Mary A, Drueke TB, Kamel S, Brazier M, Mentaverri R. Calcimimetics increase CaSR expression and reduce mineralization in vascular smooth muscle cells: mechanisms of action. Cardiovasc Res. 2014;101(2):256–65.
35. Ivanovski O, Nikolov IG, Joki N, Caudrillier A, Phan O, Mentaverri R, Maizel J, Hamada Y, Nguyen-Khoa T, Fukagawa M, et al. The calcimimetic R-568 retards uremia-enhanced vascular calcification and atherosclerosis in apolipoprotein E deficient (apoE−/−) mice. Atherosclerosis. 2009;205(1):55–62.
36. Rodriguez-Ortiz ME, Canalejo A, Herencia C, Martinez-Moreno JM, Peralta-Ramirez A, Perez-Martinez P, Navarro-Gonzalez JF, Rodriguez M, Peter M, Gundlach K, et al. Magnesium modulates parathyroid hormone secretion and upregulates parathyroid receptor expression at moderately low calcium concentration. Nephrol Dial Transplant. 2014;29(2):282–9.
37. Altura BM, Altura BT, Carella A, Gebrewold A, Murakawa T, Nishio A. Mg2+-Ca2+ interaction in contractility of vascular smooth muscle: Mg2+ versus organic calcium channel blockers on myogenic tone and agonist-induced responsiveness of blood vessels. Can J Physiol Pharmacol. 1987;65(4):729–45.
38. Zhang J, Berra-Romani R, Sinnegger-Brauns MJ, Striessnig J, Blaustein MP, Matteson DR. Role of Cav1.2 L-type Ca2+ channels in vascular tone: effects of nifedipine and Mg2+. AJP Heart Circ Physiol. 2006;292(1):H415–25.
39. Liamis G, Rodenburg EM, Hofman A, Zietse R, Stricker BH, Hoorn EJ. Electrolyte disorders in community subjects: prevalence and risk factors. Am J Med. 2013;126(3):256–63.
40. Peacock JM, Folsom AR, Arnett DK, Eckfeldt JH, Szklo M. Relationship of serum and dietary magnesium to incident hypertension: the Atherosclerosis Risk in Communities (ARIC) Study. Ann Epidemiol. 1999;9(3):159–65.
41. Akizawa Y, Koizumi S, Itokawa Y, Ojima T, Nakamura Y, Tamura T, Kusaka Y. Daily magnesium intake and serum magnesium concentration among Japanese people. J Epidemiol. 2008;18(4):151–9.
42. Abhishek A, Doherty S, Maciewicz RA, Muir K, Zhang W, Doherty M. Does chondrocalcinosis associate with a distinct radiographic phenotype of osteoarthritis in knees and hips? A case-control study. Arthritis Care Res. 2016;68(2):211–6.
43. VanderWeele TJ, Ding P. Sensitivity analysis in observational research: introducing the E-value. Ann Intern Med. 2017;167(4):268–74.
44. Zeng C, Li Y, Wei J, Xie D, Xie X, Li L, Gao S, Luo W, Xiong Y, Xiao W, et al. Analgesic effect and safety of single-dose intra-articular magnesium after arthroscopic surgery: a systematic review and meta-analysis. Sci Rep-Uk. 2016;6:38024.
45. Hunter DJ. Evidence of altered bone turnover, vitamin D and calcium regulation with knee osteoarthritis in female twins. Rheumatology. 2003; 42(11):1311–6.
46. Felson DT. The epidemiology of knee osteoarthritis: results from the Framingham Osteoarthritis Study. Semin Arthritis Rheum. 1990;20(3 Suppl 1):42–50.
47. Ledingham J, Dawson S, Preston B, Milligan G, Doherty M. Radiographic patterns and associations of osteoarthritis of the hip. Ann Rheum Dis. 1992; 51(10):1111–6.
48. Ledingham J, Regan M, Jones A, Doherty M. Radiographic patterns and associations of osteoarthritis of the knee in patients referred to hospital. Ann Rheum Dis. 1993;52(7):520–6.
49. Sanmarti R, Kanterewicz E, Pladevall M, Panella D, Tarradellas JB, Gomez JM. Analysis of the association between chondrocalcinosis and osteoarthritis: a community based study. Ann Rheum Dis. 1996;55(1):30–3.
50. Neame RL, Carr AJ, Muir K, Doherty M. UK community prevalence of knee chondrocalcinosis: evidence that correlation with osteoarthritis is through a shared association with osteophyte. Ann Rheum Dis. 2003;62(6):513–8.
51. Musacchio E, Ramonda R, Perissinotto E, Sartori L, Hirsch R, Punzi L, Zambon S, Corti M, Baggio G, Manzato E, et al. The impact of knee and hip chondrocalcinosis on disability in older people: the ProVA Study from northeastern Italy. Ann Rheum Dis. 2011;70(11):1937–43.
52. Abhishek A, Doherty S, Maciewicz R, Muir K, Zhang W, Doherty M. Evidence of a systemic predisposition to chondrocalcinosis and association between chondrocalcinosis and osteoarthritis at distant joints: a cross-sectional study. Arthritis Care Res. 2013;65(7):1052–8.

2

Association of medial meniscal extrusion with medial tibial osteophyte distance detected by T2 mapping MRI in patients with early-stage knee osteoarthritis

Shinnosuke Hada[1], Muneaki Ishijima[1,2,3*], Haruka Kaneko[1], Mayuko Kinoshita[1], Lizu Liu[1,3], Ryo Sadatsuki[1], Ippei Futami[1], Anwajan Yusup[1,4], Tomohiro Takamura[5], Hitoshi Arita[1], Jun Shiozawa[1], Takako Aoki[3], Yuji Takazawa[1], Hiroshi Ikeda[1], Shigeki Aoki[5], Hisashi Kurosawa[6], Yasunori Okada[2*] and Kazuo Kaneko[1,2,3]

Abstract

Background: Medial meniscal extrusion (MME) is associated with progression of medial knee osteoarthritis (OA), but no or little information is available for relationships between MME and osteophytes, which are found in cartilage and bone parts. Because of the limitation in detectability of the cartilage part of osteophytes by radiography or conventional magnetic resonance imaging (MRI), the rate of development and size of osteophytes appear to have been underestimated. Because T2 mapping MRI may enable us to evaluate the cartilage part of osteophytes, we aimed to examine the association between MME and OA-related changes, including osteophytes, by using conventional and T2 mapping MRI.

Methods: Patients with early-stage knee OA ($n = 50$) were examined. MRI-detected OA-related changes, in addition to MME, were evaluated according to the Whole-Organ Magnetic Resonance Imaging Score. T2 values of the medial meniscus and osteophytes were measured on T2 mapping images. Osteophytes surgically removed from patients with end-stage knee OA were histologically analyzed and compared with findings derived by radiography and MRI.

Results: Medial side osteophytes were detected by T2 mapping MRI in 98% of patients with early-stage knee OA, although the detection rate was 48% by conventional MRI and 40% by radiography. Among the OA-related changes, medial tibial osteophyte distance was most closely associated with MME, as determined by multiple logistic regression analysis, in the patients with early-stage knee OA ($\beta = 0.711$, $p < 0.001$). T2 values of the medial meniscus were directly correlated with MME in patients with early-stage knee OA, who showed ≥ 3 mm of MME ($r = 0.58$, $p = 0.003$). The accuracy of osteophyte evaluation by T2 mapping MRI was confirmed by histological analysis of the osteophytes removed from patients with end-stage knee OA.

Conclusions: Our study demonstrates that medial tibial osteophyte evaluated by T2 mapping MRI is frequently observed in the patients with early-stage knee OA, showing close association with MME, and that MME is positively correlated with the meniscal degeneration.

Keywords: Osteoarthritis, Early-stage knee osteoarthritis, Medial meniscal extrusion, Diagnosis, MRI, Osteophyte, T2 mapping

* Correspondence: ishijima@juntendo.ac.jp; ya-okada@juntendo.ac.jp
[1]Department of Medicine for Orthopaedics and Motor Organ, Juntendo University Graduate School of Medicine, 2-1-1, Hongo, Bunkyo-ku, Tokyo 113-8421, Japan
[2]Department of Pathophysiology for Locomotive and Neoplastic Diseases, Juntendo University Graduate School of Medicine, 2-1-1 Hongo, Bunkyo-ku, Tokyo 113-8421, Japan
Full list of author information is available at the end of the article

Background

Osteoarthritis of the knee (knee OA) is an important public health concern because the prevalence of the disease is increasing with the aging population, and to date there are no disease-modifying treatments [1]. An essential component of the knee joint is the meniscus, which functions as a shock absorber of local mechanical stress and maintains joint stability [2]. Dislocation and/or tears of the meniscus contribute to the development of knee OA [3]. In fact, previous studies have shown that medial meniscal extrusion (MME) [4], which is also called *medial meniscus subluxation* or *displacement* [5], is associated with the cartilage damage and disease progression of knee OA [6].

Osteophytes, one of the structural signs of knee OA, develop at the peripheries of the articular cartilage by following the processes of the endochondral ossification [7]. Osteophyte formation is generally considered to be a repair process of damaged articular cartilage and thus a late event in knee OA [7, 8]. Histologically, osteophytes are composed of the cartilage and bone parts [7, 9], but only the bone part has been clinically evaluated because the cartilage component is undetectable by radiography and difficult to evaluate by proton density-weighted magnetic resonance imaging (conventional MRI). These diagnostic methods, therefore, appear to have underestimated the rate of development and the size of osteophytes. On one hand, because T2 mapping MRI can monitor changes in water content and organization of the collagen network in articular cartilage [10], this diagnostic method is expected to be useful for detection and monitoring of the cartilage part of osteophytes in knee OA joints. On the other hand, a recent community cohort study of people without radiographic knee OA showed that osteophytes were detected by conventional MRI in 70–80% of middle-aged and old people (68%, 78%, and 80% of the people in their 50s, 60s, and 70s, respectively) [11]. These finding suggests that osteophyte formation is a common event in knee joints of aged people and may be involved in early-stage OA changes. However, the prevalence of osteophytes in patients with early-stage knee OA and relationships between osteophyte formation and MME remain elusive.

In the present study, we hypothesized that a positive relationship must be present between osteophyte formation and MME in early-stage knee OA. Thus, the purpose of this study was to examine the relationship of osteophytes and MME by introducing T2 mapping MRI to analyze OA changes in patients with early-stage knee OA. We evaluated osteophytes by measuring both cartilage and bone parts using T2 mapping MRI in patients with early-stage knee OA, and we analyzed the relationship between MME and osteophytes. We also assessed the accuracy of the T2 mapping MRI data in a combined histological study of the osteophytes. Our data demonstrate that formation of medial tibial osteophytes is a change closely associated with MME in early-stage knee OA.

Methods

Subjects

The sample size of this study was determined by the number of patients who had the following conditions during the study period (May 2012 to September 2015). Five hundred forty-five patients with knee pain visited the outpatient clinic of the authors (SH, MI, and HaK) in Juntendo University Hospital to seek therapy and underwent radiography and conventional and T2 mapping MRI during the study period. Diagnosis of knee OA was made according to the American College of Rheumatology criteria [12] and MRI criteria [13]. When the patients showed grade 0, 1, or 2 of the Kellgren-Lawrence (K/L) classification [14, 15] and fulfilled the definition of OA based on MRI criteria [13], they were classified as having early-stage knee OA. Fifty of the 545 patients had early-stage knee OA, and they were enrolled in this study. Among patients with end-stage knee OA ($n = 4$, three females and one male, average age 72.7 years, body mass index 23.2 kg/cm^2) who underwent total knee arthroplasty, the findings of histology, radiographs, and MRI scans of medial tibial osteophytes were compared.

The study protocol, which complied with the principles outlined in the Declaration of Helsinki, was approved by the Ethical Committee Review Board at Juntendo University. Written informed consent was obtained from the patients with end-stage knee OA. Because the studies of patients with early-stage knee OA were categorized as retrospective, the Ethical Committee Review Board waived the requirement for patients' informed consent because of the anonymous nature of the data.

Radiographic evaluation

Standing, extended, and anteroposterior and lateral view radiographs, as well as posteroanterior weight-bearing radiographs made with the knee in 45 degrees of flexion, were evaluated according to K/L grade [14, 15].

MRI analyses

The knee joints were analyzed using the MAGNETOM Verio MR 3.0-Tesla MRI system (Siemens Medical Solutions, Erlangen, Germany) with proton density-weighted image fast spin echo sequences (repetition time [TR] 1800 milliseconds, echo time [TE] 11 milliseconds, slice thickness 3 mm, field of view [FOV] 160 mm, matrix 384 × 384) and T2 mapping sequences (TR 1000 milliseconds; TE 13.8, 27.6, 41.4, 55.2, and 69.0 milliseconds; slice thickness 3 mm; FOV 160 mm; matrix 384 × 384) as we previously described [16, 17]. The MRI data were evaluated in the medial tibiofemoral joint, and OA morphological changes were scored according to the Whole-Organ Magnetic Resonance Imaging Score (WORMS) [18]. Each region of a compartment received its own score, and these scores were added together [16]. The diagnosis of knee OA for the subjects was made using the MRI findings according to a previously reported method [16, 19]. The regions of interest on T2 mapping MRI studies were manually drawn using a three-dimensional image analysis software program (VirtualPlace; AZE, Tokyo, Japan). T2 values of the medial meniscus were calculated as described previously [16].

Evaluation of MME and osteophytes

MME distance was defined as the distance from the outermost edge of the medial meniscus to a line connecting the femoral and tibial cortices [3] and graded according to previously described methods [19]. Thus, the knee joint was examined by proton density-weighted MRI (conventional MRI) and MME distance was measured by drawing a line connecting the femoral and tibial cortices, as shown in Fig. 1a. Although an osteophyte is composed of bone and cartilage parts [7], only the bone part of the osteophyte was detected by radiography (Fig. 1b) and conventional MRI with or without suppression of fat signals (Fig. 1c and d). Therefore, we evaluated osteophytes by T2 mapping MRI, which enabled us to detect both cartilage and bone parts of osteophyte (Fig. 1e). Because the boundary between bone parts of the osteophyte and tibial cortex was difficult to determine by T2 mapping MRI, the borderline between the osteophyte and the tibial cortex was drawn by tracing identical

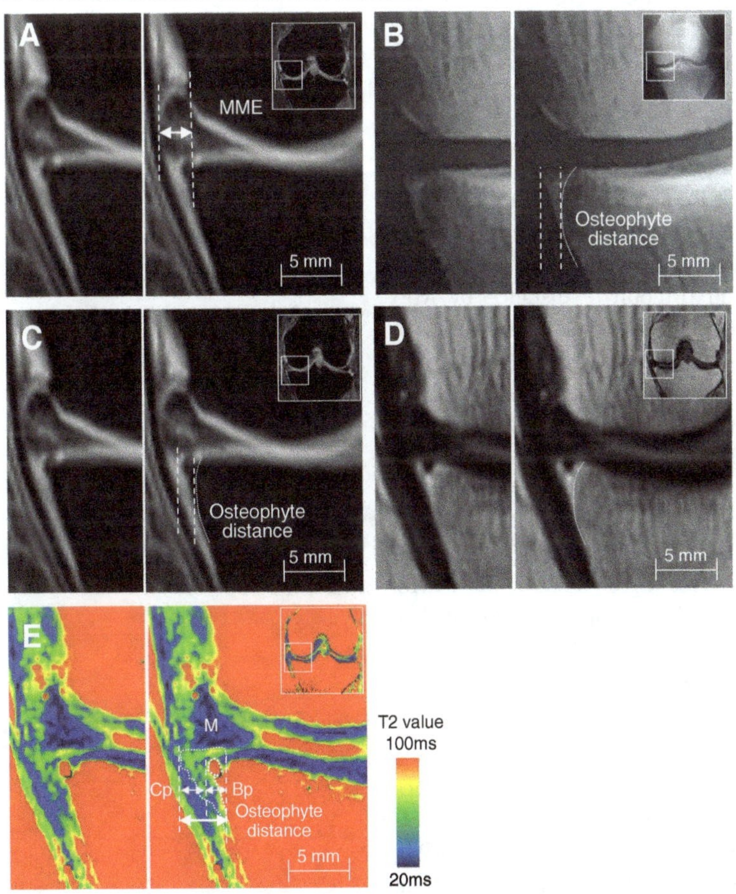

Fig. 1 Representative data derived from the measurement of medial meniscal extrusion (MME) and medial tibial osteophyte distance by radiography, proton density-weighted magnetic resonance imaging (MRI), and T2 mapping MRI in the early-stage knee osteoarthritis joint. **a** Coronal fast spin echo proton density-weighted MRI with fat suppression. MME distance was measured as the distance from the outermost edge of the medial meniscus to a line connecting the femoral and tibial cortices. **b** Osteophyte distance measurement using radiography. **c** Osteophyte distance measurement using proton density-weighted MRI with fat suppression. **d** Definition of a boundary between the tibial cortex and osteophyte (high signal zone) using proton density-weighted imaging without fat suppression. **e** Osteophyte distance measurement using T2 mapping MRI. *Dashed lines* indicate cartilage and bone parts of the osteophyte. The line between bone part of osteophyte and tibial cortex was drawn by tracing the image obtained by proton density-weighted MRI without fat suppression. *Bp* Bone part of osteophyte, *Cp* Cartilage part of osteophyte, *M* Meniscus

slices of the knee on the conventional MRI scan and the T2 mapping MRI scan. The distance of the cartilage and bone parts of the osteophyte was calculated separately on T2 mapping images (Fig. 1e). The occurrence rate of osteophytes in the medial side of the knee joint was evaluated by radiography, conventional MRI, and T2 mapping MRI, in which positive osteophyte was defined as radiographic K/L grade ≤ 2 and WORMS grade ≤ 2 as previously reported [11].

Histological examination

The medial tibial osteophytes obtained at surgery from patients with end-stage knee OA were fixed in 10% neutral buffered formalin. After decalcification, the osteophytes were cut vertically in the center from the outer border to the bottom. Serial paraffin sections were stained with hematoxylin and eosin and Safranin O and microscopically photodocumented. Distances of the osteophytes were determined by measuring the ossified and cartilage-capped areas using cellSens software (Olympus, Tokyo, Japan).

Reproducibility measurements

Two observers (SH and TT) conducted the examination to assess interobserver reproducibility. The intraobserver reproducibility of T2 value measurement, WORMS evaluation, MME distance, and osteophyte distance by MRI was as follows: interclass correlation coefficient (ICC) for interreader agreement 0.91 (95% CI 0.64–0.98) for T2 value, 0.94 (95% CI 0.91–0.96) for WORMS, 0.95 (95% CI 0.78–0.99) for MME, and 0.94 (95% CI 0.85–0.98) for osteophyte distance. Observers were blinded to any patient information during the evaluation process. The interobserver reproducibility was also high: ICC 0.91 (95% CI 0.63–0.97) for T2 value measurement, 0.90 (95% CI 0.86–0.93) for WORMS, 0.93 (95% CI 0.76–0.98) for MME, and 0.94 (95% CI 0.84–0.97) for osteophyte distance. The weighted kappa coefficients of inter- and intraobserver reliability for WORMS were 0.66 and 0.65, respectively.

Statistical analysis

All analyses were performed using IBM SPSS Statistics 21.0 software program (IBM, Armonk, NY, USA). Associations between MME- and OA-related factors, including cartilage, osteophyte, bone marrow lesion, subchondral bone cyst, subchondral bone attrition, medial meniscus lesion, medial femoral osteophyte distance, medial tibial osteophyte distance, and T2 value of medial meniscus, were determined by logistic regression and multiple logistic regression analyses. Relationships between tibial osteophyte distance and MME grade were assessed by one-way analysis of variance. Correlations between MME and T2 value of the medial meniscus were examined using

Table 1 Characteristics of patients with early-stage knee osteoarthritis

Characteristics	Data
Number of subjects	50
Age, years	57.0 (15.1)
BMI, kg/cm^2	24.1 (3.9)
Sex, M/F	23/27
Radiography	
K/L grade 0/1/2	3/27/20
Femorotibial angle, degrees	178.4 (2.6)
Medial joint space width, mm	3.7 (0.9)
Proton density-weighted MRI (MTFJ)	
WORMS	
Cartilage (0–30)	11.9 (6.8)
Osteophyte (0–35)	4.4 (5.1)
Bone marrow lesion (0–15)	1.0 (1.9)
Subchondral bone cyst (0–15)	2.5 (4.4)
Subchondral bone attrition (0–15)	1.3 (1.5)
Medial meniscus lesion (0–6)	2.2 (1.6)
Medial meniscus	
MME, mm	3.0 (1.6)
Tears, *n*	15
Root tear, *n*	0
T2 mapping MRI (MTFJ)	
T2 value of medial meniscus	22.0 (2.8)
Medial femoral osteophyte distance	
Bone part + cartilage part, mm	2.1 (1.4)
Bone part, mm	1.3 (0.9)
Cartilage part, mm	0.8 (0.8)
Medial tibial osteophyte distance	
Bone part + cartilage part, mm	3.3 (1.9)
Bone part, mm	1.8 (1.4)
Cartilage part, mm	1.5 (1.5)
Osteophyte prevalence (MTFJ)	
Radiograph	40.0%
Proton density-weighted MRI	48.0%
K/L 0	0%
K/L 1	44.4%
K/L 2	60.0%
T2 mapping MRI	98.0%
K/L 0	100%
K/L 1	96.7%
K/L 2	100%

Abbreviations: BMI Body mass index, *K/L* Kellgren-Lawrence classification, *MFTJ* Medial tibiofemoral joint, *MME* Medial meniscal extrusion, *MRI* Magnetic resonance imaging, *WORMS* Whole-Organ Magnetic Resonance Imaging Score

The femorotibial angle and the medial joint space width of the knee joints were determined at the center point of the medial femorotibial compartment on a radiograph. Osteophytes observed by radiograph and MRI were defined as the presence of K/L grade ≤ 2 and the presence of WORMS grade ≤ 2, respectively. The data are expressed as mean (SD), count, or percent

Spearman's correlation coefficients. *p* values < 0.05 were considered significant.

Results

Frequent detection of osteophytes composed of bone and cartilage parts by T2 mapping MRI in patients with early-stage knee OA

OA changes of knee joints in patients with early-stage OA ($n = 50$) were examined by radiography, conventional MRI, and T2 mapping MRI according to the methods depicted in Fig. 1. Characteristics of the patients and the findings of the medial tibiofemoral joint are summarized in Table 1. Although more than half of patients with early-stage knee OA (30 of 50 patients) showed radiographic K/L grade 0 or 1, OA changes were observed by conventional MRI (Table 1). MME distance in the patients was 3.0 ± 1.6 mm by conventional MRI (Table 1). When MME distance (Fig. 1a) and osteophyte distance (Fig. 1c) were assessed by conventional MRI, the MME distance appeared to be longer than that of osteophyte distance. However, osteophyte distance measured by T2 mapping MRI (Fig. 1e) (i.e., sum of the bone and cartilage parts) appeared to be similar to MME distance calculated by conventional MRI (3.3 ± 1.9 mm versus 3.0 ± 1.6 mm) (Table 1). Conventional MRI showed tears of the medial meniscus in 30% of the patients (15 of 50 patients), but no root tear was observed (Table 1).

On one hand, the prevalence of osteophyte in the medial side of the knee joint of the patients was 40% by radiography, and conventional MRI showed osteophytes in 48% of the patients (Table 1). On the other hand, T2 mapping MRI demonstrated osteophytes in 98% of patients with early-stage knee OA, and the prevalence of osteophytes was increased depending on the radiographic severity of knee OA (Table 1). When medial tibial and femoral osteophyte distances in the patients were calculated by separately measuring the cartilage and bone parts using T2 mapping MRI, the sums of both parts in the medial femoral and tibial osteophyte distances were 2.1 ± 1.4 mm and 3.3 ± 1.9 mm, respectively (Table 1).

Association between MME and medial tibial osteophyte distance in patients with early-stage knee OA

Associations between MME and MRI-detected OA features of the medial tibiofemoral joint were next examined. By univariate analysis, cartilage scores ($\beta = 0.472$), osteophyte ($\beta = 0.350$), subchondral bone cyst ($\beta = 0.393$), subchondral bone attrition ($\beta = 0.300$), medial meniscus lesion ($\beta = 0.445$), medial femoral osteophyte distance ($\beta = 0.429$), medial tibial osteophyte distance ($\beta = 0.711$) and T2 value of medial meniscus ($\beta = 0.397$) were associated with MME (Table 2). Multivariate analysis indicated that among these factors, the medial tibial osteophyte distance was most closely associated with MME ($\beta = 0.711$, $p < 0.001$) (Table 2).

Association between MME and medial tibial osteophyte distance was analyzed by dividing the subjects into four subgroups with MME grade 0 (distance < 2 mm), grade 1 (2–2.9 mm), grade 2 (3–4.9 mm), or grade 3 (≥5 mm) according to the degree of MME [20] (Fig. 2a). The medial tibial osteophyte distance (sum of the bone and cartilage parts of the osteophyte) in each subgroup positively correlated with the MME grades ($p < 0.0001$) (Fig. 2b). A similar positive correlation was also obtained when the distance of the cartilage part of the medial tibial osteophyte was separately evaluated ($p = 0.0002$). When the correlation between T2 values of the medial meniscus and MME was analyzed among the patient subgroups, the T2 value in the subgroup with MME

Table 2 Association between medial meniscal extrusion and magnetic resonance imaging-detected osteoarthritis features of medial tibiofemoral joint of the knee in patients with early-stage knee osteoarthritis

Factor	Univariable β	*p* Value	Multivariable β	*p* Value
Proton density-weighted MRI				
WORMS				
Cartilage	0.472	0.001	0.352	0.009
Osteophyte	0.350	0.013	−0.200	0.207
Bone marrow lesion	0.112	0.440	−0.037	0.725
Subchondral bone cyst	0.393	0.005	−0.038	0.785
Subchondral bone attrition	0.300	0.034	−0.039	0.763
Medial meniscus lesion	0.445	0.001	0.174	0.144
T2 mapping MRI				
Medial femoral osteophyte distance	0.429	0.002	−0.070	0.648
Medial tibial osteophyte distance	0.711	<0.001	0.711	<0.001
T2 value of medial meniscus	0.397	0.004	0.080	0.489

MRI Magnetic resonance imaging, *WORMS* Whole-Organ Magnetic Resonance Imaging Score
Osteophyte distance by T2 mapping is shown as the sum of the bone and cartilage parts of osteophyte distance

grade 3 was significantly higher than that in the subgroup with grade 2 ($p < 0.0001$), whereas no significant differences were observed between the subgroups with MME grade 0, 1, or 2 (Fig. 2c). The patient subgroups with MME grade 2 or 3 showed a direct correlation with the T2 value of the medial meniscus ($r = 0.58$, $p = 0.003$), whereas no such association was obtained in the subgroups of MME grade 0 or 1 ($r = 0.29$, $p = 0.15$) (Fig. 2d).

Histological demonstration of accuracy for medial tibial osteophyte distance evaluated by T2 mapping MRI

To examine the accuracy of T2 mapping MRI for the evaluation of osteophytes, we compared the findings of osteophytes by radiography, conventional MRI, T2 mapping MRI, and histology in patients with end-stage OA who underwent joint arthroplasty. The cartilage part of the osteophyte was undetectable by radiography (Fig. 3a and b) or difficult to be clearly shown by conventional MRI (Fig. 3c and d), but both cartilage and bone parts were detected by T2 mapping MRI (Fig. 3e and f). The osteophyte was isolated from the tibial plateau obtained at arthroplasty (Fig. 4a) and histologically examined. As shown in Fig. 4b and c, histology demonstrated that the bone part of the osteophyte is covered with cartilage cap. When the medial tibial osteophyte distance, which is the sum of the cartilage and bone parts, was separately measured by T2 mapping MRI and histology, the osteophyte distance measured by T2

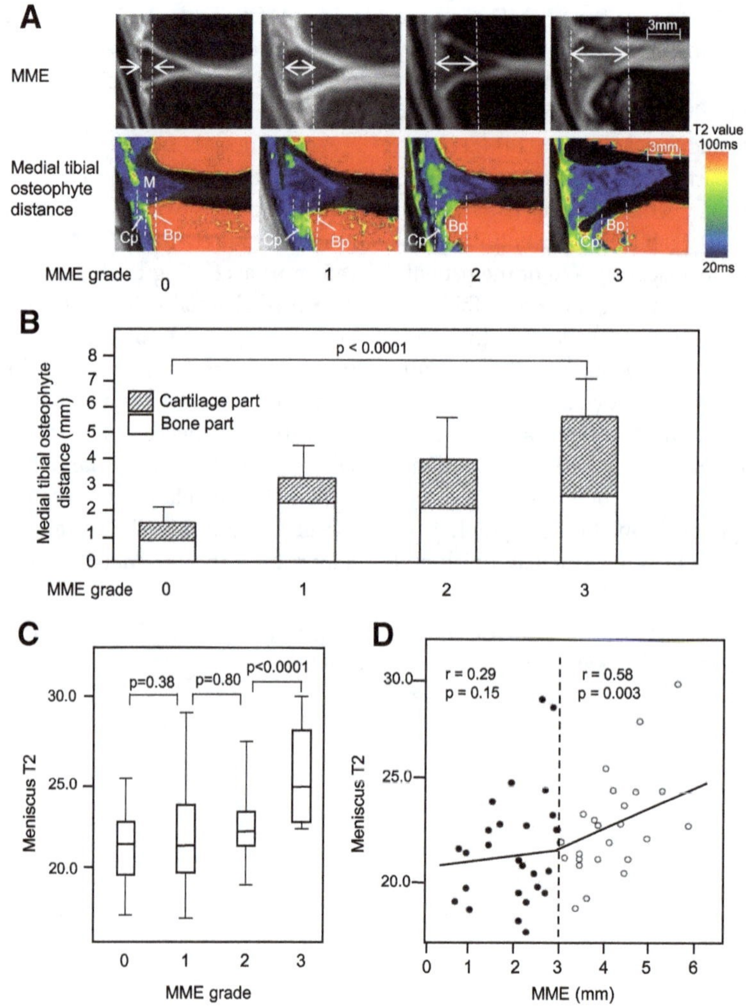

Fig. 2 Association between medial meniscal extrusion (MME) and medial tibial osteophyte distance in patients with early-stage knee osteoarthritis. **a** Representative images of proton density-weighted magnetic resonance imaging (MRI) with fat suppression and T2 mapping MRI of the medial tibiofemoral joint. The patients were classified into four subgroups with MME grade 0, 1, 2, or 3. **b** Correlation between medial tibial osteophyte distance and MME. The medial tibial osteophyte distance was compared among the subgroups with MME grade 0 ($n = 13$), 1 ($n = 13$), 2 ($n = 18$), or 3 ($n = 6$). **c** Comparison of T2 values of medial meniscus among the subgroups with MME grade 0 ($n = 13$), 1 ($n = 13$), 2 ($n = 18$), or 3 ($n = 6$). **d** Correlation between T2 values of medial meniscus and MME. *Closed circles* represent the patient subgroup with MME grade 0 or 1 ($n = 26$); *open circles* represent the patients with MME grade 2 or 3 ($n = 24$). *Bp* Bone part of osteophyte, *Cp* Cartilage part of osteophyte, *M* Medial meniscus

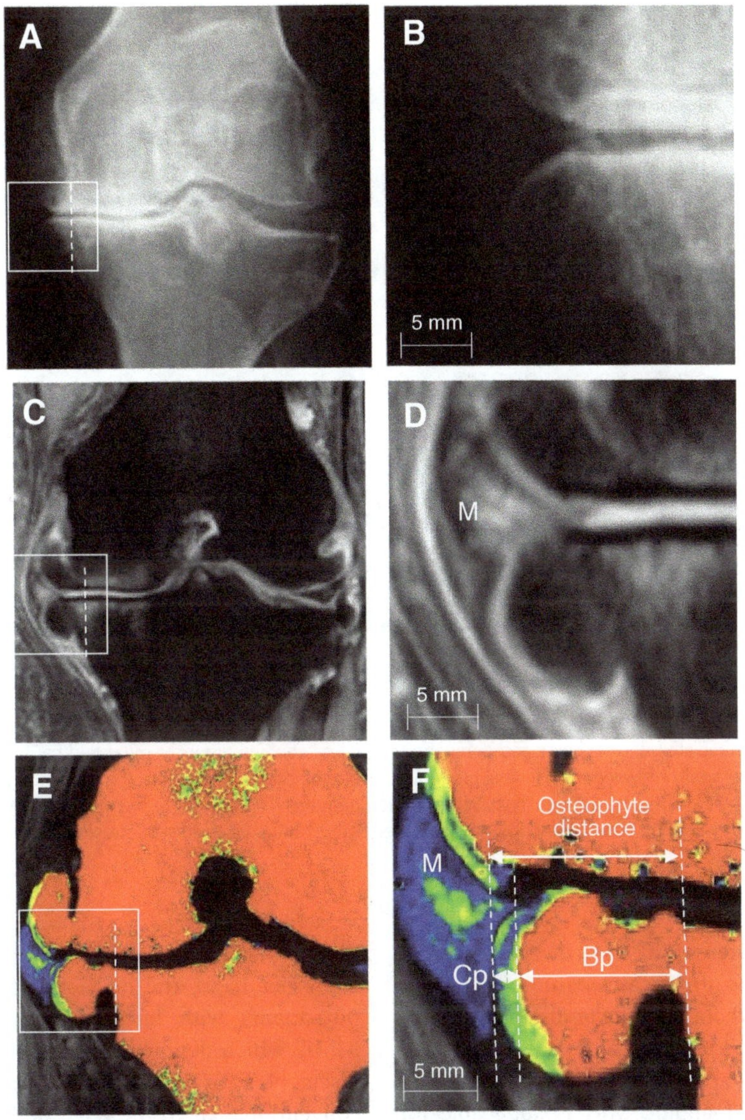

Fig. 3 Findings of medial tibial osteophytes by radiography, proton density-weighted magnetic resonance imaging (MRI), and T2 mapping MRI. **a** Representative radiograph of the end-stage knee osteoarthritis joint. **b** High-power view of the boxed area in (**a**). **c** Proton density-weighted MRI with fat suppression of the same knee joint shown in (**a**). **d** High-power view of the boxed area in (**c**). **e** T2 mapping MRI of the same knee joint shown in (**a**). **f** High-power view of the boxed area in (**e**). *Bp* bone part of osteophyte, *Cp* cartilage part of osteophyte, *M* medial meniscus

mapping MRI and histology showed a direct correlation ($r = 0.98$, $p = 0.017$) (Fig. 4d).

Discussion

In the present study, to the best of our knowledge, we have demonstrated for the first time that MME is most closely associated with the medial tibial osteophyte distance in patients with early-stage knee OA. Our data suggest a possible relationship between medial tibial osteophyte formation and MME development.

Osteophyte formation is generally thought to occur in florid stages of OA as a tissue repair process secondary to the damaged articular cartilage [7–9, 21] by following the processes of endochondral ossification [7, 9]. However, recent studies using MRI have suggested that osteophytes are commonly present within the knee joints in adults without radiographic OA [11, 16]. In this study, we have demonstrated that images of the cartilage and bone parts of osteophytes obtained by T2 mapping MRI correspond well to the histologically identified cartilage and bone parts. We have also shown that T2 mapping MRI is useful for evaluating osteophytes more accurately than conventional MRI by detecting both cartilage and bone parts. Consequently, osteophytes were found to be more frequent and larger than previously thought in patients with early-stage knee OA. Osteophytes in the medial tibial and/

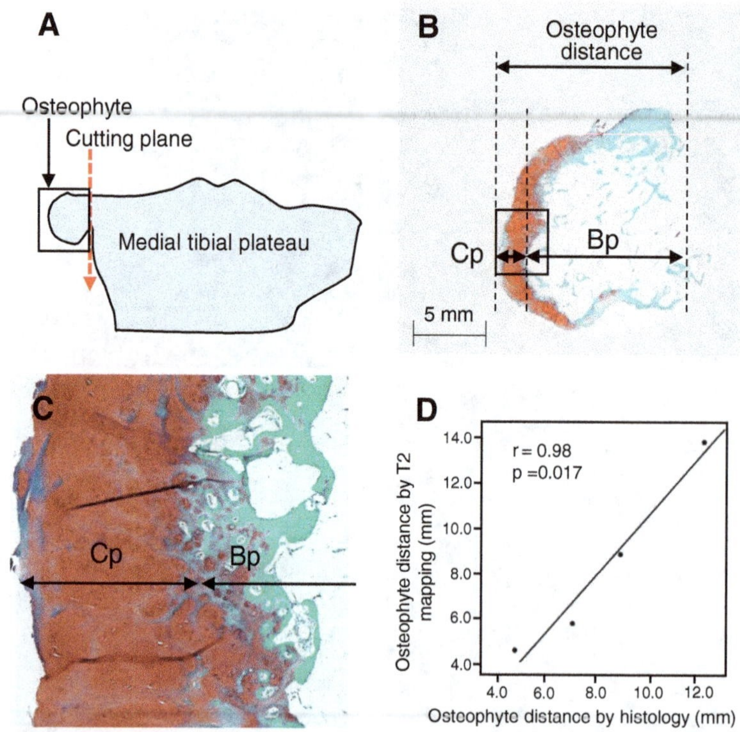

Fig. 4 Histological analysis of medial tibial osteophyte and comparison of the osteophyte distances measured by T2 mapping and histology. **a** Schematic diagram of the surgically removed medial tibial plateau including the osteophyte. **b** Histological section of the osteophyte stained with Safranin O. **c** High-power view of the boxed area in (**b**). **d** Correlation between the osteophyte distance measured by T2 mapping magnetic resonance imaging and that by histology in patients with end-stage knee osteoarthritis. *Bp* Bone part of osteophyte, *Cp* Cartilage part of osteophyte

or femoral sites were present in 98% of patients with early-stage knee OA (49 of 50 cases). Importantly, approximately half of the whole osteophyte distance was the cartilage part, which was not detected by radiography and underestimated by conventional MRI. Our data provide direct evidence that T2 mapping MRI is applicable for measurement of whole osteophyte distance and suggest that osteophyte formation is a very common event in early-stage knee OA.

Molecular mechanisms of osteophyte formation remain unknown. However, experimental studies using animal models have shown that osteophytes develop as a result of repeated mechanical stresses [22] or by an intraarticular injection of transforming growth factor-β [7, 9, 23], bone morphogenetic protein [23], fibroblast growth factor [24], or insulin-like growth factor-1 [25]. Thus, mechanical stresses and/or soluble growth factors may contribute to osteophyte formation in early-stage knee OA joints as a different reaction from cartilage repair.

One of the most intriguing findings in the present study is that the medial tibial osteophyte distance was directly correlated with MME in patients with early-stage knee OA. On one hand, under normal conditions, the medial meniscus is attached tightly to the medial tibial plateau by the coronary ligament (Fig. 5a) [26]. On the other hand, the development of MRI-based studies of patients with knee OA generated the concept of MME, which denotes the medial shift of the medial meniscus [4, 6, 27, 28]. On the basis of findings obtained by conventional MRI, the edge of the medial meniscus has been considered to be more medially located than that of the medial tibial osteophyte [3], showing that the length of MME is longer than the osteophyte distance (Fig. 5b). However, as depicted in Fig. 5c, our study using T2 mapping analysis indicates that the length of MME is almost similar to the osteophyte distance, which was calculated as the sum of bone and cartilage parts detected by T2 mapping.

MME has recently attracted attention as one of the abnormalities related to the progression of knee OA [6, 20, 29–32]. Although MME seems to be enhanced dependently on the severity of knee OA and the mechanical stresses due to weight bearing [5], the mechanism of MME formation in knee OA remains unclear [33]. MME was reported to be associated with root tear of the medial meniscus [27, 34]. However, recent studies have indicated that only a few patients with knee OA with MME (2.4%) have an

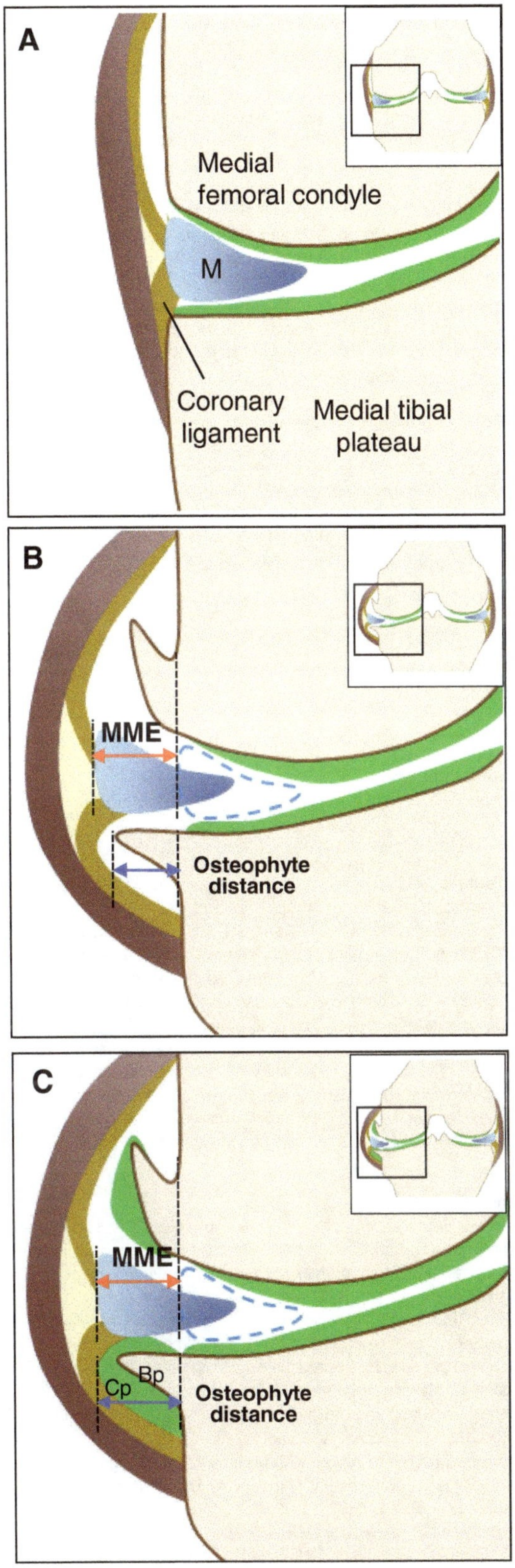

Fig. 5 Schematic illustrations of normal knee joint and osteoarthritis knee joint with osteophyte and medial meniscal extrusion (MME). **a** Normal knee joint. Medial meniscus is tightly fixed to the coronary ligament in the medial tibial plateau. **b** Relationship between MME and medial tibial osteophyte distance based on observations by conventional magnetic resonance imaging (MRI). Note that MME distance appears to be longer than osteophyte distance. **c** Relationship between MME and medial tibial osteophyte distance according to the findings obtained by T2 mapping MRI. Note that the edge of the extruded medial meniscus matches that of the cartilage part of the osteophyte. *Bp* Bone part of osteophyte, *Cp* Cartilage part of osteophyte, *M* Medial meniscus

accompanying root tear in early-stage knee OA [35], and they have suggested that the root tear itself is caused by meniscus degeneration [36]. In the present study, the root tear was not observed in patients with early-stage knee OA, and the patients with MME grade 2 or 3, but not MME grade 0 or 1, showed direct correlation with higher T2 values of the meniscus (meniscus degradation). These data suggest that MME may occur earlier than meniscus degradation.

Although MME and medial tibial osteophyte were closely associated in the present study, their causal relationship remains obscure. One can think that osteophyte develops as a result of mechanical stresses locally induced after the occurrence of MME. In fact, researchers in a previous study proposed this hypothesis, although no direct evidence has been provided [37]. However, the medial meniscus is attached tightly to the medial plateau by the coronary ligament [26]; thus, once an osteophyte is formed, it is possible to speculate that the osteophyte may contribute to medial displacement of the meniscus, leading to MME. However, further work, such as follow-up studies of patients with early-stage knee OA by T2 mapping MRI and experimental studies with animal OA models, is definitely needed to clarify this issue.

The present study has potential limitations. We confirmed the accuracy of osteophyte evaluation by T2 mapping MRI in the combined histological analysis of the osteophytes, which were removed from end-stage knee OA joints, but such information about the osteophytes in early-stage knee OA joints is not available. In animal OA models, the osteophyte is formed through several processes, which include proliferation of synovial and resident cells in the periosteum, their differentiation into chondrocytes and formation of cartilage matrix components, further differentiation of central chondrocytes into hypertrophic chondrocytes, bone formation through endochondral ossification, and fully developed osteophyte formation [7]. A similar mechanism has been proposed for human osteophyte formation [38], although to the best of our knowledge, there are no reports describing the processes of human osteophyte formation.

Therefore, further analyses of the knee joints of human subjects, including cadavers, are necessary to clarify the mechanism of osteophyte formation and the relationship between the T2 mapping MRI data and pathological changes of osteophytes. Ultrasonography has been introduced to examine OA changes of knee joints and reported to be more sensitive than radiography to detect knee osteophytes [39] and MME [40]. Cartilage is exhibited as a hypoechoic area on ultrasonograms [41], and the cartilage thickness is underestimated by ultrasonography compared with conventional MRI [42, 43]. However, because ultrasonography is easy to use and available at a much lower cost than MRI, frequent monitoring of MME and osteophytes by ultrasonography is possible, and this may provide a clue leading to better understanding of the relationship between MME and osteophytes. Although this study provides the first evidence of the close relationship between medial tibial osteophyte distance and MME, this was based on MRI data of subjects in a supine, non-weight-bearing position, which may lead to an underestimation of what would be expected in axially loaded knees. Thus, to further analyze the relationship between MME and osteophyte formation, the degree of MME should be assessed with the knee bearing a full load, the images of which can be obtained by the recently developed upright positional MRI.

Conclusions

We have demonstrated that the medial tibial osteophyte is commonly observed in patients with early-stage knee OA, showing a close association with MME, and that MME is positively correlated with medial meniscal degeneration.

Abbreviations

BMI: Body mass index; Bp: Bone part of osteophyte; Cp: Cartilage part of osteophyte; FOV: Field of view; ICC: Interclass correlation; K/L: Kellgren-Lawrence classification; M: Meniscus; MFTJ: Medial tibiofemoral joint; MME: Medial meniscal extrusion; MRI: Magnetic resonance imaging; OA: Osteoarthritis; TE: Echo time; TR: Repetition time; WORMS: Whole-Organ Magnetic Resonance Imaging Score

Acknowledgements

We thank the members of the Laboratory of Molecular and Biochemical Research, Research Support Center, Juntendo University Graduate School of Medicine, for their technical assistance. We also express our deep appreciation to Tatsuya Miyazaki and his colleagues at the Medical Scanning Hospital (Tokyo, Japan) for their help with the MRI analysis.

Funding

This study was supported by grants-in-aid for scientific research from the Japanese Society for the Promotion of Science (16 K20069 [SH], 15 K10494 [to MI], 15 K20019 [to HaK], and 16H05454 [to YO]). This study was also funded in part by a High Technology Research Center Grant and the Program for the Strategic Research Foundation at Private Universities (2014–2019) from the Ministry of Education, Culture, Sports, Science and Technology of Japan (MEXT).

Authors' contributions

SH conceived of and designed the study, had a major role in analysis and interpretation of the data, and contributed to drafting the report. MI conceived of and designed the study, collected and registered patients, had a major role in analysis and interpretation of the data, and contributed to drafting the report. HaK conceived of and designed the study, collected and registered patients, and had a role in analysis and interpretation of the data. MK had a role in analysis and interpretation of the data and contributed to drafting the report. LL had a role in analysis and interpretation of the data and contributed to drafting the report. RS had a role in analysis and interpretation of the data and contributed to drafting the report. IF had a role in interpretation of the data and contributed to drafting the report. AY had a role in interpretation of the data and contributed to drafting the report. TT had a role in analysis and contributed to drafting the report. HA had a role in interpretation of the data and contributed to drafting the report. JS had a role in interpretation of the data and contributed to drafting the report. TA had a role in analysis and contributed to drafting the report. YT and HI had a role in interpretation of the data and contributed to drafting the report. SA had a role in interpretation of the data and contributed to drafting the report. HKu had a role in interpretation of the data and contributed to drafting the report. YO conceived of and designed the study, had a role in interpretation of the data, and contributed to drafting the report. KK supervised the statistical analysis, had a role in interpretation of the data, and contributed to drafting the report. All authors read and approved the final manuscript.

Authors' information

Not applicable.

Competing interests

The authors declare that they have no competing interests.

Author details

[1]Department of Medicine for Orthopaedics and Motor Organ, Juntendo University Graduate School of Medicine, 2-1-1, Hongo, Bunkyo-ku, Tokyo 113-8421, Japan. [2]Department of Pathophysiology for Locomotive and Neoplastic Diseases, Juntendo University Graduate School of Medicine, 2-1-1 Hongo, Bunkyo-ku, Tokyo 113-8421, Japan. [3]Sportology Center, Juntendo University Graduate School of Medicine, Tokyo, Japan. [4]Research Institute for Diseases of Old Age, Juntendo University Graduate School of Medicine, Tokyo, Japan. [5]Department of Radiology, Juntendo University Graduate School of Medicine, Tokyo, Japan. [6]Department of Orthopaedics, Juntendo Tokyo Koto Geriatric Medical Center, Tokyo, Japan.

References

1. Felson DT. Osteoarthritis of the knee. N Engl J Med. 2006;354(8):841–8.
2. Kurosawa H, Fukubayashi T, Nakajima H. Load-bearing mode of the knee joint: physical behavior of the knee joint with or without menisci. Clin Orthop Relat Res. 1980;149:283–90.
3. Hunter DJ, Zhang YQ, Niu JB, Tu X, Amin S, Clancy M, Guermazi A, Grigorian M, Gale D, Felson DT. The association of meniscal pathologic changes with cartilage loss in symptomatic knee osteoarthritis. Arthritis Rheum. 2006;54(3):795–801.
4. Adams JG, McAlindon T, Dimasi M, Carey J, Eustace S. Contribution of meniscal extrusion and cartilage loss to joint space narrowing in osteoarthritis. Clin Radiol. 1999;54(8):502–6.
5. Kawaguchi K, Enokida M, Otsuki R, Teshima R. Ultrasonographic evaluation of medial radial displacement of the medial meniscus in knee osteoarthritis. Arthritis Rheum. 2012;64(1):173–80.
6. Berthiaume MJ, Raynauld JP, Martel-Pelletier J, Labonte F, Beaudoin G, Bloch DA, Choquette D, Haraoui B, Altman RD, Hochberg M, et al. Meniscal tear and extrusion are strongly associated with progression of symptomatic knee osteoarthritis as assessed by quantitative magnetic resonance imaging. Ann Rheum Dis. 2005;64(4):556–63.
7. van der Kraan PM, van den Berg WB. Osteophytes: relevance and biology. Osteoarthritis Cartilage. 2007;15(3):237–44.

8. Abramson SB, Attur M. Developments in the scientific understanding of osteoarthritis. Arthritis Res Ther. 2009;11(3):227.
9. Kaneko H, Ishijima M, Futami I, Tomikawa-Ichikawa N, Kosaki K, Sadatsuki R, Yamada Y, Kurosawa H, Kaneko K, Arikawa-Hirasawa E. Synovial perlecan is required for osteophyte formation in knee osteoarthritis. Matrix Biol. 2013; 32(3-4):178–87.
10. Mosher TJ, Dardzinski BJ, Smith MB. Human articular cartilage: influence of aging and early symptomatic degeneration on the spatial variation of T2—preliminary findings at 3 T. Radiology. 2000;214(1):259–66.
11. Guermazi A, Niu J, Hayashi D, Roemer FW, Englund M, Neogi T, Aliabadi P, McLennan CE, Felson DT. Prevalence of abnormalities in knees detected by MRI in adults without knee osteoarthritis: population based observational study (Framingham Osteoarthritis Study). BMJ. 2012;345, e5339.
12. Altman R, Asch E, Bloch D, Bole G, Borenstein D, Brandt K, Christy W, Cooke TD, Greenwald R, Hochberg M, et al. Development of criteria for the classification and reporting of osteoarthritis: classification of osteoarthritis of the knee. Arthritis Rheum. 1986;29(8):1039–49.
13. Hunter DJ, Arden N, Conaghan PG, Eckstein F, Gold G, Grainger A, Guermazi A, Harvey W, Jones G. Hellio Le Graverand MP, et al. Definition of osteoarthritis on MRI: results of a Delphi exercise. Osteoarthritis Cartilage. 2011;19(8):963–9.
14. Kellgren JH, Lawrence JS. Radiological assessment of osteo-arthrosis. Ann Rheum Dis. 1957;16(4):494–502.
15. The epidemiology of chronic rheumatism. In: The epidemiology of chronic rheumatism; a symposium organized by the Council for International Organizations of Medical Sciences. Oxford, UK: Blackwell Scientific Publications; 1963.
16. Hada S, Kaneko H, Sadatsuki R, Liu L, Futami I, Kinoshita M, Yusup A, Saita Y, Takazawa Y, Ikeda H, et al. The degeneration and destruction of femoral articular cartilage shows a greater degree of deterioration than that of the tibial and patellar articular cartilage in early stage knee osteoarthritis: a cross-sectional study. Osteoarthritis Cartilage. 2014;22(10):1583–9.
17. Yusup A, Kaneko H, Liu L, Ning L, Sadatsuki R, Hada S, Kamagata K, Kinoshita M, Futami I, Shimura Y, et al. Bone marrow lesions, subchondral bone cysts and subchondral bone attrition are associated with histological synovitis in patients with end-stage knee osteoarthritis: a cross-sectional study. Osteoarthritis Cartilage. 2015;23(11):1858–64.
18. Peterfy CG, Guermazi A, Zaim S, Tirman PFJ, Miaux Y, White D, Kothari M, Lu Y, Fye K, Zhao S, et al. Whole-Organ Magnetic Resonance Imaging Score (WORMS) of the knee in osteoarthritis. Osteoarthritis Cartilage. 2004;12(3):177–90.
19. Hunter DJ, Guermazi A, Lo GH, Grainger AJ, Conaghan PG, Boudreau RM, Roemer FW. Evolution of semi-quantitative whole joint assessment of knee OA: MOAKS (MRI Osteoarthritis Knee Score). Osteoarthritis Cartilage. 2011; 19(8):990–1002.
20. Emmanuel K, Quinn E, Niu J, Guermazi A, Roemer F, Wirth W, Eckstein F, Felson D. Quantitative measures of meniscus extrusion predict incident radiographic knee osteoarthritis – data from the Osteoarthritis Initiative. Osteoarthritis Cartilage. 2016;24(2):262–9.
21. Liu L, Ishijima M, Kaneko H, Futami I, Sadatsuki R, Hada S, Yusup A, Shimura Y, Kubota M, Saita Y, et al. Disability for daily living is a predictor for joint replacement in patients with end-stage knee osteoarthritis. J Bone Miner Metab. 2014;32(2):192–9.
22. Kawaguchi H. Endochondral ossification signals in cartilage degradation during osteoarthritis progression in experimental mouse models. Mol Cells. 2008;25(1):1–6.
23. Blaney Davidson EN, Vitters EL, van der Kraan PM, van den Berg WB. Expression of transforming growth factor-β (TGFβ) and the TGFβ signalling molecule SMAD-2P in spontaneous and instability-induced osteoarthritis: role in cartilage degradation, chondrogenesis and osteophyte formation. Ann Rheum Dis. 2006;65(11):1414–21.
24. Jingushi S, Shida J, Iwamoto Y, Kinoshita T, Hiyama Y, Tamura M, Izumi T. Transient exposure of fibroblast growth factor-2 induced proliferative but not destructive changes in mouse knee joints. Connect Tissue Res. 2006; 47(4):242–8.
25. Okazaki K, Jingushi S, Ikenoue T, Urabe K, Sakai H, Ohtsuru A, Akino K, Yamashita S, Nomura S, Iwamoto Y. Expression of insulin-like growth factor I messenger ribonucleic acid in developing osteophytes in murine experimental osteoarthritis and in rats inoculated with growth hormone-secreting tumor. Endocrinology. 1999;140(10):4821–30.
26. De Maeseneer M, Lenchik L, Starok M, Pedowitz R, Trudell D, Resnick D. Normal and abnormal medial meniscocapsular structures: MR imaging and sonography in cadavers. Am J Roentgenol. 1998;171(4):969–76.
27. Costa CR, Morrison WB, Carrino JA. Medial meniscus extrusion on knee MRI: is extent associated with severity of degeneration or type of tear? Am J Roentgenol. 2004;183(1):17–23.
28. Englund M, Guermazi A, Roemer FW, Aliabadi P, Yang M, Lewis CE, Torner J, Nevitt MC, Sack B, Felson DT. Meniscal tear in knees without surgery and the development of radiographic osteoarthritis among middle-aged and elderly persons: the Multicenter Osteoarthritis Study. Arthritis Rheum. 2009; 60(3):831–9.
29. Sharma L, Nevitt M, Hochberg M, Guermazi A, Roemer FW, Crema M, Eaton C, Jackson R, Kwoh K, Cauley J, et al. Clinical significance of worsening versus stable preradiographic MRI lesions in a cohort study of persons at higher risk for knee osteoarthritis. Ann Rheum Dis. 2015;75(9):1630–6.
30. Roemer FW, Zhang Y, Niu J, Lynch JA, Crema MD, Marra MD, Nevitt MC, Felson DT, Hughes LB, El-Khoury GY, et al. Tibiofemoral joint osteoarthritis: risk factors for MR-depicted fast cartilage loss over a 30-month period in the multicenter osteoarthritis study. Radiology. 2009;252(3):772–80.
31. Englund M, Roemer FW, Hayashi D, Crema MD, Guermazi A. Meniscus pathology, osteoarthritis and the treatment controversy. Nat Rev Rheumatol. 2012;8(7):412–9.
32. Badlani JT, Borrero C, Golla S, Harner CD, Irrgang JJ. The effects of meniscus injury on the development of knee osteoarthritis: data from the osteoarthritis initiative. Am J Sports Med. 2013;41(6):1238–44.
33. Driban JB, Ward RJ, Eaton CB, Lo GH, Price LL, Lu B, McAlindon TE. Meniscal extrusion or subchondral damage characterize incident accelerated osteoarthritis: data from the Osteoarthritis Initiative. Clin Anat. 2015;28(6):792–9.
34. Bhatia S, LaPrade CM, Ellman MB, LaPrade RF. Meniscal root tears: significance, diagnosis, and treatment. Am J Sports Med. 2014;42(12):3016–30.
35. Crema MD, Roemer FW, Felson DT, Englund M, Wang K, Jarraya M, Nevitt MC, Marra MD, Torner JC, Lewis CE, et al. Factors associated with meniscal extrusion in knees with or at risk for osteoarthritis: the Multicenter Osteoarthritis Study. Radiology. 2012;264(2):494–503.
36. Park DY, Min BH, Choi BH, Kim YJ, Kim M, Suh-Kim H, Kim JH. The degeneration of meniscus roots is accompanied by fibrocartilage formation, which may precede meniscus root tears in osteoarthritic knees. Am J Sports Med. 2015;43(12):3034–44.
37. Ding C, Martel-Pelletier J, Pelletier JP, Abram F, Raynauld JP, Cicuttini F, Jones G. Knee meniscal extrusion in a largely non-osteoarthritic cohort: association with greater loss of cartilage volume. Arthritis Res Ther. 2007;9(2):R21.
38. Di Cesare PE, Haudenschild DR, Samuels J, Abramson SB. Pathogenesis of osteoarthritis. In: Firestein GS, Budd RC, Gabriel SE, McInnes IB, O'Dell JR, editors. Kelley & Firestein's textbook of rheumatology. Vol. II. 10th ed. Philadelphia: Elsevier; 2017. p. 1685–704.
39. Koski JM, Kamel A, Waris P, Waris V, Tarkiainen I, Karvanen E, Szkudlarek M, Aydin SZ, Alasaarela E, Schmidt W, et al. Atlas-based knee osteophyte assessment with ultrasonography and radiography: relationship to arthroscopic degeneration of articular cartilage. Scand J Rheumatol. 2016; 45(2):158–64.
40. Ko CH, Chan KK, Peng HL. Sonographic imaging of meniscal subluxation in patients with radiographic knee osteoarthritis. J Formos Med Assoc. 2007; 106(9):700–7.
41. Saarakkala S, Waris P, Waris V, Tarkiainen I, Karvanen E, Aarnio J, Koski JM. Diagnostic performance of knee ultrasonography for detecting degenerative changes of articular cartilage. Osteoarthritis Cartilage. 2012;20(5):376–81.
42. Schmitz RJ, Wang HM, Polprasert DR, Kraft RA, Pietrosimone BG. Evaluation of knee cartilage thickness: a comparison between ultrasound and magnetic resonance imaging methods. Knee. 2017;24(2):217–23.
43. Keshava SN, Gibikote SV, Mohanta A, Poonnoose P, Rayner T, Hilliard P, Lakshmi KM, Moineddin R, Ignas D, Srivastava A, et al. Ultrasound and magnetic resonance imaging of healthy paediatric ankles and knees: a baseline for comparison with haemophilic joints. Haemophilia. 2015;21(3):e210–222.

Levels of serum biomarkers from a two-year multicentre trial are associated with treatment response on knee osteoarthritis cartilage loss as assessed by magnetic resonance imaging

Johanne Martel-Pelletier[1], Jean-Pierre Raynauld[1], François Mineau[1], François Abram[2], Patrice Paiement[3], Philippe Delorme[3] and Jean-Pierre Pelletier[1*]

Abstract

Background: There is an obvious need to identify biomarkers that could predict patient response to an osteoarthritis (OA) treatment. This post hoc study explored in a 2-year randomized controlled trial in patients with knee OA, the likelihood of some serum biomarkers to be associated with a better response to chondroitin sulfate in reducing cartilage volume loss.

Methods: Eight biomarkers were studied: hyaluronic acid (HA), C reactive protein (CRP), adipsin, leptin, N-terminal propeptide of collagen IIα (PIIANP), C-terminal crosslinked telopeptide of type I collagen (CTX-1), matrix metalloproteinase-1 (MMP-1), and MMP-3. Patients were treated with chondroitin sulfate (1200 mg/day; $n = 57$) or celecoxib (200 mg/day; $n = 62$). Serum biomarkers were measured at baseline. The cartilage volume at baseline and its loss at 2 years were assessed by quantitative magnetic resonance imaging (MRI). Statistical analysis included analysis of covariance.

Results: As data from the original MOSAIC trial showed no differences in cartilage volume and loss in the lateral compartment of the knee joint between the two treatment groups in any comparison, only the medial compartment and its subregions were studied. Stratification according to the median biomarker levels was used to discriminate treatment effect. In patients with levels of biomarkers of inflammation (HA, leptin and adipsin) lower than the median, those treated with chondroitin sulfate demonstrated less cartilage volume loss in the medial compartment, condyle, and plateau ($p \leq 0.047$). In contrast, patients treated with chondroitin sulfate with higher levels of MMP-1 and MMP-3, biomarkers of cartilage catabolism, had less cartilage volume loss in the medial compartment, condyle, and plateau ($p \leq 0.050$). Patients with higher levels of PIIANP and CTX-1, biomarkers related to collagen anabolism and bone catabolism, respectively, had reduced cartilage volume loss in the medial condyle ($p \leq 0.026$) in the chondroitin sulfate group.

Conclusion: This study is suggestive of a potentially greater response to chondroitin sulfate treatment on cartilage volume loss in patients with knee OA with low level of inflammation and/or greater level of cartilage catabolism.

(Continued on next page)

* Correspondence: dr@jppelletier.ca
[1]Osteoarthritis Research Unit, University of Montreal Hospital Research Centre (CRCHUM), 900 Saint-Denis, Suite R11.412, Montreal, Quebec H2X 0A9, Canada
Full list of author information is available at the end of the article

(Continued from previous page)

Keywords: Knee, Osteoarthritis, Biomarkers, Clinical trial

Background

Osteoarthritis (OA) is one of the most highly prevalent joint diseases characterized by progressive articular structural changes and cartilage degradation. This disease represents an increasing burden from a medical, social and economic point of view, as it affects the majority of people in the second half of their lifespan, having a significant negative impact on quality of life. The primary etiological factors may be numerous; hence, in the majority of patients the disease is considered to be idiopathic. At present, pharmacologic therapies only reduce symptoms, and they have adverse events. For this reason, attention has been focused on the investigation and development of new types of drugs that in addition to improving the clinical symptoms of OA and having better safety profiles can also decrease cartilage volume loss.

One such product is chondroitin sulfate, which is a sulfated glycosaminoglycan that has been shown to play a role not only in the metabolism of the proteoglycans (a major macromolecule in the cartilage), but also in OA joint tissues and cells, to improve the anabolic/catabolic balance of the extracellular cartilage matrix, and to reduce some pro-inflammatory and catabolic factors and the resorptive properties of subchondral bone osteoblasts [1–5]. In addition to its ability to reduce OA symptoms, similar to that of non-steroidal anti-inflammatory drugs (NSAIDs) [6, 7], in clinical trials and studies [6, 8, 9] it has also been shown to decrease cartilage volume loss as assessed by quantitative magnetic resonance imaging (qMRI). However, as mentioned in the original trial publication [6], although it has been recommended in some guidelines [10, 11], a general consensus has not been reached on the use of chondroitin sulfate [12, 13], due in part to the unavailability of prescription-quality products, indicated for use in OA, which have been evaluated by the US Food and Drug Administration (FDA) [12]. Over the years, several studies have looked into identifying biomarkers with predictive value to assess the risk of OA progression, particularly in patients with knee OA (see reviews [14–18]). A number of such biomarkers have been identified, predominantly in observational patient cohort studies, yet none has qualified for use in clinical practice for the follow up of patients with knee OA [14, 19]. There is an obvious need to identify prognostic biomarkers, but an even greater need to identify biomarkers that could predict patient response to potential disease-modifying OA drug treatments [14, 16, 20, 21].

Recently, the Osteoarthritis Research Society International-FDA (OARSI-FDA) Biomarkers Group identified twelve distinct biochemical biomarkers of bone and cartilage turnover that could be of interest and included in the BIPEDS classification system [17]. This group further looked at the predictive validity of eighteen biomarkers as OA-related predictors of radiographic and persistent pain progression [18]. They identified nine such biomarkers that were individually able to predict clinically relevant progression over 48 months; eight catabolic and one anabolic biomarker.

Most studies assessing biomarkers in relation to articular changes have used radiographic parameters, a technology that is not sensitive for the validation of biomarkers [14, 19, 20]. Converging data argue for the use of qMRI, another imaging technology that may assist in delineating the predictive value of biomarkers with regard to OA joint structural changes [14, 16, 22]. A few trials have used this technology to identify biomarkers that would be of value in predicting drug efficacy in cartilage volume loss and clinical outcomes such as total knee replacement [23, 24].

The present study aimed to explore whether biomarkers could identify patients with knee OA most likely to benefit from a chondroitin sulfate treatment, a commonly used treatment for knee OA. The information gathered from the present study could be very useful in the context of personalized medicine, as targeting responders would reduce the cost of treatment for OA patients and, importantly, improve patient benefits.

Using the knee OA patient cohort from a phase III clinical trial [6], eight serum biomarkers (C reactive protein (CRP), hyaluronic acid (HA), leptin, adipsin, matrix metalloproteinase-1 (MMP-1), MMP-3, N-terminal propeptide of collagen IIα (PIIANP) and C-terminal crosslinked telopeptide of type I collagen (CTX-1)) were assessed for their predictive value in determining the evolution of changes in cartilage in OA over a 2-year period by qMRI, and in relation to the effect of chondroitin sulfate treatment on cartilage volume loss. The rationale behind the selection of biomarkers was to use those that are representative of the most important pathways related to OA progression: inflammation (CRP, HA, leptin, and adipsin), cartilage catabolism (MMP-1, MMP-3) and anabolism (PIIANP), and bone remodeling (CTX-1), which have been found promising [16–18, 23, 24]. We reasoned that the biomarkers chosen for the study covered a broad range of pathways including the major pathological pathways of OA and were therefore likely to provide new information about biomarkers that could be associated with a treatment effect on cartilage volume loss.

Methods

Patients and treatments

This post hoc study used the patient cohort from a 2-year phase-III comparative, double-blind clinical trial (ClinicalTrials.gov Identifier NCT01354145) [6]. In brief, patients with symptomatic knee OA, diagnosed according to the clinical and radiological criteria of the American College of Rheumatology [25], and clinical synovitis, were randomized to explore the effects of chondroitin sulfate (Condrosan®; Bioibérica S.A.U., Barcelona, Spain) (1200 mg daily; $n = 97$) compared to celecoxib (200 mg daily; $n = 97$) on cartilage volume loss in knee OA. Celecoxib was chosen as the comparator since, among many other reasons, it was shown to have no effect on the progression of cartilage volume loss in patients with knee OA [26].

The original study protocol was approved by a central review board (Institutional Review Board (IRB) Services, Toronto, ON, Canada) and the IRB of the Centre hospitalier de l'Université de Sherbrooke (CHUS), Sherbrooke, QC, Canada. The original trial [6] was conducted in compliance with the ethical principles that have their origin in the Declaration of Helsinki (2000) and are consistent with "Good Clinical Practice" International Conference of Harmonization (ICH) Tripartite Guideline (January 1997) and the applicable laws and regulations of Canada, whichever afforded the greater protection to the individual. Ethical approval for this post hoc study was obtained with the original study, thus further approval was not required. All patients provided informed consent.

The according-to-protocol (ATP) population (chondroitin sulfate $n = 57$; celecoxib $n = 62$) was chosen as it included patients who fully complied with the study's 2-year protocol and for whom serum and MRI at baseline and at 2 years were available. Of note, compared to the original ATP population [6], one serum sample was missing in the celecoxib group. These patients had taken the study medication throughout the entire study period (compliance ≥75%) and had no major protocol violations.

Outcome

The primary outcome of the study was the usefulness of some serum biomarkers to indicate patients who are most likely to have reduction in cartilage volume loss in response to chondroitin sulfate. Of note, pain was not considered as an outcome because in the original MOSAIC trial [6] both therapeutic groups experienced a comparable reduction in disease-associated pain at 2 years. Moreover, data from the original trial [6] showed no difference between the two treatment groups in cartilage volume in the lateral compartment of the knee at baseline or loss of cartilage volume in any comparison; therefore, only the medial compartment of the knee (condyle plus plateau) and its sub-regions (condyle and plateau) were studied.

Clinical, structural and biomarker assessments

Clinical evaluation at baseline

Clinical evaluation at baseline is shown in Table 1.

Clinical evaluation at baseline included assessment of knee pain on a visual analog scale (VAS), the Western Ontario and McMaster Universities Osteoarthritis Index (WOMAC) scores, the quality of life Short Form 36 General Health (SF-36), and clinical examination (swelling, visual examination; effusion, bulge sign).

MRI evaluation at baseline

Assessment using MR images included, in addition to cartilage volume [27, 28] (see subsequent description), the extent of synovitis assessed by measuring synovial thickness (mm) in four regions of interest (ROIs): the medial and lateral articular recess and the medial and lateral outer wall of the suprapatellar bursa [29]. The synovial fluid was determined using a fully automated system as previously described [30]. Bone marrow lesions were assessed in the same MRI sequences used for the cartilage assessment [31], and their extent was evaluated using the following scale: 0, absence; 1, <25%; 2, 25–50%; 3, >50% of the surface. The readers were blinded to treatment and to MRI examination time point except for baseline [6].

Cartilage volume assessment

Cartilage volume was assessed by MRI, which was performed on 1.5 T scanners (Siemens, Erlangen, Germany; General Electric, Milwaukee, WI, USA) using a standard knee coil, and the sequence acquisitions were as previously described [32]. The cartilage volume was measured by two experienced readers trained by musculoskeletal radiologists using the computer program Cartiscope™ (ArthroLab, Montreal, QC, Canada) as previously described [27, 28]. The change (percentage) in knee cartilage volume was obtained by subtracting the follow-up volume from the initial (baseline) volume divided by the initial (baseline) volume multiplied by 100. The percent coefficient of variation (CV%) is excellent as described [27].

Biomarker assessment

Blood samples were obtained after subjects fasted overnight. The samples were first allowed to coagulate and

Table 1 Patient characteristics

	Chondroitin sulfate (*n* = 57)	Celecoxib (*n* = 62)	*P* value
Male, *n* (%)	26 (46)	29 (47)	0.899*
Age, years	61 ± 8	61 ± 8	0.909
Body mass index, kg/m^2	30.3 ± 6.42	32.5 ± 5.9	*0.020*
Synovial membrane thickness, mm	1.04 ± 0.23	1.01 ± 0.22	0.528
Bone marrow lesion, score	2.49 ± 3.20	2.63 ± 2.33	0.291
Synovial fluid volume, mL	14.8 ± 15.9	11.2 ± 12.3	0.210
Joint swelling and effusion, *n* (%)	37 (65)	32 (52)	0.142*
Pain VAS, mm	60.6 ± 15.9	57.2 ± 18.6	0.252
WOMAC			
Total score (0–240)	121 ± 38	120 ± 46	0.934
Pain score (0–50)	24 ± 8	24 ± 9	0.909
Stiffness score (0–20)	11 ± 4	11 ± 4	0.694
Physical function score (0–170)	86 ± 29	85 ± 34	0.842
Quality of life (SF-36)			
Physical component summary	36.31 ± 7.82	36.33 ± 8.13	0.610
Cartilage volume (mm^3)			
Medial			
Compartment	4586 ± 1517	4324 ± 1309	0.445
Condyle	2881 ± 1020	2682 ± 833	0.448
Plateau	1705 ± 545	1642 ± 532	0.529

Data shown are number of patients (%) or mean ± SD. Continuous variables were compared using the Student's *t* test/Mann-Whitney test; *p* values in italics are statistically significant. *Proportions were compared using the chi-squared test/Fisher's exact test. *VAS* visual analog scale, *WOMAC* Western Ontario and McMaster Universities Osteoarthritis Index, *SF-36* Short Form 36

were then centrifuged (2200 rpm/1000 g, 10 minutes). Samples were stored at −80 °C until analyzed.

CTX-1 (Neo Scientific, Cambridge, MA, USA), HA (R&D Systems, Minneapolis, MN, USA) and PIIANP (EMD Millipore Corporation, Billerica, MA, USA) were assessed using specific ELISAs. Each assay is highly sensitive (sensitivity for CTX-1, 0.1 ng/mL; HA, 0.027 ng/mL; and PIIANP, 30.0 ng/mL) and designed to eliminate interference by other factors present in biological samples. Factors were read with a spectrophotometer (Multiskan Spectrum; Thermo Fisher Scientific, Mississauga, ON, Canada) and analyses performed with SkanIt sofware (Thermo). The CRP data (absolute values) available from the clinical trial report were used. The levels of the adipokines leptin and adipsin, and of MMP-1 and MMP-3 were assessed using the Human Magnetic Luminex Performance Assay kits (R&D Systems) in accordance with the manufacturer's instructions with the minimum detectable dose (MDD) of 7.69 ng/mL; 1.8 pg/mL; 0.57 pg/mL and 1.8 pg/mL, respectively. The assessment was performed using a multiplex immunoassay (Luminex Corporation, Austin, TX, USA) on a LiquiChip 200. Analyte-specific antibodies were read using a Luminex analyzer, which discriminates each different analyte, and quantitated using LiquidChip Analyzer (QIAGEN, Toronto, ON, Canada). For each factor, an 8-point standard curve and appropriate controls were included, and samples were done in duplicate.

Statistical analyses

Descriptive variables at baseline were presented as number, percentage, or mean ± standard deviation (SD) (Table 1). Differences between the two treatment groups were assessed using Student's *t* test or the Mann-Whitney test for continuous variables with a non-normal distribution, and the chi-squared or Fisher's exact test for categorical variables (Tables 1 and 2). Correlation between all biomarker levels at baseline were carried out using Pearson's correlation analysis in all subjects (Table 3).

Linear regressions adjusting for age, gender and body mass index (BMI) were also carried out to assess associations between baseline serum levels of the biomarkers and cartilage volume at baseline, and volume loss over 2 years within the medial compartment, medial condyle and medial plateau in all subjects (Table 4).

Since serum biomarkers are relatively new to the OA field in the context of a clinical trial, the median baseline biomarker levels were used to discriminate for the overall cohort (Additional file 1: Table S1) and within

Table 2 Biomarker levels at baseline

	Chondroitin sulfate (*n* = 57)	Celecoxib (*n* = 62)	*P* value*
CRP, μg/mL[†]	4.02 ± 5.41 (*n* = 48)	5.56 ± 5.54 (*n* = 46)	*0.042*
HA, ng/mL	62.46 ± 44.81	72.46 ± 60.45	0.267
Leptin, ng/mL	37.60 ± 43.78	44.23 ± 38.53	0.214
Adipsin, μg/mL	4.05 ± 1.07	4.19 ± 1.07	0.638
MMP-1, ng/mL	5.11 ± 4.13	4.69 ± 3.15	0.827
MMP-3, ng/mL	13.03 ± 6.31	13.85 ± 11.04	0.720
PIIANP, μg/mL	4.10 ± 1.92	4.10 ± 1.61	0.468
CTX-1, ng/mL	0.59 ± 0.18	0.53 ± 0.12	*0.035*

Data shown are mean ± SD. *CRP* C reactive protein, *HA* hyaluronic acid, *MMP* matrix metalloproteinase, *PIIANP* N-terminal propeptide of collagen IIα, *CTX*-1 C-terminal crosslinked telopeptide of type I collagen. *Mann-Whitney test; *p* values in italics are statistically significant. [†]Data missing for 25 patients at baseline

the treatment groups (chondroitin sulfate vs. celecoxib) (Table 5, Additional file 1: Table S2) to assess associations with baseline cartilage volume (medial compartment, medial condyle and medial plateau) and the predictive power of change in cartilage volume in the same regions at 2 years. The difference between mean cartilage volume within the three knee areas for lower vs. higher median biomarker levels was assessed by univariate analysis using Student's *t* test or the Mann-Whitney test if the distribution was non-normal distribution (Additional file 1: Table S2).

Multivariate analyses (ANCOVA) were performed adjusting for the potential confounding factors at the onset of the study, including age, gender, BMI, and baseline cartilage volume for HA only (Table 5), as it is the only biomarker that showed, in patients with levels lower than the median, a statistically significant difference in the medial condyle between treatment groups (see Additional file 1: Table S2).

All tests were two-sided and a *p* value <0.05 was considered statistically significant. Since this was an exploratory study, no statistical corrections were made for multiple comparisons. All statistical analyses were performed using SAS software, version 9.3 (SAS Institute, Cary, NC, USA).

Results

Baseline demographic, clinical, and imaging data

The two therapeutic groups were balanced with the exception of BMI, which was slightly higher in the

Table 3 Correlations between the biomarker levels at baseline in all subjects

		CRP (*n* = 94*)	HA (*n* = 119)	Leptin (*n* = 119)	Adipsin (*n* = 119)	MMP-1 (*n* = 119)	MMP-3 (*n* = 119)	PIIANP (*n* = 119)	CTX-1 (*n* = 117**)
CRP	*r*	-	-	-	-	-	-	-	-
	p value[†]	-	-	-	-	-	-	-	-
HA	*r*	<0.0001	-	-	-	-	-	-	-
	p value	>0.999	-	-	-	-	-	-	-
Leptin	*r*	0.344	-0.006	-	-	-	-	-	-
	p value	*0.001*	0.947	-	-	-	-	-	-
Adipsin	*r*	-0.016	0.188	0.343	-	-	-	-	-
	p value	0.881	*0.040*	*0.001*	-	-	-	-	-
MMP-1	*r*	0.045	-0.009	0.036	0.234	-	-	-	-
	p value	0.664	0.922	0.702	*0.010*	-	-	-	-
MMP-3	*r*	0.051	0.195	-0.245	0.049	-0.064	-	-	-
	p value	0.627	*0.033*	*0.007*	0.594	0.489	-	-	-
PIIANP	*r*	0.025	-0.042	0.015	-0.059	-0.277	-0.070	-	-
	p value	0.813	0.650	0.875	0.524	*0.002*	0.451	-	-
CTX-1	*r*	-0.093	0.063	0.016	-0.105	-0.049	-0.099	0.075	-
	p value	0.380	0.497	0.862	0.262	0.601	0.287	0.422	-

CRP C reactive protein, *HA* hyaluronic acid, *MMP* matrix metalloproteinase, *PIIANP* N-terminal propeptide of collagen IIα, *CTX*-1 C-terminal crosslinked telopeptide of type I collagen. *Data missing for 25 patients at baseline; **data missing for 2 patients at baseline
[†]Pearson's correlation; *p* values in italics are statistically significant

Table 4 Associations between cartilage volume and its loss and biomarker levels at baseline for all subjects

		CRP ($n = 94$*)	HA ($n = 119$)	Leptin ($n = 119$)	Adipsin ($n = 119$)	MMP-1 ($n = 119$)	MMP-3 ($n = 119$)	PIIANP ($n = 119$)	CTX-1 ($n = 117$**)
Cartilage volume at baseline									
Medial compartment	β	-49.24	-1.66	-4.26	101.26	-2.49	9.35	-40.65	-773.37
	p value†	*0.045*	0.409	0.385	0.315	0.931	0.454	0.489	0.256
Medial condyle	β	-37.09	-0.75	-2.62	74.50	-1.99	7.41	-38.66	-407.44
	p value	*0.030*	0.591	0.441	0.287	0.920	0.392	0.342	0.389
Medial plateau	β	-12.15	-0.91	-1.63	26.77	-0.50	1.94	-1.99	-365.94
	p value	0.170	0.215	0.361	0.468	0.962	0.671	0.926	0.141
Cartilage volume loss at 2 years									
Medial compartment	β	-0.179	0.001	0.009	0.334	0.049	-0.022	-0.546	3.418
	p value	*0.029*	0.905	0.590	0.342	0.622	0.615	*0.007*	0.150
Medial condyle	β	-0.184	0.004	-0.012	0.275	0.137	-0.038	-0.606	2.792
	p value	*0.050*	0.643	0.560	0.501	0.235	0.455	*0.010*	0.313
Medial plateau	β	-0.164	-0.005	0.049	0.415	-0.100	-0.001	-0.420	4.532
	p value	0.102	0.512	*0.016*	0.321	0.402	0.989	0.083	0.106

CRP C reactive protein, *HA* hyaluronic acid, *MMP* matrix metalloproteinase, *PIIANP* N-terminal propeptide of collagen IIα, *CTX-1* C-terminal crosslinked telopeptide of type I collagen, *β* regression parameter estimate of the biomarker. *Data missing for 25 patients at baseline; **data missing for 2 patients at baseline. †Linear regression adjusted for age, gender and body mass index; *p* values in italics are statistically significant

celecoxib group than in the chondroitin sulfate group (Table 1).

Biomarkers

Baseline levels

In the study population, with the exception of lower values of CRP and higher values of CTX-1 in the chondroitin sulfate group, there was no significant difference between the two groups (Table 2). The differences in the levels of CTX-1, although statistically significant, were very small and unlikely to be clinically relevant. Moreover, those differences found for CRP and CTX-1 no longer existed when the data were stratified by the median value (data not shown).

Correlations between biomarker levels

There was positive correlation between levels (Table 3) of CRP and leptin, HA and adipsin, HA and MMP-3, leptin and adipsin, and adipsin and MMP-1. There was negative correlation between MMP-1 and PIIANP, and between leptin and MMP-3.

Associations between biomarkers and cartilage volume

A statistically significant negative adjusted (age, gender, BMI) linear association was found between the level of CRP and cartilage volume in the medial compartment and condyle at baseline ($p = 0.045$ and $p = 0.030$, respectively) (Table 4). A statistically significant negative adjusted association was also found between the levels of CRP and PIIANP and cartilage volume loss: medial compartment ($p = 0.029$ and $p = 0.007$, respectively) and condyle ($p = 0.050$ and $p = 0.010$, respectively). A statistically significant positive adjusted association was found between the level of leptin and cartilage volume loss in the plateau ($p = 0.016$).

Biomarker and cartilage volume levels at baseline and treatment effects

Since this work is among the first attempts to assess the impact of the studied biomarkers on knee OA structure as assessed by qMRI in relation to OA treatment, and no a priori cutoff values were available, we elected, as mentioned in "Statistical analysis", to stratify the biomarkers at baseline according to their median levels. First, there were no differences in the cartilage volume between the two stratifications for any of the biomarkers (Additional file 1: Table S1). There were also no significant differences between the two treatment groups for each biomarker with the exception of HA, which, at baseline levels lower than the median, showed a statistically significant increase ($p = 0.030$) in volume for chondroitin sulfate vs. celecoxib (Additional file 1: Table S2).

Of all of the biomarkers studied (Table 5), only CRP did not show any difference in the extent of cartilage volume loss between the treatment groups, in either the lower or higher median group. The levels of all the other biomarkers were able to discriminate the extent of cartilage degradation between the treatment groups.

With regard to the biomarkers of inflammation (Table 5), compared to celecoxib, patients with levels of HA lower than the median treated with chondroitin sulfate demonstrated less cartilage volume loss in the medial

Table 5 Two-year medial region cartilage volume loss (%) according to median value of baseline biomarker levels per treatment group

	Lower than median			Higher than median		
	Chondroitin Sulfate	Celecoxib	*P* value[†]	Chondroitin Sulfate	Celecoxib	*P* value[†]
CRP[a] (*n* = 94)* Median 3.2 μg/mL						
n	28	19		20	27	
Medial compartment	-6.00 ± 3.31	-7.40 ± 3.81	0.237	-7.21 ± 3.49	-8.63 ± 4.65	0.510
Medial condyle	-5.13 ± 4.05	-6.99 ± 4.46	0.188	-6.05 ± 4.22	-8.28 ± 4.90	0.211
Medial plateau	-7.40 ± 3.90	-7.91 ± 4.49	0.745	-9.10 ± 5.12	-9.14 ± 5.56	0.642
HA[a] (*n* = 119) Median 50.2 ng/mL						
n	31	28		34	26	
Medial compartment	-5.85 ± 3.24	-8.90 ± 3.95	0.083	-7.45 ± 3.11	-8.10 ± 4.46	0.629
Medial condyle	-4.99 ± 4.03	-8.57 ± 4.79	*0.047*	-6.61 ± 3.89	-7.73 ± 4.74	0.334
Medial clateau	-7.12 ± 3.74	-9.32 ± 4.32	0.275	-8.98 ± 4.50	-8.71 ± 5.33	0.671
LEPTIN[b] (*n* = 119) Median 24.9 ng/ml						
n	30	30		27	32	
Medial compartment	-6.58 ± 3.12	-9.42 ± 4.50	*0.011*	-6.58 ± 3.45	-7.61 ± 3.89	0.445
Medial condyle	-5.90 ± 3.93	-9.16 ± 5.40	*0.014*	-5.54 ± 4.17	-7.16 ± 3.99	0.227
Medial plateau	-7.64 ± 3.08	-9.90 ± 4.90	*0.037*	-8.34 ± 5.17	-8.20 ± 4.85	0.846
ADIPSIN[b] (n = 119) Median 4.1 μg/mL						
n	31	29		26	33	
Medial compartment	-6.48 ± 3.06	-8.76 ± 4.40	*0.040*	-6.70 ± 3.53	-8.20 ± 4.11	0.161
Medial condyle	-5.16 ± 3.83	-8.38 ± 4.97	*0.007*	-6.42 ± 4.19	-7.88 ± 4.60	0.249
Medial plateau	-8.64 ± 4.14	-9.35 ± 5.21	0.701	-7.16 ± 4.15	-8.67 ± 4.61	0.190
MMP-1[c] (*n* = 119) Median 3.6 ng/mL						
n	25	34		32	28	
Medial compartment	-7.12 ± 3.38	-8.44 ± 3.68	0.239	-6.16 ± 3.14	-8.49 ± 4.86	*0.050*
Medial condyle	-6.29 ± 4.47	-8.20 ± 4.41	0.165	-5.30 ± 3.63	-8.01 ± 5.20	*0.028*
Medial plateau	-8.53 ± 3.48	-8.77 ± 4.46	0.908	-7.53 ± 4.65	-9.26 ± 5.40	0.269
MMP-3[c] (*n* = 119) Median 11.2 ng/mL						
n	27	32		30	30	
Medial compartment	-7.10 ± 3.26	-7.29 ± 4.26	0.945	-6.12 ± 3.23	-9.72 ± 3.86	*0.001*
Medial condyle	-6.39 ± 3.81	-6.94 ± 4.45	0.765	-5.15 ± 4.16	-9.37 ± 4.79	*0.001*
Medial plateau	-8.21 ± 4.53	-7.67 ± 5.04	0.736	-7.75 ± 3.89	-10.40 ± 4.34	*0.048*
PIIANP[d] (*n* = 119) Median 3.9 μg/mL						
n	28	31		29	31	
Medial compartment	-5.59 ± 2.96	-7.45 ± 4.02	0.115	-7.54 ± 3.28	-9.48 ± 4.23	0.070
Medial condyle	-4.91 ± 4.00	-6.97 ± 4.43	0.164	-6.52 ± 3.93	-9.25 ± 4.84	*0.026*
Medial plateau	-6.52 ± 3.23	-8.27 ± 5.04	0.129	-9.37 ± 4.54	-9.71 ± 4.67	0.829
CTX-1[d] (*n* = 117)** Median 0.53 ng/mL						
n	23	35		33	26	
Medial compartment	-7.11 ± 3.46	-8.83 ± 4.14	0.170	-6.15 ± 3.13	-7.83 ± 4.37	0.085
Medial condyle	-6.43 ± 4.08	-8.38 ± 4.65	0.186	-5.20 ± 4.01	-7.67 ± 5.00	*0.025*
Medial plateau	-8.03 ± 4.14	-9.56 ± 4.78	0.237	-7.87 ± 4.29	-7.99 ± 4.89	0.931

Data are cartilage volume loss (%) expressed as mean ± SD. *CRP* C reactive protein, *HA* hyaluronic acid, *MMP* matrix metalloproteinase, *PIIANP* N-terminal propeptide of collagen IIα, *CTX*-1 C-terminal crosslinked telopeptide of type I collagen. Biomarkers related to [a]inflammation; [b]adipokines; [c]matrix metalloproteinases; [d]collagen metabolism. [†]Analysis of covariance adjusted for age, gender, body mass index and, for HA only, cartilage volume at baseline; *p* values in italics are statistically significant. *Data missing for 25 patients at baseline; **data missing for 2 patients at baseline condyle ($p = 0.047$), with a numerical trend toward significance in the compartment ($p = 0.083$).

Similarly, the lower levels of the two studied adipokines (Table 5), factors involved in inflammation and in cartilage catabolism, showed differentiation between the two treatment groups, with patients treated with chondroitin sulfate having less cartilage volume loss than with celecoxib. This was found in all medial sub-regions for leptin ($p \leq 0.037$), and in the compartment ($p = 0.040$) and condyle ($p = 0.007$) for adipsin.

In contrast, for MMP-1 and MMP-3 (Table 5), it was in patients with the higher levels that differences between the two treatment groups were found: for MMP-1, patients treated with chondroitin sulfate had less cartilage volume loss than with celecoxib in the medial compartment ($p = 0.050$) and condyle ($p = 0.028$), and for MMP-3 in the medial compartment ($p = 0.001$) and both the condyle ($p = 0.001$) and plateau ($p = 0.048$).

For PIIANP and CTX-1 (Table 5), which are biomarkers related to collagen anabolism and catabolism, respectively, patients with higher baseline levels that were treated with chondroitin sulfate had less cartilage volume loss in the medial condyle compared to the celecoxib group ($p \leq 0.026$).

Discussion

Disease-modifying OA drug trials would benefit from the availability of biomarkers that could predict patients who are most likely to be responsive to a given treatment. The present study, although exploratory, provides important and novel information about the association of some serum biomarker levels with cartilage degradation, which could help to identify such patients. The original trial [6] demonstrated that chondroitin sulfate treatment in patients with knee OA had a significant beneficial effect on cartilage volume loss in the medial compartment (condyle). Here, we further showed that higher baseline values of the biomarkers PIIANP, CTX-1, MMP-1, and MMP-3, and lower baseline values of HA, leptin and adipsin seem to be associated with response to chondroitin sulfate treatment in reducing cartilage loss in patients with knee OA.

Data first showed that the extent of systemic inflammation at baseline, assessed by the levels of CRP and HA, positively correlated with the levels of cartilage catabolic factors such as leptin, adipsin, and MMP-3. Moreover, the level of leptin, an adipokine associated with inflammation, was found to positively correlate with the level of another adipokine, adipsin, which was also shown to be associated with cartilage degradation [24]. Interestingly, the inverse correlation between the levels of PIIANP and MMP-1 could likely reflect increased turnover and loss of type II collagen in cartilage, as PIIANP is associated with collagen formation/repair and MMP-1 with this macromolecule's degradation. From these data, it can be hypothesized that joint inflammation often seen in knee OA and reflected by an increased level of CRP or HA, may induce an increase in the level of leptin and, secondarily, catabolic factors such as adipsin and MMPs [33], leading to cartilage degradation and loss, the latter reflected by negative correlation with PIIANP levels. Such a hypothesis is supported by the findings of this study, which show a negative association between the level of CRP at baseline and the cartilage volume at baseline, and cartilage loss at 2 years. This is well in line with a recent review on several related studies [34]. Our findings also concur with previous reports in which the level of CRP is correlated with disease progression in patients with knee OA assessed by X-rays and MRI, and an elevated level is associated with poorer disease outcome [23, 35–38]. However, these findings have not yet attained unanimity [39].

This study also showed that lower baseline values of leptin, adipsin and HA, and higher values of MMP-3 and MMP-1, were associated with greater reduction in cartilage volume loss with chondroitin sulfate than celecoxib. This suggests that patients with a milder level of inflammation, yet sufficient to induce the synthesis of cartilage catabolic factors (MMPs), and greater cartilage catabolism and disease progression [23], are more likely to be responsive to treatment with chondroitin sulfate. These findings are in line with those of previous studies [9, 40] that reported that OA patients who had a better response to glucosamine plus chondroitin sulfate treatment were those with less severe disease but greater cartilage degradation.

HA was found to be more strongly associated with the response to treatment with chondroitin sulfate than CRP. It could be speculated that HA may be more specific than CRP at assessing synovial inflammation. One might argue that the celecoxib treated patients had significantly higher CRP values at baseline and therefore a more severe degree of inflammation, which could have precluded a response to treatment. However, the stratification of patients based on the median value of CRP, which did not differ between treatment subgroups, does not provide support for such a hypothesis. HA has been found to be correlated with symptoms (WOMAC score) and with the degree of radiographic evidence of the disease (Kellgren-Lawrence (KL) grade) [41]. In the present study, patients with lower HA were more responsive to treatment with chondroitin sulfate, which, from the aforementioned findings and those in the review by Singh et al. [41], could mean that patients with less cartilage damage had a better response to this treatment.

The aforementioned data also agree with those from the adipokines, in that patients treated with chondroitin sulfate who had lower baseline levels of adipokines had less pronounced cartilage loss and likely less synovial inflammation [42], a finding that is in line with those related to HA. This has potential clinical relevance because leptin and adipsin have been associated not only with synovial inflammation but also with OA progression and cartilage degradation in both knee and hip OA as assessed by qMRI [24, 43, 44] and with the incidence of total knee replacement [24].

There was also evidence that the level of type II collagen synthesis in OA cartilage, assessed by measuring PIIANP, was clearly associated with response to treatment. The beneficial effect of chondroitin sulfate observed in patients with higher PIIANP values, which is usually indicative of less advanced disease [45], also supports the aforementioned assumption that the response to such treatment may be more pronounced in these patients.

The protective effect of chondroitin sulfate in patients with higher levels of CTX-I, reflecting an increase in the turnover of type I collagen in bone, is interesting and may possibly be related to the positive effect of chondroitin sulfate on bone marrow lesions [8] and on mechanisms related to the remodeling of bone in OA patients [2, 5, 46].

This study has limitations, the main one being related to the fact that the original study [6] was exploratory and therefore the analysis was performed on the available samples, which were from a limited number of patients. The absence of correction for multiple comparisons is also a study limitation, but should be taken in the context of an exploratory trial. Nevertheless, findings from this study agree with some [8, 47–54], but not all [55–58], previous trials/studies and meta-analyses. Pain could not be considered as a variable, as in the original MOSAIC trial [6] chondroitin sulfate showed a beneficial effect comparable to that of celecoxib. The data on CTX-1 were obtained from serum samples as, unfortunately, urine samples were not available. This could have had an impact on the correlation with other biomarkers. The absence of correlation between CRP and HA was somewhat surprising; the smaller number of samples for CRP could potentially have impacted the results of the analysis. Finally, the use of qMRI to assess the overall cartilage loss over time in knee OA provides a global appreciation of the change in knee cartilage volume in specific anatomical areas and represents a summation of cartilage loss (negative value) and areas of cartilage swelling (positive value), both of which are part of the OA cartilage changes observed during the evolution of knee OA.

Conclusion

Although this study is exploratory and should be replicated with a larger number of patients to fully confirm the findings, data indicate that higher baseline values of the biomarkers related to collagen metabolism, PIIANP and CTX-1, and those related to cartilage degradation, MMP-1 and MMP-3, and lower baseline values of biomarkers related to inflammation, HA, leptin and adipsin, seem to be related to better response to chondroitin sulfate treatment in patients with knee OA. This is supportive of a potentially better response to treatment with chondroitin sulfate on cartilage volume loss in patients with knee OA with greater levels of cartilage catabolism and/or lower levels of inflammation.

Abbreviations

ANCOVA: Analysis of covariance; ATP: According-to-protocol; BMI: Body mass index; CRP: C reactive protein; CTX-1: C-terminal crosslinked telopeptide of type I collagen; ELISA: Enzyme-linked immunosorbent assay; HA: Hyaluronic acid; KL: Kellgren-Lawrence; MDD: Minimum detectable dose; MMP: Matrix metalloproteinase; NSAID: Non-steroidal anti-inflammatory drug; OA: Osteoarthritis; PIIANP: N-terminal propeptide of collagen IIα; qMRI: Quantitative magnetic resonance imaging; SD: Standard deviation; VAS: Visual analog scale; WOMAC: Western Ontario and McMaster Universities Osteoarthritis Index

Acknowledgements

The authors thank André Pelletier and Josée Thériault for the MRI reading and Virginia Wallis for her assistance with the manuscript preparation.

Funding

The original trial was funded by Bioibérica SAU, Barcelona, Spain. The sponsor provided all of the study medication free of charge and met the expenses that arose during the course of the study and post hoc analysis. This study was funded by an unrestrictive grant from Bioibérica. The sponsor had no role in the design or conduct of the study, the management, analysis, or interpretation of the data, or the preparation, review, or approval of the manuscript. The sponsor had no access to the data and did not perform any of the study analysis.

Authors' contributions

JM-P and J-PP designed the study and J-PR participated in the study design. PP was responsible for the collection and integrity of the serum. FM conducted the biomarker experiments and the related data interpretation. FA performed the MRI determination and the related data interpretation. PD performed the statistical analyses and related data interpretation. JM-P, J-PP, J-PR, and PD performed the overall data analysis and interpretation. JM-P and J-PP drafted the manuscript and J-PR assisted with drafting the manuscript. All of the authors read and approved the final manuscript.

Competing interests

JM-P and J-PP are consultants for Bioiberica, SAU and shareholders in ArthroLab Inc. J-PR is a consultant for ArthroLab Inc. FA, PP and PD are employees of ArthroLab Inc. FM has no conflict of interest. No non-financial conflicts of interest exist for any of the authors.

Author details

[1]Osteoarthritis Research Unit, University of Montreal Hospital Research Centre (CRCHUM), 900 Saint-Denis, Suite R11.412, Montreal, Quebec H2X 0A9, Canada. [2]Medical Imaging Research & Development, ArthroLab Inc, Montreal, Quebec, Canada. [3]ArthroLab Inc, Montreal, Quebec, Canada.

References

1. Chan PS, Caron JP, Orth MW. Effect of glucosamine and chondroitin sulfate on regulation of gene expression of proteolytic enzymes and their inhibitors in interleukin-1-challenged bovine articular cartilage explants. Am J Vet Res. 2005;66(11):1870–6.
2. Tat SK, Pelletier JP, Vergés J, Montell E, Lajeunesse D, Fahmi H, Lavigne M, Martel-Pelletier J. Chondroitin and glucosamine sulfate in combination decrease the pro-resorptive properties of human osteoarthritis subchondral bone osteoblasts. Arthritis Res Ther. 2007;9:R117.
3. Monfort J, Pelletier J-P, Garcia-Giralt N, Martel-Pelletier J. Biochemical basis of the effect of chondroitin sulfate on osteoarthritis articular tissues. Ann Rheum Dis. 2008;67:735–40.
4. du Souich P, Garcia AG, Verges J, Montell E. Immunomodulatory and anti-inflammatory effects of chondroitin sulphate. J Cell Mol Med. 2009;13(8A): 1451–63.
5. Martel-Pelletier J, Kwan Tat S, Pelletier JP. Effects of chondroitin sulfate in the pathophysiology of the osteoarthritic joint: a narrative review. Osteoarthritis Cartilage. 2010;18 Suppl 1:S7–11.
6. Pelletier JP, Raynauld JP, Beaulieu AD, Bessette L, Morin F, de Brum-Fernandes AJ, Delorme P, Dorais M, Paiement P, Abram F, et al. Chondroitin sulfate efficacy versus celecoxib on knee osteoarthritis structural changes using magnetic resonance imaging: a 2-year multicentre exploratory study. Arthritis Res Ther. 2016;18(1):256.
7. Hochberg MC, Martel-Pelletier J, Monfort J, Moller I, Castillo JR, Arden N, Berenbaum F, Blanco FJ, Conaghan PG, Domenech G, et al. Combined chondroitin sulfate and glucosamine for painful knee osteoarthritis: a multicentre, randomised, double-blind, non-inferiority trial versus celecoxib. Ann Rheum Dis. 2016;75(1):37–44.
8. Wildi LM, Raynauld JP, Martel-Pelletier J, Beaulieu A, Bessette L, Morin F, Abram F, Dorais M, Pelletier JP. Chondroitin sulphate reduces both cartilage volume loss and bone marrow lesions in knee osteoarthritis patients starting as early as 6 months after initiation of therapy: a randomised, double-blind, placebo-controlled pilot study using MRI. Ann Rheum Dis. 2011;70(6):982–9.
9. Martel-Pelletier J, Roubille C, Abram F, Hochberg MC, Dorais M, Delorme P, Raynauld JP, Pelletier JP. First-line analysis of the effects of treatment on progression of structural changes in knee osteoarthritis over 24 months: data from the osteoarthritis initiative progression cohort. Ann Rheum Dis. 2015;74(3):547–56.
10. Jordan KM, Arden NK, Doherty M, Bannwarth B, Bijlsma JW, Dieppe P, Gunther K, Hauselmann H, Herrero-Beaumont G, Kaklamanis P, et al. EULAR recommendations 2003: an evidence based approach to the management of knee osteoarthritis: Report of a Task Force of the Standing Committee for International Clinical Studies Including Therapeutic Trials (ESCISIT). Ann Rheum Dis. 2003;62(12):1145–55.
11. Bruyere O, Cooper C, Pelletier JP, Branco J, Luisa Brandi M, Guillemin F, Hochberg MC, Kanis JA, Kvien TK, Martel-Pelletier J, et al. An algorithm recommendation for the management of knee osteoarthritis in Europe and internationally: a report from a task force of the European Society for Clinical and Economic Aspects of Osteoporosis and Osteoarthritis (ESCEO). Semin Arthritis Rheum. 2014;44(3):253–63.
12. Hochberg MC, Altman RD, April KT, Benkhalti M, Guyatt G, McGowan J, Towheed T, Welch V, Wells G, Tugwell P. American College of Rheumatology 2012 recommendations for the use of nonpharmacologic and pharmacologic therapies in osteoarthritis of the hand, hip, and knee. Arthritis Care Res (Hoboken). 2012;64(4):465–74.
13. McAlindon TE, Bannuru RR, Sullivan MC, Arden NK, Berenbaum F, Bierma-Zeinstra SM, Hawker GA, Henrotin Y, Hunter DJ, Kawaguchi H, et al. OARSI guidelines for the non-surgical management of knee osteoarthritis. Osteoarthritis Cartilage. 2014;22(3):363–88.
14. Lotz M, Martel-Pelletier J, Christiansen C, Brandi ML, Bruyere O, Chapurlat R, Collette J, Cooper C, Giacovelli G, Kanis JA, et al. Value of biomarkers in osteoarthritis: current status and perspectives. Ann Rheum Dis. 2013;72(11):1756–63.
15. Daghestani HN, Kraus VB. Inflammatory biomarkers in osteoarthritis. Osteoarthritis Cartilage. 2015;23(11):1890–6.
16. Hunter DJ, Nevitt M, Losina E, Kraus V. Biomarkers for osteoarthritis: current position and steps towards further validation. Best Pract Res Clin Rheumatol. 2014;28(1):61–71.
17. Kraus VB, Blanco FJ, Englund M, Henrotin Y, Lohmander LS, Losina E, Onnerfjord P, Persiani S. OARSI clinical trials recommendations: soluble biomarker assessments in clinical trials in osteoarthritis. Osteoarthritis Cartilage. 2015;23(5):686–97.
18. Kraus VB, Collins JE, Hargrove D, Losina E, Nevitt M, Katz JN, Wang SX, Sandell LJ, Hoffmann SC, Hunter DJ, et al. Predictive validity of biochemical biomarkers in knee osteoarthritis: data from the FNIH OA Biomarkers Consortium. Ann Rheum Dis. 2016. doi:10.1136/annrheumdis-2016-209252.
19. Arden N, Richette P, Cooper C, Bruyere O, Abadie E, Branco J, Brandi ML, Berenbaum F, Clerc C, Dennison E, et al. Can we identify patients with high risk of osteoarthritis progression who will respond to treatment? A focus on biomarkers and frailty. Drugs Aging. 2015;32(7):525–35.
20. Attur M, Krasnokutsky-Samuels S, Samuels J, Abramson SB. Prognostic biomarkers in osteoarthritis. Curr Opin Rheumatol. 2013;25(1):136–44.
21. Kraus VB, Hargrove DE, Hunter DJ, Renner JB, Jordan JM. Establishment of reference intervals for osteoarthritis-related soluble biomarkers: the FNIH/OARSI OA Biomarkers Consortium. Ann Rheum Dis. 2016. doi:10.1136/annrheumdis-2016-209253.
22. Pelletier JP, Cooper C, Peterfy C, Reginster JY, Brandi ML, Bruyere O, Chapurlat R, Cicuttini F, Conaghan PG, Doherty M, et al. What is the predictive value of MRI for the occurrence of knee replacement surgery in knee osteoarthritis? Ann Rheum Dis. 2013;72(10):1594–604.
23. Pelletier JP, Raynauld JP, Caron J, Mineau F, Abram F, Dorais M, Haraoui B, Choquette D, Martel-Pelletier J. Decrease in serum level of matrix metalloproteinases is predictive of the disease-modifying effect of osteoarthritis drugs assessed by quantitative MRI in patients with knee osteoarthritis. Ann Rheum Dis. 2010;69(12):2095–101.
24. Martel-Pelletier J, Raynauld JP, Dorais M, Abram F, Pelletier JP. The levels of the adipokines adipsin and leptin are associated with knee osteoarthritis progression as assessed by MRI and incidence of total knee replacement in symptomatic osteoarthritis patients: a post hoc analysis. Rheumatology (Oxford). 2016;55(4):680–8.
25. Altman R, Asch E, Bloch D, Bole G, Borenstein D, Brandt K, Christy W, Cooke TD, Greenwald R, Hochberg M, et al. Development of criteria for the classification and reporting of osteoarthritis. Classification of osteoarthritis of the knee. Diagnostic and Therapeutic Criteria Committee of the American Rheumatism Association. Arthritis Rheum. 1986;29(8):1039–49.
26. Raynauld JP, Martel-Pelletier J, Beaulieu A, Bessette L, Morin F, Choquette D, Haraoui B, Abram F, Pelletier JP. An open-label pilot study evaluating by magnetic resonance imaging the potential for a disease-modifying effect of celecoxib compared to a modelized historical control cohort in the treatment of knee osteoarthritis. Semin Arthritis Rheum. 2010;40(3):185–92.
27. Raynauld JP, Martel-Pelletier J, Berthiaume MJ, Labonté F, Beaudoin G, de Guise JA, Bloch DA, Choquette D, Haraoui B, Altman RD, et al. Quantitative magnetic resonance imaging evaluation of knee osteoarthritis progression over two years and correlation with clinical symptoms and radiologic changes. Arthritis Rheum. 2004;50:476–87.
28. Kauffmann C, Gravel P, Godbout B, Gravel A, Beaudoin G, Raynauld JP, Martel-Pelletier J, Pelletier JP, de Guise JA. Computer-aided method for quantification of cartilage thickness and volume changes using MRI: validation study using a synthetic model. IEEE Trans Biomed Eng. 2003;50(8):978–88.
29. Pelletier JP, Raynauld JP, Abram F, Haraoui B, Choquette D, Martel-Pelletier J. A new non-invasive method to assess synovitis severity in relation to symptoms and cartilage volume loss in knee osteoarthritis patients using MRI. Osteoarthritis Cartilage. 2008;16 Suppl 3:S8–13.
30. Li W, Abram F, Pelletier JP, Raynauld JP, Dorais M, d'Anjou MA, Martel-Pelletier J. Fully automated system for the quantification of human osteoarthritic knee joint effusion volume using magnetic resonance imaging. Arthritis Res Ther. 2010;12(5):R173.
31. Raynauld JP, Martel-Pelletier J, Berthiaume MJ, Beaudoin G, Choquette D, Haraoui B, Tannenbaum H, Meyer JM, Beary JF, Cline GA, et al. Long term evaluation of disease progression through the quantitative magnetic resonance imaging of symptomatic knee osteoarthritis patients: correlation with clinical symptoms and radiographic changes. Arthritis Res Ther. 2006;8(1):R21.
32. Wildi LM, Martel-Pelletier J, Abram F, Moser T, Raynauld JP, Pelletier JP. Assessment of cartilage changes over time in knee osteoarthritis disease-modifying osteoarthritis drug trials using semiquantitative and quantitative methods: pros and cons. Arthritis Care Res (Hoboken). 2013;65(5):686–94.
33. Koskinen A, Vuolteenaho K, Nieminen R, Moilanen T, Moilanen E. Leptin enhances MMP-1, MMP-3 and MMP-13 production in human osteoarthritic

cartilage and correlates with MMP-1 and MMP-3 in synovial fluid from OA patients. Clin Exp Rheumatol. 2011;29(1):57–64.
34. Bay-Jensen AC, Reker D, Kjelgaard-Petersen CF, Mobasheri A, Karsdal MA, Ladel C, Henrotin Y, Thudium CS. Osteoarthritis year in review 2015: soluble biomarkers and the BIPED criteria. Osteoarthritis Cartilage. 2016;24(1):9–20.
35. Smith JW, Martins TB, Gopez E, Johnson T, Hill HR, Rosenberg TD. Significance of C-reactive protein in osteoarthritis and total knee arthroplasty outcomes. Ther Adv Musculoskelet Dis. 2012;4(5):315–25.
36. Sharif M, Shepstone L, Elson CJ, Dieppe PA, Kirwan JR. Increased serum C reactive protein may reflect events that precede radiographic progression in osteoarthritis of the knee. Ann Rheum Dis. 2000;59:71–4.
37. Wang X, Hunter D, Xu J, Ding C. Metabolic triggered inflammation in osteoarthritis. Osteoarthritis Cartilage. 2015;23(1):22–30.
38. Saberi Hosnijeh F, Siebuhr AS, Uitterlinden AG, Oei EH, Hofman A, Karsdal MA, Bierma-Zeinstra SM, Bay-Jensen AC, van Meurs JB. Association between biomarkers of tissue inflammation and progression of osteoarthritis: evidence from the Rotterdam study cohort. Arthritis Res Ther. 2015;18:81.
39. Jin X, Beguerie JR, Zhang W, Blizzard L, Otahal P, Jones G, Ding C. Circulating C reactive protein in osteoarthritis: a systematic review and meta-analysis. Ann Rheum Dis. 2015;74(4):703–10.
40. Roubille C, Martel-Pelletier J, Abram F, Dorais M, Delorme P, Raynauld JP, Pelletier JP. Impact of disease treatments on the progression of knee osteoarthritis structural changes related to meniscal extrusion: Data from the OAI progression cohort. Semin Arthritis Rheum. 2015;45(3):257–67.
41. Singh S, Kumar D, Sharma NR. Role of hyaluronic acid in early diagnosis of knee osteoarthritis. J Clin Diagn Res. 2014;8(12):LC04–07.
42. de Boer TN, van Spil WE, Huisman AM, Polak AA, Bijlsma JW, Lafeber FP, Mastbergen SC. Serum adipokines in osteoarthritis; comparison with controls and relationship with local parameters of synovial inflammation and cartilage damage. Osteoarthritis Cartilage. 2012;20(8):846–53.
43. Stannus OP, Jones G, Quinn SJ, Cicuttini FM, Dore D, Ding C. The association between leptin, interleukin-6, and hip radiographic osteoarthritis in older people: a cross-sectional study. Arthritis Res Ther. 2010;12(3):R95.
44. Stannus OP, Cao Y, Antony B, Blizzard L, Cicuttini F, Jones G, Ding C. Cross-sectional and longitudinal associations between circulating leptin and knee cartilage thickness in older adults. Ann Rheum Dis. 2015;74(1):82–8.
45. Berry PA, Maciewicz RA, Wluka AE, Downey-Jones MD, Forbes A, Hellawell CJ, Cicuttini FM. Relationship of serum markers of cartilage metabolism to imaging and clinical outcome measures of knee joint structure. Ann Rheum Dis. 2010;69(10):1816–22.
46. Raynauld JP, Pelletier JP, Delorme P, Dodin P, Abram F, Martel-Pelletier J. Bone curvature changes can predict in knee osteoarthritis the impact of treatment on cartilage volume loss: data from a two-year clinical trial. Rheumatology (Oxford). 2017;56(6):989-98.
47. Uebelhart D, Malaise M, Marcolongo R, DeVathaire F, Piperno M, Mailleux E, Fioravanti A, Matoso L, Vignon E. Intermittent treatment of knee osteoarthritis with oral chondroitin sulfate: a one-year, randomized, double-blind, multicenter study versus placebo. Osteoarthritis Cartilage. 2004;12(4):269–76.
48. Michel BA, Stucki G, Frey D, De Vathaire F, Vignon E, Bruehlmann P, Uebelhart D. Chondroitins 4 and 6 sulfate in osteoarthritis of the knee: a randomized, controlled trial. Arthritis Rheum. 2005;52(3):779–86.
49. Kahan A, Uebelhart D, De Vathaire F, Delmas PD, Reginster JY. Long-term effects of chondroitins 4 and 6 sulfate on knee osteoarthritis: the study on osteoarthritis progression prevention, a two-year, randomized, double-blind, placebo-controlled trial. Arthritis Rheum. 2009;60(2):524–33.
50. Hochberg MC. Structure-modifying effects of chondroitin sulfate in knee osteoarthritis: an updated meta-analysis of randomized placebo-controlled trials of 2-year duration. Osteoarthritis Cartilage. 2010;18 Suppl 1:S28–31.
51. Lee YH, Woo JH, Choi SJ, Ji JD, Song GG. Effect of glucosamine or chondroitin sulfate on the osteoarthritis progression: a meta-analysis. Rheumatol Int. 2010;30(3):357–63.
52. Hochberg M, Chevalier X, Henrotin Y, Hunter DJ, Uebelhart D. Symptom and structure modification in osteoarthritis with pharmaceutical-grade chondroitin sulfate: what's the evidence? Curr Med Res Opin. 2013;29(3):259–67.
53. Gallagher B, Tjoumakaris FP, Harwood MI, Good RP, Ciccotti MG, Freedman KB. Chondroprotection and the prevention of osteoarthritis progression of the knee: a systematic review of treatment agents. Am J Sports Med. 2015; 43(3):734–44.
54. Singh JA, Noorbaloochi S, MacDonald R, Maxwell LJ. Chondroitin for osteoarthritis. Cochrane Database Syst Rev. 2015;1:CD005614.
55. Richy F, Bruyere O, Ethgen O, Cucherat M, Henrotin Y, Reginster JY. Structural and symptomatic efficacy of glucosamine and chondroitin in knee osteoarthritis: a comprehensive meta-analysis. Arch Intern Med. 2003;163(13):1514–22.
56. Clegg DO, Reda DJ, Harris CL, Klein MA, O'Dell JR, Hooper MM, Bradley JD, Bingham 3rd CO, Weisman MH, Jackson CG, et al. Glucosamine, chondroitin sulfate, and the two in combination for painful knee osteoarthritis. N Engl J Med. 2006;354(8):795–808.
57. Reichenbach S, Sterchi R, Scherer M, Trelle S, Burgi E, Burgi U, Dieppe PA, Juni P. Meta-analysis: chondroitin for osteoarthritis of the knee or hip. Ann Intern Med. 2007;146(8):580–90.
58. Wandel S, Juni P, Tendal B, Nuesch E, Villiger PM, Welton NJ, Reichenbach S, Trelle S. Effects of glucosamine, chondroitin, or placebo in patients with osteoarthritis of hip or knee: network meta-analysis. BMJ. 2010;341:c4675.

4

Anabolic role of lysyl oxidase like-2 in cartilage of knee and temporomandibular joints with osteoarthritis

Weam Alshenibr[1†], Mustafa M. Tashkandi[1†], Saqer F. Alsaqer[1], Yazeed Alkheriji[1], Amelia Wise[2], Sadanand Fulzele[3], Pushkar Mehra[4], Mary B. Goldring[5,6], Louis C. Gerstenfeld[2] and Manish V. Bais[1*]

Abstract

Background: Lysyl oxidase like-2 (LOXL2) is a copper-dependent amine oxidase. Our previous studies showed that LOXL2 is elevated during mouse fracture healing. The goal of this study was to evaluate the potential of LOXL2 to act as an anabolic agent in cartilage affected by osteoarthritis (OA).

Methods: LOXL2 was visualized in tissues from human knee and hip joints and temporomandibular joints (TMJ) by immunofluorescence. The activity of LOXL2 in human articular and TMJ chondrocytes was assessed by cell-based assays, microarray analysis, and RT-qPCR, and LOXL2-mediated activation of NF-κB and extracellular signal-related kinase (ERK) signaling pathways was measured by western blotting. To examine LOXL2-induced effect in vivo, we implanted Matrigel-imbedded human chondrocytes into nude mice and exposed them to exogenous LOXL2 for 6 weeks. Finally, LOXL2-induced effects on collagen type 2 α1 (COL2A1) and phospho-SMAD2/3 were evaluated by immunofluorescence analysis.

Results: LOXL2 staining was detected in damaged regions of human TMJ, hip and knee joints affected by OA. Stimulation with transforming growth factor (TGF)-β1 upregulated LOXL2 expression, while pro-inflammatory cytokines IL-1β and TNF-α downregulated LOXL2, in human chondrocytes. Viral transduction of LOXL2 in OA chondrocytes increased the mRNA levels of chondroitin sulfate proteoglycan (CSPG4), aggrecan (ACAN), sex determining region Y-box containing gene 9 (SOX9), and COL2A1 but reduced the levels of extracellular matrix (ECM)-degrading enzymes matrix metalloproteinase (MMP)1, MMP3, and MMP13. Further, forced expression of LOXL2 promoted chondrogenic lineage-specific gene expression, increased the expression of *COL2A1* in the presence of TNF-α, and inhibited chondrocyte apoptosis. LOXL2 expression also inhibited IL-1β-induced phospho-NF-κB/p65 and TGF-β1-induced ERK1/2 phosphorylation. Matrigel constructs of human chondrocytes from the knee joint and TMJ implanted in nude mice showed anabolic responses after LOXL2 transduction, including increased expression of *SOX9*, *ACAN*, and *COL2A1*. Finally, immunofluorescence staining revealed co-localization of LOXL2 with SOX9 in the nuclei of cells in the implants, decreased phospho-SMAD2/3, and increased COL2A1 staining.

Conclusion: Our results suggest that although LOXL2 is upregulated in cartilage affected by OA, this may be a protective response that promotes anabolism while inhibiting specific catabolic responses in the pathophysiology of OA.

Keywords: LOXL2, Anabolic response, Cartilage, Osteoarthritis

* Correspondence: bmanish@bu.edu
†Equal contributors
[1]Department of Molecular and Cell Biology, Boston University Henry M. Goldman School of Dental Medicine, W-216, 700 Albany Street, Boston, MA 02118, USA
Full list of author information is available at the end of the article

Background

Osteoarthritis (OA), the most common degenerative joint disease, leads to structural damage and ultimately loss of function and disability. Progressive, irreversible destruction of the joints in OA is driven by defective cartilage extracellular matrix (ECM) remodeling and the loss of chondrocytes due to apoptosis [1]. Knee pain and symptomatic knee OA have increased in prevalence [2], and similar manifestations of the disease process are seen in temporomandibular joint (TMJ) disorders [3]. Advances in understanding the disease pathogenesis are critical to OA prevention and treatment.

Lysyl oxidase (LOX) family members (LOX, LOXL1-4) are copper-dependent amine oxidases that function in ECM remodeling and collagen cross-linking. LOX activity is required for the formation of immature and mature pyrodinoline (PYR) cross-links in native and engineered cartilage. Hypoxia-induced LOX increases PYR cross-links and tensile properties of the articular cartilage, knee meniscus, patellar tendon, and anterior and posterior cruciate ligaments, while exogenously applied LOX proteins are capable of enhancing collagen cross-linking and cartilage tissue functional properties [4]. Our previous studies showed that a member of the LOX family, LOXL2, is elevated during fracture healing in mice and that it promotes chondrogenesis and the formation of cartilage ECM [5, 6]. Whether LOXL2 plays any role in the pathophysiology of OA and the effect on cartilage is not known.

Pro-inflammatory cytokines such as tumor necrosis factor (TNF)-α and interleukin (IL)-1β are catabolic cytokines [7] involved in chondrocyte apoptosis and matrix proteolysis; they contribute to the pathophysiology of OA [8]. Anti-cytokine agents have been evaluated for OA therapy, but with limited success [9, 10]. Anabolic factors that have roles in chondrogenesis and articular cartilage maintenance have been used as additive factors in tissue engineering strategies and are considered as candidate structure-modifying agents for OA therapy [11]. Examples are fibroblast growth factor-18 [12] and members of the bone morphogenetic protein 2 (BMP)/transforming growth factor β1 (TGF-β) family. Differential chondrocyte responses due to aging and OA may account for off-target effects in joints treated with pro-anabolic agents; such effects can result in cartilage calcification, osteophyte formation, angiogenesis, and synovial fibrosis [13, 14]. Thus, alternative approaches to regulating these inflammatory cytokines could lead to improved therapies.

To better understand the role of LOXL2 in OA cartilage, we used global gene expression, immunohistochemical, and mouse xenotransplantation studies to assess the effects of LOXL2 overexpression in OA chondrocytes in vitro and in vivo. Our findings indicate that LOXL2 may act as a pro-anabolic agent in OA cartilage, providing a foundation for future work on OA therapy.

Methods

Human tissues and animal experiments

Human tissues were obtained with Institutional Review Board (IRB) approval and informed consent from all subjects. TMJ tissues were obtained from Boston University (IRB H33300). TMJ tissues were selected on the basis of clinical features such as TMJ pain and mobility and confirmed by pathological diagnostic findings as healthy or TMJ-OA, at the Department of Pathology, Boston University. The exclusion criteria included a history of any rheumatic disease or cancer. Histological slides from 16 patients (8/condition) including TMJ normal (Osteoarthritis Research Society International (OARSI) grade I) and TMJ-OA (OARSI grade V) from right and left joints were obtained. Freshly isolated cells from TMJ-OA cartilage from five patients were used for animal experiments. Histological slides of tissues from hip joints were obtained from the Department of Orthopaedic Surgery, School of Medicine, Boston University, Boston, MA, USA (IRB H-32517). Tissue sections included both uninvolved and involved regions of the femoral head based on micro computed tomography (microCT) mapping of the regions of cartilage erosion relative to bone cysts. Histological sample slides were obtained from six individuals. The OA cartilage histological tissue slides from the knee joints were obtained from Georgia Medical College, Augusta, GA, USA under IRB approval (657441-5). Tibial epiphyses from OA-affected regions (OARSI grade V) and the adjacent healthy region (OARSI grade I) were collected from five patients. All mouse experiments were performed with guidance and regulations through Boston University Institutional Animal Care and Use Committee (IACUC), approval number AN-15387.

Immunofluorescence of human tissue sections

Human tissues were fixed in 4% paraformaldehyde overnight, paraffin-embedded, and sectioned for subsequent immunofluorescence by standard procedures. The tissue sections were exposed to anti-LOXL2-specific antibodies (GeneTex) or isotype control antibody; primary antibodies were detected with anti-biotin antibody combined with streptavidin-conjugated Texas red. Anti-fade reagent with 4′,6-diamidino-2-phenylindole (DAPI) was added to all the samples. Sections were viewed under epifluorescence microscopy (Zeiss 710). Quantification of images was performed using Image J software (NIH), as shown in an earlier study [15]. Briefly, the region of interest was selected by drawing the margins. Parameters were set to measure area, integrated density, and mean fluorescence for stained regions, and data were obtained from several regions. Next, the same measurements were obtained from adjacent regions as a background control. We calculated the total corrected cellular fluorescence (TCCF):

$$\begin{aligned}\text{TCCF} = \text{Integrated density} - (&\text{Area of selected cell} \\ &\times \text{Mean fluorescence of background readings})\end{aligned}$$

Data are reported as the fold-change expression compared to respective controls.

RNA isolation and analysis

Total RNA was extracted from paraffin-embedded sections of the femur, tibia, and TMJ condyle using Trizol (Qiagen) and FFPE RNA isolation kit (Qiagen), according to the manufacturer's instructions. Briefly, tissue sections were deparaffinized with Xylenes for 10 min, washed with Xylenes then ethanol, and air-dried. Tissues were treated with proteinase K and RNAase inhibitor overnight and extracted with Trizol. Finally, RNA was precipitated using 10 μg glycogen and isopropanol, washed with ethanol, and reconstituted in nuclease-free water. Quantitative real-time PCR (RT-qPCR) analysis was performed using TaqMan gene expression assays from Life Technologies, according to a standard protocol [16]. TaqMan® Gene Expression Assay IDs for human and mouse primers were: Sex determining region Y-box containing gene 9 (SOX9) (Hs01001343_g1 and Mm00448840_m1), matrix metalloproteinase (MMP)13 (Hs00233992_m1 and Mm00439491_m1), aggrecan (ACAN) (Hs00153936_m1 and Mm00545794_m1), collagen type II α1 (COL2A1) (Hs00264051_m1 and Mm01309565_m1), and LOXL2 (Hs00158757_m1).

Human cell cultures

Human articular chondrocytes (HAC) from three OA patients (HAC-OA) (Cell Application Inc. from lot no. 2356, 1777, and 2881) were used. Normal HAC (HAC-N) cells were from Lonza (CC-2550). Cell lines were grown in chondrocyte growth medium (CGM™ BulletKit™, CC-3216, Lonza Inc.) or in chondrocyte differentiation medium (CDM BulletKit, CC-3225, Lonza), both of which contain 5% fetal bovine serum (FBS), R3-insulin-like growth factor-1, human recombinant fibroblast growth factor-beta; insulin-transferrin-selenium (ITS), and gentamycin/amphotericin-B for in vitro studies. The chondrocyte differentiation medium also contains TGF-β3. These supplements have been optimized for HAC [17, 18]. The medium, with a similar composition, from Lonza and Cell Applications optimized for HAC (HAC-O and HAC) has been used in several in vitro and in vivo studies [19, 20] and in our experiments. Primary TMJ cells were obtained as outgrowths from explants of TMJ condylar cartilage within 24 h after collection as 1-mm to 3-mm punch biopsies, and cultured in chondrocyte growth medium with 5% FBS (Lonza Inc.).

Preparation of lentivirus and adenovirus

Adenoviruses for transient expression of LOXL2 (Ad-CMV-RFP-CMV-hLOXL2-His; referred to as Ad-RFP-LOXL2), and its empty vector (EV) control (Ad-RFP-EV) were custom-synthesized (ADV-214438) by Vector Biolabs. These adenovirus particles were amplified in 293 T cells and quantified using an adenovirus quantification kit (Cell Biolabs). The lentivirus packaging was performed using the 3-plasmid protocol [16]. Lentiviral vector for LOXL2 (CMV-LOXL2) and CMV-EV)) were purchased from Genecopoeia Inc. (EX-Y2020-Lv128 and LV128;). The expression of LOXL2 protein was evaluated by western blotting of the medium and cell layer, and enzymatic activity of purified LOXL2 was evaluated by the Amplex Red assay [21].

Cell proliferation

The CyQuant cell proliferation reagent assay (Molecular Probes), was used to measure the cell proliferation. HAC or HAC-OA cells were seeded at a density of 20,000 cells per well in 24-well plates and transduced with Adv-RFP-EV or Adv-RFP-LOXL2 in the respective group. After 24 h, they were washed with PBS, and the plates with cell layer were stored at −80 °C. For measurements, plates were thawed at room temperature for 30 min and 200 μl of CyQuant GR dye/cell-lysis buffer added to each well. Fluroscence measured as per manufacturer's instructions with excitation at 420 nm and emission detection at 535 nm.

Apoptosis assay

HAC-N or HAC-OA were infected with the Ad-RFP-EV or ad-RFP-LOXL2 at a multiplicity of infection (MOI) of 50 in triplicate wells. The next day, cells were treated with 10 ng/mL of IL-1β, 10 ng/mL of TNF-α, or vehicle for 24 h in serum-free medium. Cells were lysed using lysis buffer provided in the kit and were analyzed with a bioluminescence-based caspase-3/7 glow apoptosis assay (Promega) according to manufacturer's instructions.

Molecular signaling analysis

HAC-OA, transduced with either Ad-RFP-LOXL2 or Ad-RFP-EV at MOI 25, were incubated in serum-free growth medium for at least 16 h and then left untreated (vehicle) or treated for 10 min with 10 ng/mL of IL-1β or TGF-β1. Proteins were extracted for western blot analysis.

Western blotting

Tissue or cell layers were extracted with SDS-PAGE sample buffer (0.1 mM Tris-HCl, 4% SDS, 10% glycerol, 5% β-mercaptoethanol) and boiled for 3–5 minutes. Protein concentrations were determined using Nano Orange assay kits (Molecular Probes, Eugene, OR, USA). From tumors, approximately 20 μg of protein per experimental group were then subjected to 10% SDS-PAGE and western blotting with primary antibodies (Cell Signaling Technology). The antibodies used were for evaluation of phospho-NF-κB-p65 (S536) and NF-κB-p65 (total), phospho-ERK1/2, total extracellular signal-related kinase (ERK) and β-actin. Anti-rabbit and anti-mouse secondary antibodies were purchased from Cell Signaling Technology. Quantification was performed using a digital densitometry system (Versadoc; BioRad, Hercules, CA, USA) and Image J software.

Gene array experiments

To evaluate the genes that were differentially regulated by LOXL2, HAC-OA from three different OA patients were cultured in chondrocyte growth medium (Lonza)

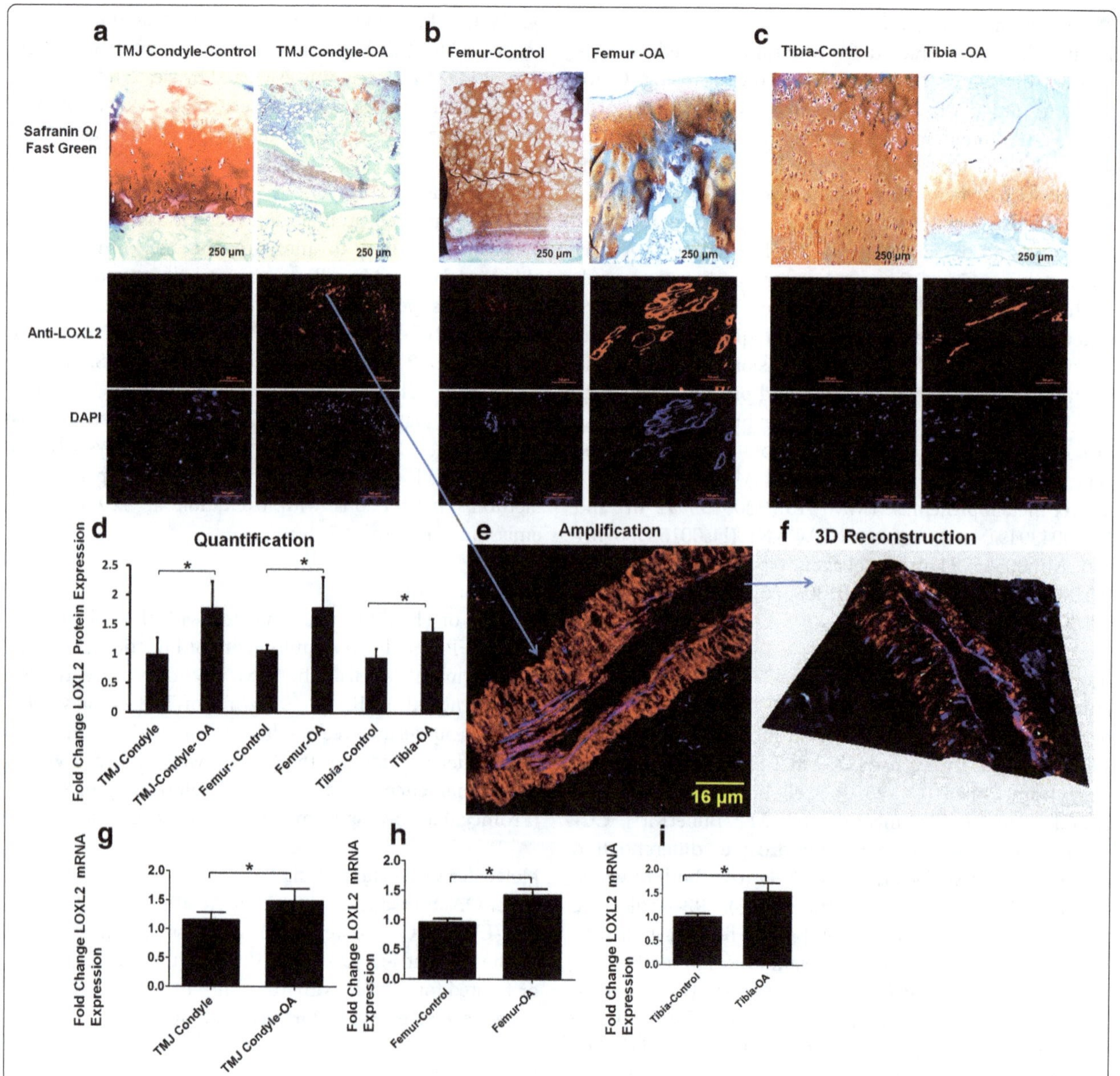

Fig. 1 Immunolocalization of LOXL2 protein in the human temporomandibular joints (*TMJ*) and hip and knee joints: Safranin O/Fast green staining of cartilage (*orange/green, upper panels*), immunofluorescence staining with LOXL2 antibody (*red, middle panels*), and 4′,6-diamidino-2-phenylindole (*DAPI*) staining (*blue, lower panels*) in human TMJ condyles from normal and TMJ-osteoarthritis (*TMJ-OA*) patients **a** and unaffected and OA-affected regions of the femoral head from the same patient (**b**), unaffected and OA-affected regions of the tibial plateau from the same patient (**c**), with quantification of staining intensities in OA tissues (fold-change) compared to normal/unaffected (set at 1.0) (**d**). **e** Higher magnification of a damaged region from a TMJ-OA specimen, where LOXL2 is expressed. **f** Three-dimensional reconstruction of the LOXL2-expressing region. RT-qPCR analysis of LOXL2 mRNA in a normal TMJ condyle compared to a TMJ-OA condyle (**g**), unaffected control compared to hip OA (femoral head) (**h**), and unaffected control compared to knee OA (tibial plateau) (**i**). *Scale bar* = 250, 50, or 16 µm as indicated in *panel*; n = 5/condition; *$P < 0.001$ (Student's *t* test)

until they reached confluence and were infected with Ad-RFP-EV or Ad-RFP-LOXL2 at MOI of 25 in medium supplemented with 5% FBS. After overnight incubation, cells were washed once with PBS and cultured overnight in the fresh serum-free medium. Cells were processed for total RNA extraction using the RNeasy kit (Qiagen). The sample integrity was verified using RNA 6000 Nano Assay RNA chips run in an Agilent 2100 Bioanalyzer (Agilent Technologies). Analysis of mRNA was performed on microarrays and by TaqMan RT-qPCR. All microarray procedures were performed at the Boston University Microarray Resource Facility, according to the protocol for the GeneChip® WT Plus Kit Reagent Manual (Affymetrix,). The total RNA (100 ng) was reverse-transcribed using GeneChip® WT Plus Reagent Kit (Affymetrix,). The cDNA was used as a template for in vitro transcription to antisense cRNA, which was purified using Purification Beads (Affymetrix,) and then used as a template for reverse transcription to produce single-stranded DNA in the sense orientation. Microarrays were immediately scanned using Affymetrix Gene Array Scanner 3000 7G Plus (Affymetrix). Log2 (expression) was computed across all samples and laid over a colored representation (heatmap), which was scaled so that red and blue indicated expression values ≥2 standard deviations above and below, respectively, the row-wise mean (white).

Gene array analysis

Affymetrix GeneChip Human Gene 2.0 ST CEL files were normalized to produce gene-level expression values using the implementation of the Robust Multiarray Average (RMA) [22] in the Affymetrix package (version 1.36.1) [23] included in the Bioconductor software suite (version 2.12) [24] and an Entrez gene-specific probeset mapping (version 17.0.0) from the Molecular and Behavioral Neuroscience Institute (Brainarray) at the University of Michigan [25]. Array quality was assessed by computing relative log expression (RLE) and normalized unscaled standard error (NUSE) using the affyPLM Bioconductor package (version 1.34.0). Principal component analysis (PCA) was performed using the "prcomp R" function with expression values that had been normalized across all samples to a mean of zero and a standard deviation of one. Pairwise differential expression was assessed using the moderated (empirical Bayesian) t test implemented in the limma package (version 3.14.4) (i.e., creating simple linear models with lmFit, followed by empirical Bayesian adjustment with eBayes). Fold changes are indicated as 2 = twofold higher or −2 = twofold lower in Ad-RFP-LOXL2- than in Ad-RFP-EV-transduced cells. Correction for multiple hypothesis testing was accomplished using the Benjamini-Hochberg false discovery rate (FDR) and represented as FDR q values. All statistical analyses were performed using the R environment for statistical computing (version 2.15.1).

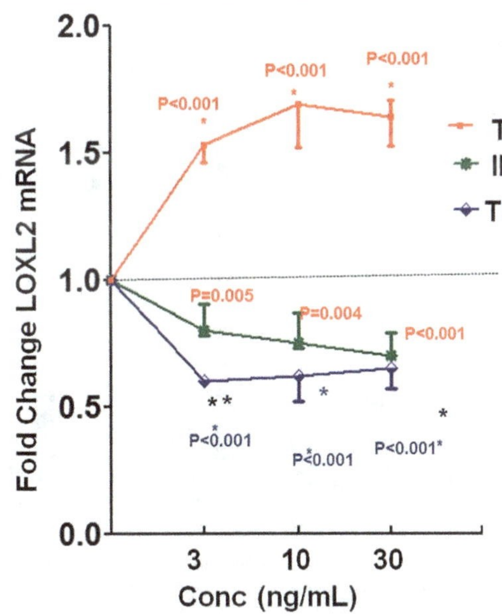

Fig. 2 Regulation of LOXL2 gene expression by osteoarthritis (OA)-related mediators: Human articular OA chondrocytes (HAC-OA) were treated with TNF-α, IL-1β, or transforming growth factor-β1 (*TGF-β1*) at 10 or 30 ng/mL for 24 h, and LOXL2 mRNA levels were assessed by RTqPCR. Data are represented as mean ± SEM of three independent experiments with 95% confidence interval (CI) (*$P < 0.001$; Student's t test). LOXL2 gene expression was significantly upregulated by TGF-β1 ($P < 0.001$) and downregulated by TNF-α ($P < 0.001$) and IL-1β ($P < 0.001$).

In vivo implantation of human articular and TMJ chondrocytes in nude mice

As an alternative to various models based on human chondrocytes [26–28], we established a model using implants of primary TMJ-OA or HAC-OA chondrocytes embedded in Matrigel. For in vivo applications, freshly isolated TMJ-OA cells or frozen cells obtained from Cell Application Inc., were expanded only once to maintain their phenotype prior to preparation of implants. Freshly prepared 10^6 TMJ-OA or HAC-OA chondrocytes in 50 μL medium, from TMJ or knee joints of three different patients with OA, were mixed with Matrigel at a 1:1 ratio. The total 100 μL of Matrigel:chondrocyte suspension were implanted subcutaneously in the backs of nude mice (three implants/mouse) and allowed to grow for a week. These implants were treated locally with weekly injections of 30-μL suspensions of Ad-RFP-LOXL2 or Ad-RFP-EV ($n = 5$/condition), for 6 weeks. Transduction was confirmed by visualization of RFP by in vitro imaging systems (IVIS) each week. One implant from each mouse was then processed for RNA isolation, and the other two were prepared for histologic analysis and stained with Safranin O/Fast Green (American Mastertek Inc.).

Immunofluorescence analysis of human cartilage implants extracted from mice

Paraffin-embedded tissue sections were labeled with mouse SOX9 antibody (Abcam) or its isotype control (Vector Biolabs) detected with anti-mouse IgG conjugated to Alexa 488. To detect LOXL2 expression, the tissues were subjected to rabbit anti-LOXL2 (GeneTex), anti-RFP (Abcam), anti-phospho-SMAD2/3 (Cell Signaling Technology), anti-COL2A1 (Abcam) or its isotype control antibody and detected with anti-rabbit Alexa 488-conjugated antibody or biotin antibody followed by streptavidin-conjugated Texas red, in respective samples. Anti-fade reagent with DAPI was added to all samples. A Zeiss 710 dual scanner confocal microscope with a Plan-Apochromat objective, oil immersion lens, and a CCD detector was used to obtain confocal images. Image acquisition was performed with Zeiss Zen image analysis software (Carl Zeiss Micro Imaging). The image analysis was performed using Zeiss LSM viewer and Image J software (NIH). Z-stack images analysis and 3-dimensional reconstruction was performed by using LOCI and the 3D viewer plug-in of Image J software. Quantification was performed using Image J software as described [15].

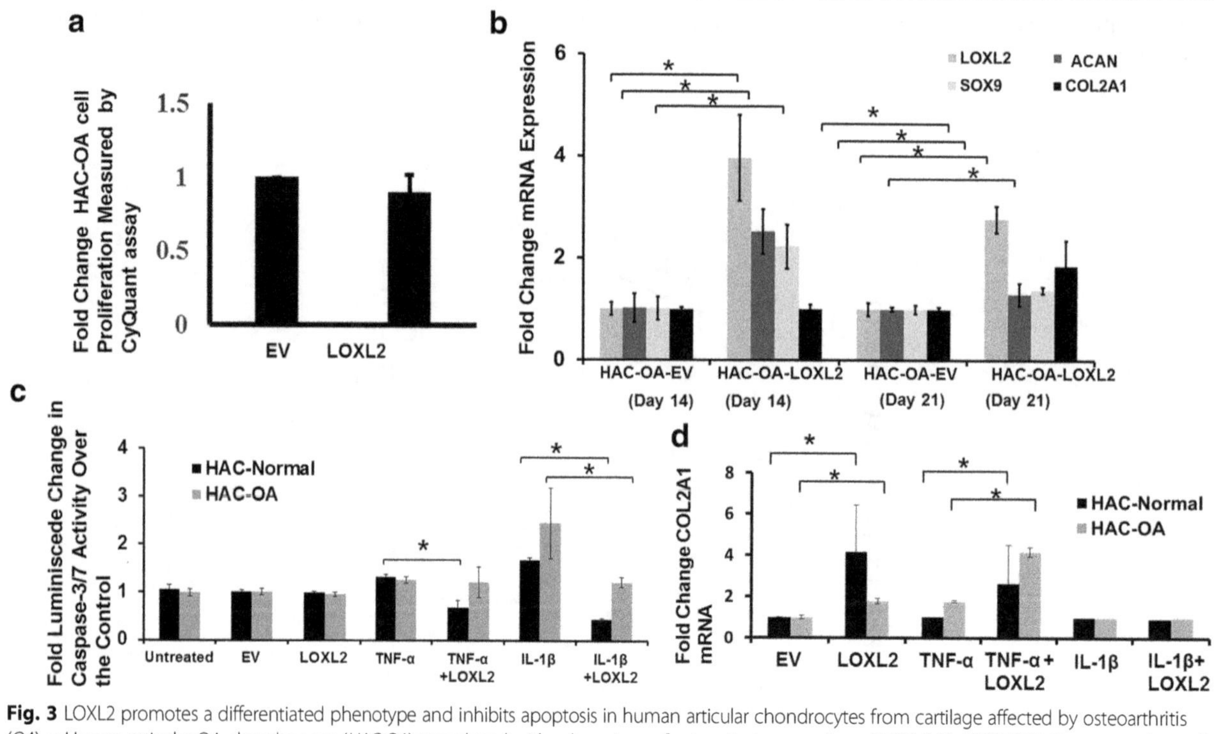

Fig. 3 LOXL2 promotes a differentiated phenotype and inhibits apoptosis in human articular chondrocytes from cartilage affected by osteoarthritis (*OA*). **a** Human articular OA chondrocytes (*HAC-OA*) transduced with adenoviruses for transient expression of LOXL2 (Ad-RFP-LOXL2) compared to cells transduced with its empty vector (*EV*) control (Ad-FP-EV) did not affect chondrocyte proliferation after 24 h. **b** Lentiviral cytomegalovirus (CMV)-LOXL2 transduction of HAC-OA compared to CMV-EV increased the mRNA levels of collagen type II α1 (*COL2A1*) ($P = 0.043$), sex determining region Y-box containing gene 9 (*SOX9*) (*$P < 0.001$), and aggrecan (*ACAN*) ($P = 0.002$). **c** Ad-RFP-LOXL2 transduction inhibited caspase 3/7 activity induced by TNF-α or IL-1β (*$P = 0.006$) compared to Ad-RFP-EV in HAC-normal (*HAC-N*) and HAC-OA cells in serum-free medium after 24 h. **d** Adenoviral transduction (Ad-RFP-LOXL2) HAC-OA in serum-free medium increased COL2A1 mRNA levels (*$P < 0.001$) compared to control (Ad-RFP-EV) in the presence of TNF-α (*$P = 0.001$)

Data analysis

Data analyses were performed using two-way analysis of variance (ANOVA) with Bonferroni post-hoc analysis or Student's t test (Graph Pad Prism 5 software). All experiments were performed three times each using cells derived from a different HAC-N, HAC-OA, or TMJ patient sample. Each data point is represented in the graphs as mean ± SEM of three experiments with significance set at $P < 0.05$.

Results

Immunolocalization of LOXL2 protein in human TMJ and hip and knee joints

To determine whether LOXL2 is present in OA tissues, we evaluated its localization by immunohistochemistry in healthy (OARSI, grade I) and OA tissues (OARSI grade V) from multiple joints, including the TMJ condyle, the femoral head, and the tibial plateau of the knee joint. Safranin O/Fast green staining was used to identify the cartilage region (Fig. 1a). LOXL2 was detectable in damaged parts of cartilage, compared to the negligible LOXL2 in the healthy regions of tissues from all three joints (Fig. 1). Thus, LOXL2 is upregulated in damaged joints, similar to other anabolic factors such as BMP2 [29], fibroblast growth factor (FGF)18 [30], insulin-like growth factor (IGF)1, and TGF-β1 [31], compared to cartilage not affected by OA.

Regulation of LOXL2 mRNA by OA-related factors

Whether LOXL2 expression is modulated by anabolic and catabolic factors involved in OA [7] has not been defined. Therefore, we investigated the effects of anabolic factors (TGF-β1, IGF-1, BMP-2, and BMP-7) and catabolic factors (TNF-α, and IL-1β) on LOXL2 gene expression in chondrocytes treated for 24 h. Compared to vehicle stimulation, LOXL2 mRNA levels in HAC-OA were induced significantly by TGF-β1 (twofold) stimulation, whereas they were downregulated 0.5-fold and 0.7-fold, respectively, by TNF-α and IL-1β (Fig. 2). However, treatment with IGF-1, BMP-2, or BMP-7 produced no significant effect on LOXL2 mRNA levels in HAC-OA (not shown). These results indicate that LOXL2 gene expression can be modulated by key factors affecting OA-related processes in cartilage.

LOXL2 promotes the differentiated chondrocyte phenotype and inhibits apoptosis in human chondrocytes from OA cartilage

To evaluate if LOXL2 promotes the differentiated chondrocyte phenotype, we examined proliferation,

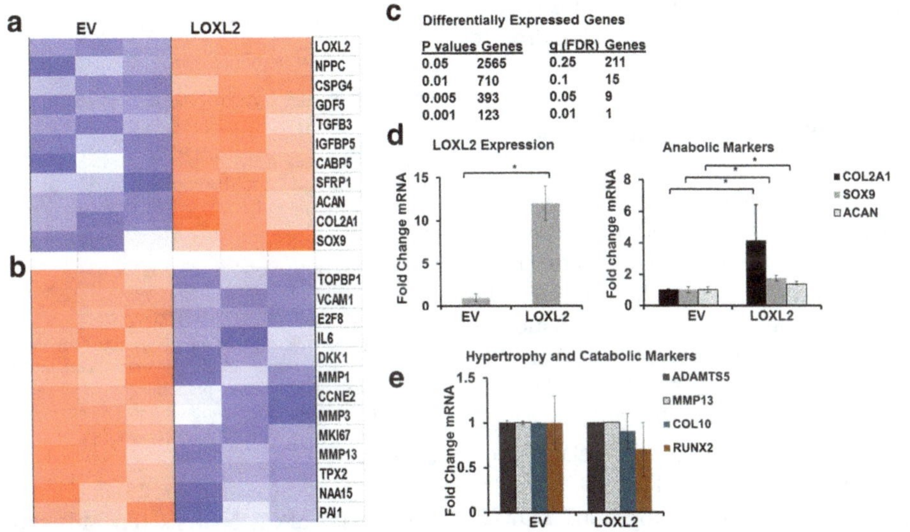

Fig. 4 LOXL2 overexpression differentially regulates genes in osteoarthritis (OA) chondrocytes. Human articular chondrocytes from OA cartilage (HAC-OA) were transduced with adenoviruses for transient expression of LOXL2 (Ad-RFP-LOXL2) or Ad-RFP-empty vector (*EV*), and total RNA extracts were subjected to global gene expression analysis. LOXL2 overexpression in HAC-OA induced the upregulated gene signature (**a**) and the downregulated gene signature (**b**). **c** Statistical significance for differential gene expression. **d** Exogenous LOXL2 expression increased anabolic markers in HAC-OA chondrocytes, whereas genes related to chondrocyte hypertrophy and catabolic markers were not changed as validated by RT-qPCR (**e**) (*$P < 0.001$; Student's t test). LOXL2 transduction increased the expression of collagen type II α1 (*COL2A1*) ($P = 0.063$), Sex determining region Y-box containing gene 9 (*SOX9*) ($P = 0.002$), and aggrecan (*ACAN*) ($P = 0.003$). *NPPC* natriuretic peptide C, *CSPG* chondroitin sulfate proteoglycan, *GDF5* growth differentiation factor 5, *TGFB3* transforming growth factor B3, *IGFBP3* insulin-like growth factor binding protein, *CABP5* calcium binding protein 5, *SFRP1* secreted frizzled-related protein 1, *TOBP1* topoisomerase II binding protein 1, *VCAM1* vascular cell adhesion molecule 1, *E2F8* E2F transcription factor 8, *DKK1* Dickkopf WNT signaling inhibitor 1, *CCNE2* cyclin E2, *TPX* microtubule-associated homolog, *NAA* N(alpha)-acetyltransferase, *FDR* false discovery rate, *MMP* matrix metalloproteinase

chondrocyte phenotypic markers, and TNF-α-induced and IL-1β-induced effects on COL2A1 mRNA and apoptosis using chondrocytes isolated from healthy cartilage (HAC-N) or OA cartilage (HAC-OA) and transduced with viral vectors. HAC-OA cells infected with Ad-RFP-LOXL2 and cultured for 24 h showed no significant difference in cell proliferation compared to those transduced with Ad-RFP-EV (Fig. 3a). To permit long-term expression of the transduced LOXL2 in the HAC-OA cultures for evaluation of chondrogenic differentiation, we used lentiviral vectors lenti-CMV-LOXL2 and lenti-CMV-EV (control). HAC-OA-LOXL2 cells showed increased SOX9, ACAN, and COL2A1 mRNA levels on days 14 and 21 after lenti-CMV-LOXL2 transduction and culture in chondrogenic differentiation medium compared to cells transduced with lenti-CMV-EV vector (Fig. 3b). Next, we determined that LOXL2 transduction inhibits IL-1β-induced caspase 3/7 activity as a measure of apoptosis in both HAC-N and HAC-OA cells (Fig. 3c). However, LOXL2 transduction inhibited caspase 3/7 activity induced by TNF-α in HAC-N but not in HAC-OA cells. Finally, transduction with Ad-RFP-LOXL2, compared to Ad-RFP-EV, increased COL2A1 mRNA levels in both healthy HAC-N and HAC-OA cells treated with TNF-α for 24 h (Fig. 3d). Thus, exogenous expression of LOXL2 does not affect chondrocyte proliferation, but promotes chondrogenic lineage-specific gene expression, increases *COL2A1* expression in the presence of TNF-α, and inhibits chondrocyte apoptosis.

LOXL2 overexpression differentially regulates genes in OA chondrocytes

To determine the consequences of LOXL2 overexpression on potential OA-related targets, we performed global gene expression analysis on total RNA extracted from HAC-OA after transduction with Ad-RFP-LOXL2 or Ad-RFP-EV. LOXL2 overexpression resulted in the upregulation of genes such as natriuretic peptide C (*NPPC*), *CSPG4*, growth differentiation factor 5 (*GDF5*), *TGFB3*, insulin-like growth factor binding protein 5 (*IGFBP5*), calcium binding protein 5 (*CABP5*), secreted frizzled-related protein 1 (*SFRP1*), *ACAN*, *COL2A1*, and *SOX9* (Fig. 4a, arranged by decreasing FDR value). Exogenous LOXL2 expression reduced the expression of genes (Fig. 4b) such as topoisomerase (DNA) II binding protein 1 (*TOPBP1*), vascular cell adhesion molecule 1 (*VCAM1*), E2F transcription factor 8 (*E2F8*), *IL6*, Dickkopf WNT signaling inhibitor 1 (*DKK1*), matrix metalloproteinase (*MMP*) 1, cyclin E2 (*CCNE2*), *MMP3*, antigen identified by monoclonal antibody Ki-67 (*Ki67*), *MMP13*, microtubule-associated homolog (*TPX2*), and N(alpha)-acetyltransferase (NAA)15. These expression changes were statistically significant (Fig. 4c). Validation of the global gene expression data by RT-qPCR analysis (Fig. 4d) showed that the key genes related to anabolic responses such as *COL2A1*, *SOX9*, and *ACAN* were increased after LOXL2 transduction, whereas those related to catabolic responses and chondrocyte hypertrophy such as ADAMTS5, MMP13, COL10, and RUNX2 were unchanged (Fig. 4e). Thus, our gene array analysis suggests that LOXL2 may be involved in promoting chondrogenic lineage maintenance, acting as an anabolic factor that also inhibits catabolic and angiogenic factors.

Table 1 GSEA of selected pathways on the basis of OA-related functions from chondrocytes transduced with ADV-LOXL2 compared to empty vector (control)

Name	Size	NES	Nom *P* value	FDR q value
Reactome cell cycle checkpoints	109	−2.478	0.0001	0.00
Reactome activation of genes by ATF4	24	−2.234	0.000	0.00
Reactome SMAD2 SMAD3 SMAD4 heterotrimer regulates transcription	25	−1.880	0.002	0.01
Reactome signaling by TGF Beta receptor complex	59	−1.748	0.0001	0.03
Reactome MAPK targets nuclear events mediated by MAP kinases	30	−1.620	0.010	0.07
ttccgtt, MIR-191	29	−1.604	0.012	0.07
Cell proliferation GO 0008283	495	−1.578	0.000	0.08
Biocarta TNFR1 pathway	29	−1.533	0.033	0.11
Negative regulation of cell proliferation	153	−1.508	0.002	0.12
aagcact, MIR-520 F	238	−1.493	0.000	0.13
Regulation of angiogenesis	26	−1.476	0.061	0.14
Reactome muscle contraction	46	2.023	0.0001	0.19
Regulation of apoptosis	332	−1.373	0.006	0.21
Regulation of cell proliferation	298	−1.371	0.010	0.21
IκB kinase NF-κB cascade	109	−1.36	0.06	0.23
Vasculature development	55	−1.346	0.072	0.24
Reactome platelet calcium homeostasis	16	1.768	0.001	0.24
Reactome antigen activates b cell receptor leading to the generation of second messengers	29	1.750	0.001	0.24
Negative regulation of developmental process	189	−1.335	0.022	0.25

A positive NES indicates that the genes in the set are predominantly upregulated with respect to the reference group, and a negative NES indicates that the genes in the set are predominantly downregulated with respect to the reference group. *GSEA* gene set enrichment analysis, *OA* osteoarthritis, *FDR* false discovery rate, *MAP* mitogen-activated protein, TGF transforming growth factor

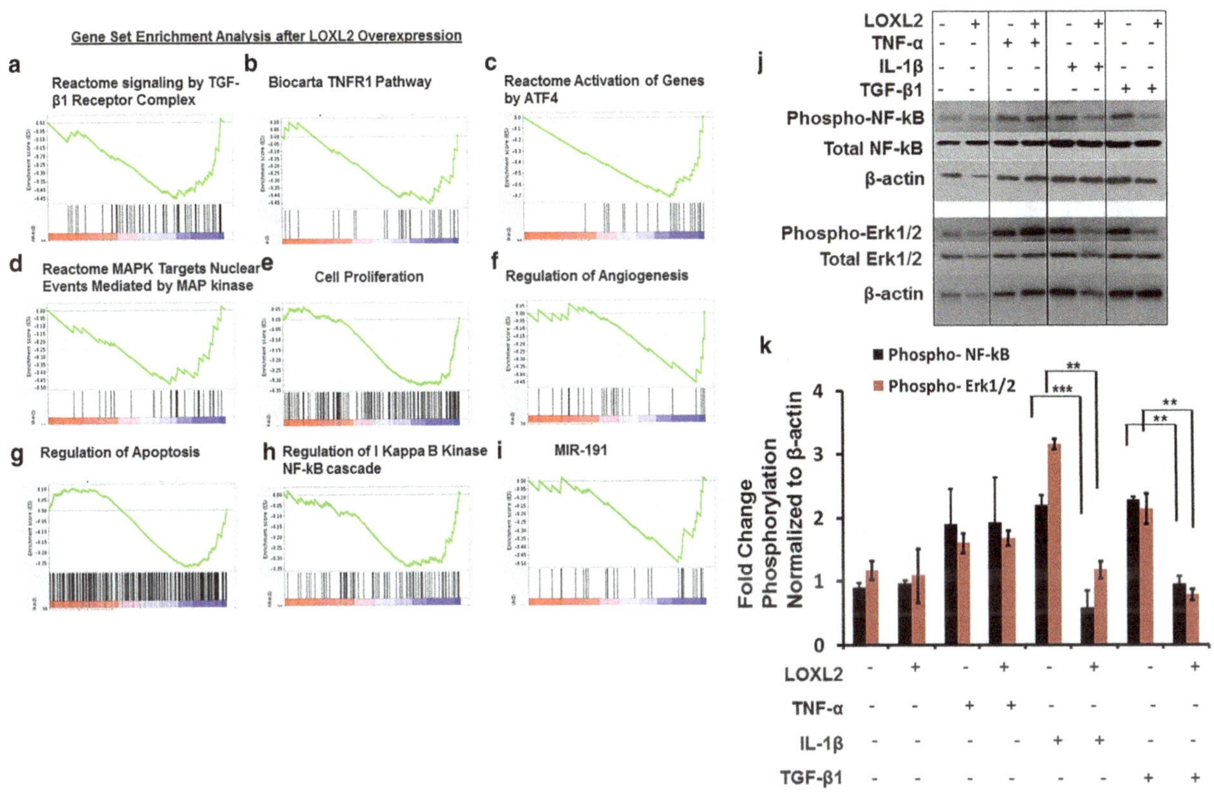

Fig. 5 LOXL2 overexpression differentially regulates signaling pathways in osteoarthritis chondrocytes. Gene set enrichment analysis data shown are reactome signaling by transforming growth factor -β1 (*TGF-β1*) receptor complex (**a**), Biocarta TNF-α receptor 1 pathway (**b**), reactome activation genes by ATF4 (**c**), reactome mitogen-activated protein kinase (*MAPK*) targets nuclear events mediated by MAPK (**d**), negative regulation of cell proliferation (**e**), regulation of angiogenesis (**f**), regulation of apoptosis (**g**), regulation of IkB kinase NF-κB cascade (**h**), and signaling by MiR-191 **i** compared to control (EV). **j** LOXL2 inhibits IL-1β-induced phospho-NF-κB and TGF-β1-induced phospho-ERK1/2 shown by western blot analysis, whereas TNF-α induced phospho-NF-κB and phospho-ERK1/2 are not affected. **k** Quantification is shown as fold-change normalized to β-actin (*$P < 0.001$; Student's *t* test; n = 3)

LOXL2 regulates specific gene sets

In HAC-OA transduced with Ad-RFP-LOXL2 and Ad-RFP-EV, 43 (*P* value <0.01) and 106 (*P* value <0.05) gene sets were enriched significantly; only 3 gene sets were enriched significantly at FDR <25% (0.25) (Table 1). LOXL2 transduction compared to the EV control down-regulated genes known to be involved in TGF-β1 and TNF-α signaling and apoptosis (Fig. 5a-i); these include reactome signaling by TGF-β1 receptor complex, Biocarta TNF-α receptor 1 pathway, reactome activation genes by ATF4, negative regulation of cell proliferation, regulation of angiogenesis regulation of apoptosis, reactome mitogen-activated protein (MAP) kinase nuclear events mediated by MAP kinases, regulation of IkB kinase NF-κB cascade, and signaling by miR-191.

LOXL2 inhibits signaling pathways induced by IL-1β and TGF-β1

We next validated the inhibitory effects of LOXL2 on signaling pathways detected by gene set enrichment analysis (GSEA) (Fig. 5a-i), focusing on those involving NF-κB and ERK. Transduction of HAC-OA with Ad-RFP-LOXL2 inhibited IL-1β-induced phospho-NF-κB/p65 and TGF-β1-induced phospho-ERK1/2 levels compared to cells transduced with Ad-RFP-EV, as shown by western blotting (Fig. 5j and k).

LOXL2 promotes anabolic responses in implants of the human knee and TMJ-OA chondrocytes in vivo and co-expresses with SOX9

To evaluate if LOXL2 can maintain the human cartilage phenotype long term (6 weeks) and induce specific chondrogenic differentiation in vivo, we produced a model of OA using chondrocyte/Matrigel constructs implanted subcutaneously in the backs of nude mice. We used adenoviral delivery of LOXL2 to evaluate the expression in implants of critical genes such as *SOX9*, *ACAN*, and *COL2A1*, which are involved in chondrogenesis. This model is an effective alternative to the human-cell-based models used previously [26–28]: it replicates the 3-dimensional cartilage environment in vivo, uses specific growth factors that preserve the differentiated

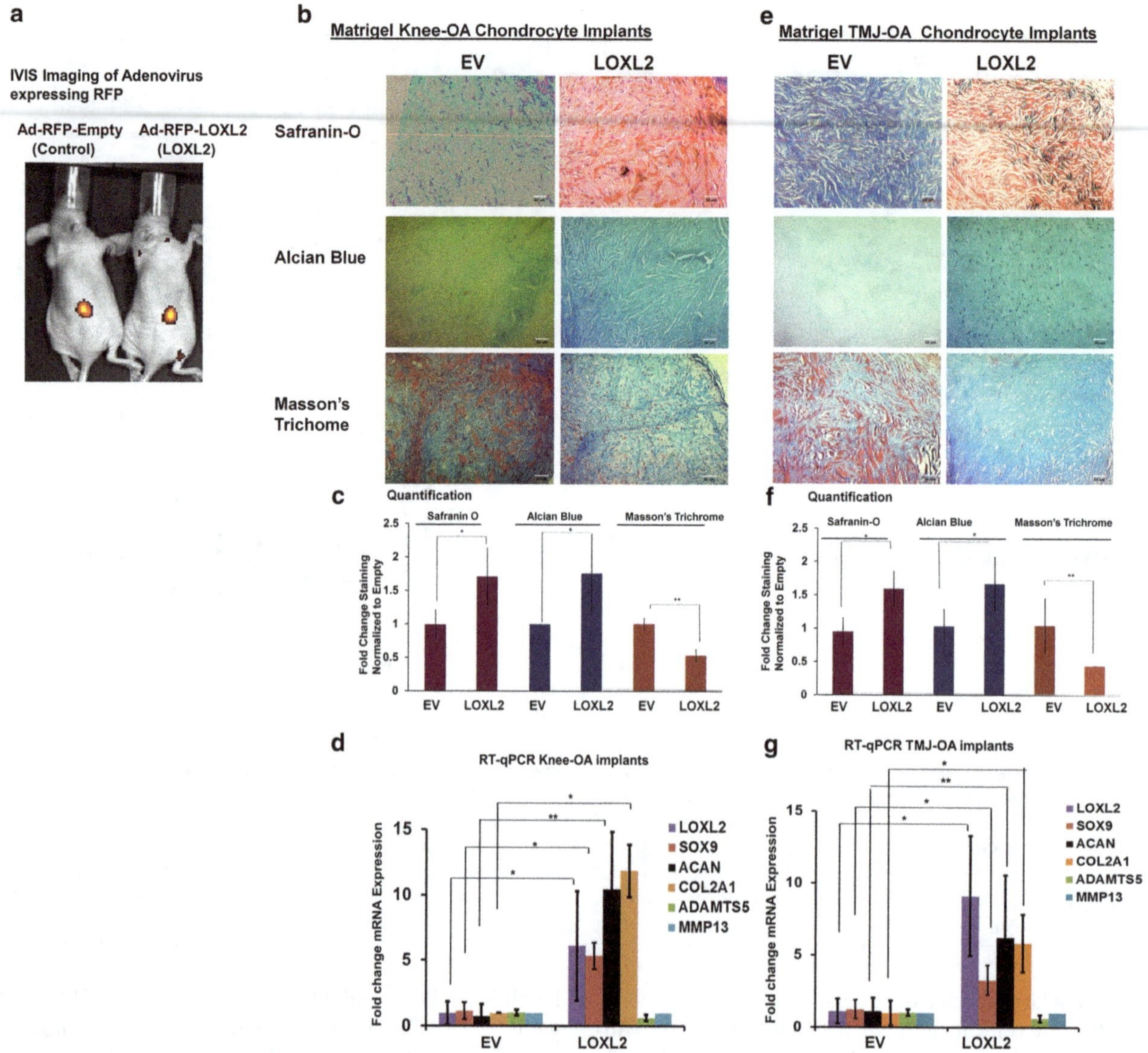

Fig. 6 LOXL2 promotes anabolic responses in implants of the human knee and osteoarthritic temporomandibular joint (*TMJ-OA*) chondrocytes in vivo. **a** In vitro imaging systems (*IVIS*) imaging of human articular chondrocytes (HAC)/Matrigel implants in nude mice after local injection every week for 6 weeks with adenoviruses for transient expression of LOXL2 (*Ad-RFP-LOXL2*) or Ad-RFP-empty vector (*EV*) (*Ad-RFP-empty*). Knee HAC-OA/Matrigel implants were injected weekly with Ad-RFP-LOXL2 or Ad-RFP-EV, harvested after 6 weeks, and analyzed by Safranin O/Fast Green, Alcian blue, and Masson's trichrome staining (**b**) with relative quantification (**c**), and RT-qPCR using human primers (**d**). TMJ-OA/Matrigel implants were injected weekly with Ad-RFP-LOXL2 or Ad-RFP-EV, harvested after 6 weeks, and analyzed by Safranin O/Fast Green, Alcian blue, and Masson's Trichrome staining (**e**) with relative quantification (**f**), and RT-qPCR (**g**) using human primers (n = 5/condition; $^{*}P < 0.05$ and $^{**}P < 0.01$; Student's *t* test). *SOX9* sex determining region Y-box containing gene 9, *ACAN* aggrecan, *COL2A1* collagen type II α1, *MMP* matrix metalloproteinase

phenotype for cartilage regeneration [32], and prevents the tissues from becoming fibrotic after 6–9 weeks [33] and myogenic [34]. Weekly injections of Ad-RFP-EV or Ad-RFP-LOXL2 near the chondrocyte-Matrigel implants were performed for up to 6 weeks. IVIS imaging confirmed successful transduction by Ad-RFP-EV or Ad-RFP-LOXL2 (Fig. 6a). After 6 weeks, histological sections of the retrieved implants stained with Safranin O/Fast Green and Alcian blue showed that LOXL2 transduction increased proteoglycan deposition and cartilage formation. However, implants after transduction with Ad-RFP-EV did not show Safranin O or Alcian blue staining, consistent with loss of chondrogenic phenotype and proteoglycan deposition (Fig. 6b). Masson's trichrome staining was reduced in LOXL2-transduced implants, showing that LOXL2 promotes specific chondrogenic changes and these implants lacked mineralization and fibrosis. In contrast, implants transduced with EV appeared fibrous (Fig. 6b). Molecular analysis of implants by RT-qPCR showed that LOXL2 treatment increased the levels of

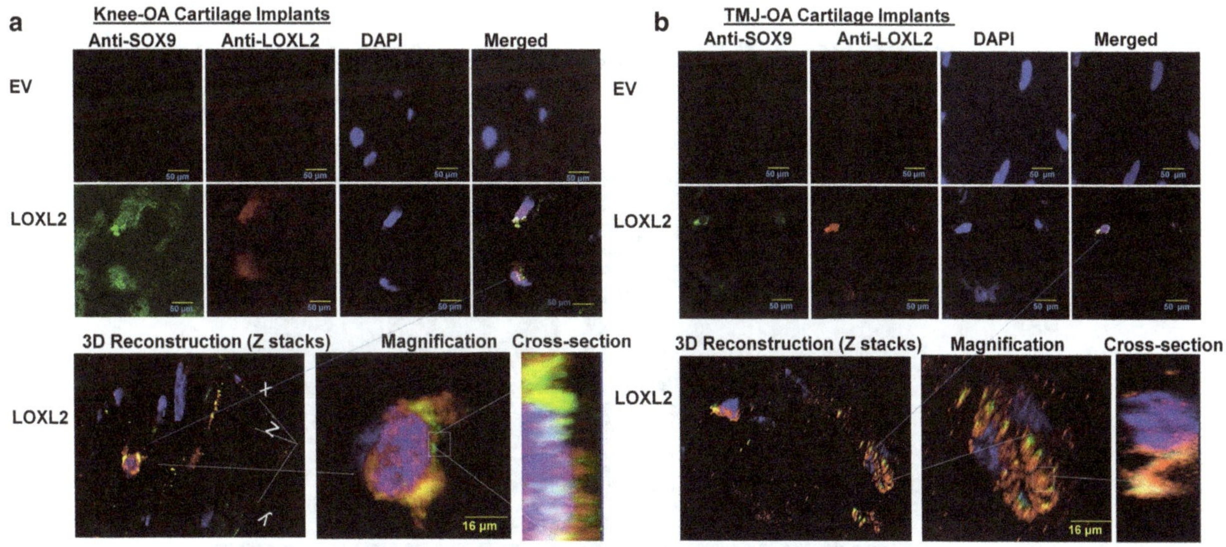

Fig. 7 LOXL2 co-expresses with sex determining region Y-box containing gene 9 (*SOX9*) in the knee joint and osteoarthritic temporomandibular joint (*TMJ-OA*) chondrocytes implants in nude mice. **a** Human knee articular chondrocytes in osteoarthritis (*HAC-OA*)/Matrigel implants or TMJ-OA/implants (**b**) from nude mice after treatments as described in Fig. 6. In the *image*, localization of proteins is shown with different *colors* such as LOXL2 (*red*), 4′,6-diamidino-2-phenylindole (*DAPI*) (*blue*), and LOXL2 and SOX9 co-localization (*yellow*). *EV* empty vector

LOXL2, SOX9, COL2A1, and ACAN mRNA compared to control, whereas MMP13 and ADAMTS5 mRNA levels were not affected significantly in HAC-OA implants (Fig. 6c) and TMJ-OA implants (Fig. 6d). Finally, we evaluated LOXL2 and SOX9 by immunofluorescence staining in HAC-OA and TMJ-OA implant tissue sections. LOXL2 co-localized with nuclear SOX9 (Fig. 7). Adv-RFP-LOXL2 transduction promoted SOX9 gene expression, which was not detected in Ad-RFP-EV-transduced implants, suggesting that LOXL2 maintains the chondrogenic phenotype via SOX9. However, a co-immunoprecipitation assay did not show direct interaction of LOXL2 with SOX9 (Additional file 1: Figure S1). Finally, forced LOXL2 expression resulted in downregulation of phospho-SMAD2/3 and upregulation of COL2A1 compared to Ad-RFP-EV-transduced HAC-OA (Fig. 8a) and TMJ-OA implants (Fig. 8b), which showed lower expression of COL2A1. Thus, LOXL2 transduction may be critical for expression of cartilage-specific matrix genes such as *COL2A1* (Fig. 8a, b). Taken together, our results show that LOXL2 induces an anabolic response in HAC-OA and TMJ-OA chondrocytes in vivo and maintains the chondrogenic phenotype, indicating its essential involvement in cartilage formation and maintenance.

Discussion

Pro-inflammatory cytokines such as TNF-α and IL-1β act as catabolic factors, promoting synovitis and altering chondrocyte differentiation, function, and viability [35–37]. We showed that LOXL2 attenuated the signaling pathways induced by TGF-β1, TNF-α, and IL-1β. In chondrocytes, IL-1β and TNF-α activate the canonical NF-κB pathway, leading to catabolic and inflammatory responses [38, 39], whereas non-canonical NF-kB signaling promotes chondrocyte hypertrophy [40, 41]. Recent studies showed that TGF-β1 expression in subchondral bone induces OA [42], and TGF-β1 inhibitors are chondroprotective in knee-OA and TMJ-OA in animal models [42–44]. We found that LOXL2 inhibits IL-1β-induced phosphorylation of the NF-κB/p65 subunit, which permits translocation of the p65/p50 complex to the nucleus, and TGF-β1-induced ERK1/2 phosphorylation, which is required for many anabolic responses in cartilage. LOX can directly interact with TGF-β1 and inhibit TGF-β1 activity [45]. Thus, LOXL2 could interact with TGF-β1 to negatively regulate its activity, or influence TNF-α and IL-1β-induced signaling pathways. LOXL2 could also induce amine oxidation at TGF-β1 receptor, inhibiting its activity, or attenuate downstream inflammatory signaling pathways NF-kB and ERK1/2. Indeed, LOXL2 overexpression reduces the expression of the TGF-β-responsive gene PAI1 and negatively regulates TGF-β1-responsive gene sets and SMAD 2/3 phosphorylation. We conclude that LOXL2 could inhibit TGF-β1 signaling, though, alternatively, LOXL2 could be a downstream target of TGF-β1 and act through feedback inhibition of TGF-β1-induced signaling.

LOXL2 is a naturally occurring enzyme and could have potential application in anabolic therapies. The ECM regulates diverse cellular functions, including proliferation, migration, and differentiation, and ECM remodeling is crucial for the development of normal organs. In contrast,

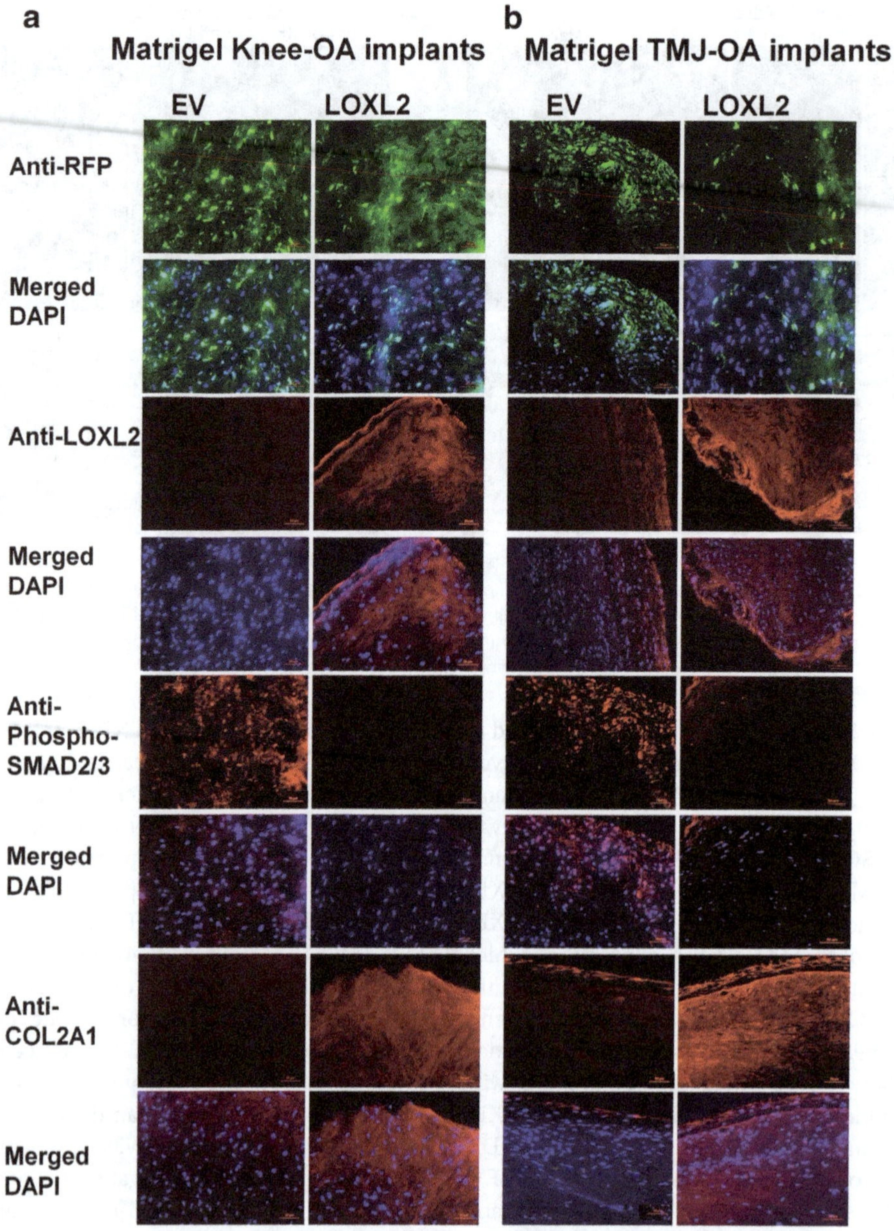

Fig. 8 LOXL2 transduction inhibits phospho-SMAD2/3 and increases type II collagen (*COL2A1*). **a** Human knee articular chondrocytes in osteoarthritis (*HAC-OA*)/Matrigel implants and osteoarthritic temporomandibular joint (*TMJ-OA*)/Matrigel implants **b** were stained with antibodies against RFP, LOXL2, phspho-SMAD2/3, or COL2A1 with respective 4′,6-diamidino-2-phenylindole (*DAPI*) staining

dysregulation of the ECM increases LOXL2 expression and contributes to several pathological conditions such as fibrosis and invasive cancer [46–48]. LOXL2 is increased in cancer and fibrosis as a consequence of aberrant signaling pathways and inflammatory mediators leading to remodeling of ECM [49]. Although LOXL2 is present in the damaged regions, the concentration of LOXL2 may be overcome by catabolic mediators such as IL-1β and TNF-α present in degenerative cartilage, which prevent anabolic effects induced by LOXL2 during late stages of OA. These possibilities are under investigation in mouse models to evaluate LOXL2 as a potential therapeutic agent by the early vs. delayed administration, frequency, and dose of application. Current approaches in the development of disease-modifying OA drugs are to: (1) inhibit the ECM-degrading enzymes to prevent erosion of cartilage, (2) inhibit catabolic pro-inflammatory cytokines to protect chondrocytes against stress and inflammatory insults, and (3) develop anabolic agents to promote chondrocyte proliferation and selective differentiation [50]. Unlike other agents that affect one or two targets, our preliminary studies show

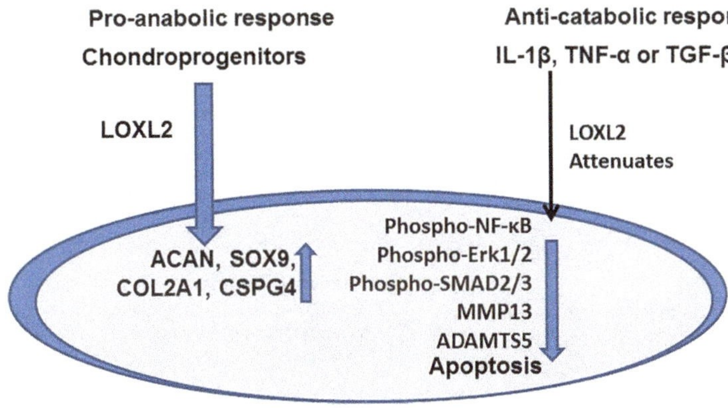

Fig. 9 Potential mechanism of LOXL2-induced anabolic effects in osteoarthritis. *TGF* transforming growth factor, ACAN aggrecan, *COL2A1* collagen type II alpha 1, *SOX9* sex determining region Y-box containing gene 9

that LOXL2 could have direct and indirect effects on all of these processes in OA as a potential pro-anabolic and anti-catabolic factor.

Long-term in vivo implanted human chondrocytes lose their chondrogenic phenotype and differentiation potential or become fibrous in the absence of specific stimulating anabolic factors or scaffolds [32, 33]. Our microarray data from both in vitro and in vivo experiments demonstrate that LOXL2 expression is critical for expression of chondrocyte-specific genes such as *SOX9*, *ACAN*, and *COL2A1*. Thus, LOXL2 could have a specific function in maintaining the chondrogenic phenotype. This is also supported by earlier studies showing that LOXL2 knockdown in chondrocytes in vitro inhibits expression of these genes and proteoglycan deposition [6].

We investigated both TMJ and knee joints affected by OA. The TMJ differs in structure compared to other joints [51], with a secondary cartilage distinct from the articular cartilage of limbs and cartilage in the cranial base. However, despite structural and functional differences in the cartilage between the knee joint and TMJ, our findings show that LOXL2 could have roles in the pathophysiology of OA in both types of joint.

Further, we show that LOXL2 co-expresses with SOX9 in the nuclei of both knee OA and TMJ OA chondrocytes in Matrigel implants in nude mice. In other cell types, LOXL2 can localize to the nucleus, perinuclear region, and cytoplasm [52, 53]. LOXL2 interacts physically and functionally with SNAIL to attenuate GSK3β-dependent SNAIL degradation [54] and to downregulate E-cadherin expression [55, 56]. Cytoplasmic/perinuclear localization is associated with distant metastasis of breast cancer cell line [57], while nuclear LOXL2 has a role in epithelial-to-mesenchymal transition [58]. Recent findings also suggest a critical intracellular role for LOXL2 in transcriptional regulation and epigenetic changes [52, 53]. Thus, nuclear LOXL2 could co-localize with SOX9 to cooperatively regulate gene expression. A recent study showed that LOXL2 induces epigenetic changes during neural progenitor differentiation [53]. LOXL2 could, therefore, regulate transcription factors such as SOX9 through direct interactions or indirectly through epigenetic changes. Future investigations of LOXL2-induced epigenetic modifications through enzymatic amine oxidation and other novel mechanisms in OA chondrocytes will provide an additional foundation for understanding its role in OA pathogenesis and for the development of disease-modifying OA drugs.

Conclusions

This is the first study to suggest a potential role for LOXL2 in the pathophysiology of OA (Fig. 9). Our hypothesis that LOXL2 acts as a specific anabolic factor in chondrocytes is supported by data showing that: (1) LOXL2 gene expression is regulated by OA-related mediators; (2) LOXL2 overexpression in chondrocytes inhibits apoptosis induced by TNF-α or IL-1β; (3) LOXL2 overexpression increases SOX9, COL2A1, and ACAN mRNA levels, which are related to the differentiated chondrocyte phenotype, without increasing MMP13 or ADAMTS5; (4) LOXL2 promotes a differentiated phenotype, unlike the dual global effects seen in TGF-β1 [42, 44] and (5) LOXL2 promotes a differentiated phenotype and maintains the chondrogenic lineage in vivo. Taken together, LOXL2 promotes anabolic responses, chondrocyte differentiation, and ECM production. We are evaluating the role of LOXL2 in mouse OA models, which will provide a basic understanding of LOXL2 function for future clinical applications.

Additional file

Additional file 1: Figure S1. LOXL2 pull-down assay: HAC-OA cells were transduced with Adv-EV or Adv-LOXL2 vector for overnight. The next day, transduced cells were replenished with fresh chondrocyte growth media and cultured for 24 h, and extracted into non-denaturing cell lysis RIPA buffer. The cell lysates were incubated with cobalt chelate NT beads overnight at 4 °C to pull down LOXL2. The beads were washed and eluted according to kit instructions (Pull-Down PolyHis Protein: Protein Interaction Kit Thermo Scientific, Waltham, MA, USA). Eluted samples were analyzed by western blotting on denaturing SDS-PAGE probed with an LOXL2 (Genetex) or SOX9 (Abcam) antibody, and the input (5% aliquots) of initial extracts taken before the immunoprecipitation was analyzed on the same gels. The figure shows pull-down of LOXL2 in IP analysis; however, co-IP with SOX9 does not show any corresponding band. (TIF 50990 kb)

Abbreviations

ACAN: Aggrecan; Ad-RFP-LOXL2: Adenoviruses for transient expression of LOXL2; BMP: Bone morphogenetic protein; CMV: Cytomegalovirus; COL2A1: Collagen type II alpha 1; CSPG: Chondroitin sulfate proteoglycan; DAPI: 4′,6-Diamidino-2-phenylindole; ECM: Extracellular matrix; ERK: Extracellular signal-related kinase; EV: Empty vector; FBS: Fetal bovine serum; FDR: False discovery rate; GSEA: Gene set enrichment analysis; HAC: Human articular chondrocytes; IL: Interleukin; IRB: Institutional Review Board; IVIS: In vivo imaging systems; LOXL2: Lysyl oxidase like-2; MAP: Mitogen-activated protein; MOI: multiplicity of infection; NES: Normalized enrichment score; Nom *p*-value: Nominal *p*-value; OA: Osteoarthritis; OARSI: Osteoarthritis Research Society International; PBS: Phosphate-buffered saline; RT-qPCR: Quantitative real-time PCR; TGF: Transforming growth factor; SOX9: Sex determining region Y-box containing gene 9; TMJ: Temporomandibular joints; TNF: Tumor necrosis factor

Acknowledgements

The authors acknowledge the funding support from NIH/NIDCR (R03DE025274) to Manish V. Bais, and the gene array analysis support provided by CTSA grant U54-TR001012A and CTSI pilot funding to Manish V. Bais. The authors also acknowledge the gift of human articular chondrocytes from three different patients from Cell Applications Inc., and IVIS spectrum imaging core for providing imaging resources. The authors acknowledge Philip Trackman for suggestions for the manuscript and resources and are thankful to Yuriy Alekseyev and Adam Gower for the gene array and its analysis.

Funding

NIH/NIDCR (R03DE025274) and CTSI pilot funding to Manish V. Bais.

Authors' contributions

MB conceived and designed the study, and performed data collection, experimentation, data analysis and interpretation, and manuscript writing. WA performed the experiments and analysis. MT performed the animal experiments, immunofluorescence analysis, and data analysis. SA performed the animal experiments, immunofluorescence analysis, and data analysis. YA performed the animal experiments and data analysis. AW performed the histology sections, validated by microCT, and data analysis. SF provided knee tissue sections, validated staining, and performed data analysis. PM identified subjects with TMJ-OA, performed surgical procedures, and provided samples for further analysis. LCG provided resources and manuscript editing. MBG conceived and designed the study, interpreted data, provided resources during the study, and edited the manuscript. All authors read and approved the final manuscript.

Authors' information

Not applicable.

Ethical approval and consent to participate

Animal experiments: all animal experiments and respective informed consent were obtained in accordance with relevant guidelines and regulations with Institutional Animal Care and Use Committee (IACUC) approval. All mouse experimental methods were performed with guidance and regulations and approved through Boston University Medical Center Boston, MA IACUC committee with approval number AN-15387.

Human experiments: all experiments and respective informed consent from all the subjects were obtained in accordance with relevant guidelines and regulations through IRB approval from Boston University and Georgia Medical College, Augusta, GA. TMJ tissues were obtained through IRB approval number H33300, and femur slides were obtained through IRB approval number H-32517 from Boston University Medical Center Boston, MA. Knee joint tissues and slides were obtained from Georgia Medical College, Augusta, GA under IRB approval number 657441-5.

Competing interests

All authors declare that they have no financial interest regarding the contents of this manuscript.

Author details

[1]Department of Molecular and Cell Biology, Boston University Henry M. Goldman School of Dental Medicine, W-216, 700 Albany Street, Boston, MA 02118, USA. [2]Department of Orthopaedic Surgery, School of Medicine, Boston University, Boston, MA 02118, USA. [3]Department of Orthopaedic Surgery and Institute of Regenerative and Reparative Medicine, Georgia Regents University, Augusta, GA 30912, USA. [4]Department of Oral and Maxillofacial Surgery, Boston University Henry M. Goldman School of Dental Medicine, 100 East Newton Street, Boston, MA 02118, USA. [5]Hospital for Special Surgery Research Institute, Weill Cornell Medical College, New York, NY 10021, USA. [6]Department of Cell and Developmental Biology, Weill Cornell Medical College, New York, NY 10021, USA.

References

1. Zamli Z, Sharif M. Chondrocyte apoptosis: a cause or consequence of osteoarthritis? Int J Rheum Dis. 2011;14(2):159–66.
2. Nguyen US, Zhang Y, Zhu Y, Niu J, Zhang B, Felson DT. Increasing prevalence of knee pain and symptomatic knee osteoarthritis: survey and cohort data. Ann Intern Med. 2011;155(11):725–32.
3. Scrivani SJ, Keith DA, Kaban LB. Temporomandibular disorders. N Engl J Med. 2008;359(25):2693–705.
4. Makris EA, Responte DJ, Paschos NK, Hu JC, Athanasiou KA. Developing functional musculoskeletal tissues through hypoxia and lysyl oxidase-induced collagen cross-linking. Proc Natl Acad Sci U S A. 2014;111(45): E4832–4841.
5. Ravindra PV, Tiwari AK, Ratta B, Bais MV, Chaturvedi U, Palia SK, Sharma B, Chauhan RS. Time course of Newcastle disease virus-induced apoptotic pathways. Virus Res. 2009;144(1-2):350–4.
6. Iftikhar M, Hurtado P, Bais MV, Wigner N, Stephens DN, Gerstenfeld LC, Trackman PC. Lysyl oxidase-like-2 (LOXL2) is a major isoform in chondrocytes and is critically required for differentiation. J Biol Chem. 2011; 286(2):909–18.
7. Mueller MB, Tuan RS. Anabolic/catabolic balance in pathogenesis of osteoarthritis: identifying molecular targets. PM R. 2011;3(6 Suppl 1):S3–11.
8. Cho TJ, Lehmann W, Edgar C, Sadeghi C, Hou A, Einhorn TA, Gerstenfeld LC. Tumor necrosis factor alpha activation of the apoptotic cascade in murine articular chondrocytes is associated with the induction of metalloproteinases and specific pro-resorptive factors. Arthritis Rheum. 2003; 48(10):2845–54.
9. Calich AL, Domiciano DS, Fuller R. Osteoarthritis: can anti-cytokine therapy play a role in treatment? Clin Rheumatol. 2010;29(5):451–5.
10. Kapoor M, Martel-Pelletier J, Lajeunesse D, Pelletier JP, Fahmi H. Role of proinflammatory cytokines in the pathophysiology of osteoarthritis. Nat Rev Rheumatol. 2011;7(1):33–42.
11. Goldring MB, Berenbaum F. Emerging targets in osteoarthritis therapy. Curr Opin Pharmacol. 2015;22:51–63.
12. Lohmander LS, Hellot S, Dreher D, Krantz EF, Kruger DS, Guermazi A, Eckstein F. Intraarticular sprifermin (recombinant human fibroblast growth factor 18) in knee osteoarthritis: a randomized, double-blind, placebo-controlled trial. Arthritis Rheumatol. 2014;66(7):1820–31.

13. Blaney Davidson EN, Vitters EL, van der Kraan PM, van den Berg WB. Expression of transforming growth factor-beta (TGFbeta) and the TGFbeta signalling molecule SMAD-2P in spontaneous and instability-induced osteoarthritis: role in cartilage degradation, chondrogenesis and osteophyte formation. Ann Rheum Dis. 2006;65(11):1414–21.
14. van Beuningen HM, Glansbeek HL, van der Kraan PM, van den Berg WB. Differential effects of local application of BMP-2 or TGF-beta 1 on both articular cartilage composition and osteophyte formation. Osteoarthr Cartil. 1998;6(5):306–17.
15. McCloy RA, Rogers S, Caldon CE, Lorca T, Castro A, Burgess A. Partial inhibition of Cdk1 in G 2 phase overrides the SAC and decouples mitotic events. Cell Cycle. 2014;13(9):1400–12.
16. Bais M, McLean J, Sebastiani P, Young M, Wigner N, Smith T, Kotton DN, Einhorn TA, Gerstenfeld LC. Transcriptional analysis of fracture healing and the induction of embryonic stem cell-related genes. PLoS One. 2009;4(5):e5393.
17. van der Kraan PM, Buma P, van Kuppevelt T, van den Berg WB. Interaction of chondrocytes, extracellular matrix and growth factors: relevance for articular cartilage tissue engineering. Osteoarthr Cartil. 2002;10(8):631–7.
18. Pei M, He F, Vunjak-Novakovic G. Synovium-derived stem cell-based chondrogenesis. Differentiation. 2008;76(10):1044–56.
19. Dua R, Comella K, Butler R, Castellanos G, Brazille B, Claude A, Agarwal A, Liao J, Ramaswamy S. Integration of stem cell to chondrocyte-derived cartilage matrix in healthy and osteoarthritic states in the presence of hydroxyapatite nanoparticles. PLoS One. 2016;11(2):e0149121.
20. Samavedi S, Diaz-Rodriguez P, Erndt-Marino JD, Hahn MS. A three-dimensional chondrocyte-macrophage coculture system to probe inflammation in experimental osteoarthritis. Tissue Eng A. 2017;23(3-4):101–14.
21. Palamakumbura AH, Trackman PC. A fluorometric assay for detection of lysyl oxidase enzyme activity in biological samples. Anal Biochem. 2002;300(2):245–51.
22. Irizarry RA, Hobbs B, Collin F, Beazer-Barclay YD, Antonellis KJ, Scherf U, Speed TP. Exploration, normalization, and summaries of high density oligonucleotide array probe level data. Biostatistics. 2003;4(2):249–64.
23. Gautier L, Cope L, Bolstad BM, Irizarry RA. affy–analysis of Affymetrix GeneChip data at the probe level. Bioinformatics. 2004;20(3):307–15.
24. Gentleman RC, Carey VJ, Bates DM, Bolstad B, Dettling M, Dudoit S, Ellis B, Gautier L, Ge Y, Gentry J, et al. Bioconductor: open software development for computational biology and bioinformatics. Genome Biol. 2004;5(10):R80.
25. Dai M, Wang P, Boyd AD, Kostov G, Athey B, Jones EG, Bunney WE, Myers RM, Speed TP, Akil H, et al. Evolving gene/transcript definitions significantly alter the interpretation of GeneChip data. Nucleic Acids Res. 2005;33(20):e175.
26. Schuller GC, Tichy B, Majdisova Z, Jagersberger T, van Griensven M, Marlovits S, Redl H. An in vivo mouse model for human cartilage regeneration. J Tissue Eng Regen Med. 2008;2(4):202–9.
27. Endres M, Neumann K, Schroder SE, Vetterlein S, Morawietz L, Ringe J, Sittinger M, Kaps C. Human polymer-based cartilage grafts for the regeneration of articular cartilage defects. Tissue Cell. 2007;39(5):293–301.
28. Yahara Y, Takemori H, Okada M, Kosai A, Yamashita A, Kobayashi T, Fujita K, Itoh Y, Nakamura M, Fuchino H, et al. Pterosin B prevents chondrocyte hypertrophy and osteoarthritis in mice by inhibiting Sik3. Nat Commun. 2016;7:10959.
29. Fukui N, Zhu Y, Maloney WJ, Clohisy J, Sandell LJ. Stimulation of BMP-2 expression by pro-inflammatory cytokines IL-1 and TNF-alpha in normal and osteoarthritic chondrocytes. J Bone Joint Surg Am. 2003;85-A Suppl 3:59–66.
30. Snelling S, Rout R, Davidson R, Clark I, Carr A, Hulley PA, Price AJ. A gene expression study of normal and damaged cartilage in anteromedial gonarthrosis, a phenotype of osteoarthritis. Osteoarthr Cartil. 2014;22(2):334–43.
31. Karlsson C, Dehne T, Lindahl A, Brittberg M, Pruss A, Sittinger M, Ringe J. Genome-wide expression profiling reveals new candidate genes associated with osteoarthritis. Osteoarthr Cartil. 2010;18(4):581–92.
32. Vinatier C, Bouffi C, Merceron C, Gordeladze J, Brondello JM, Jorgensen C, Weiss P, Guicheux J, Noel D. Cartilage tissue engineering: towards a biomaterial-assisted mesenchymal stem cell therapy. Curr Stem Cell Res Ther. 2009;4(4):318–29.
33. Peretti GM, Randolph MA, Villa MT, Buragas MS, Yaremchuk MJ. Cell-based tissue-engineered allogeneic implant for cartilage repair. Tissue Eng. 2000;6(5):567–76.
34. Cairns DM, Liu R, Sen M, Canner JP, Schindeler A, Little DG, Zeng L. Interplay of Nkx3.2, Sox9 and Pax3 regulates chondrogenic differentiation of muscle progenitor cells. PLoS One. 2012;7(7):e39642.
35. Chevalier X, Eymard F, Richette P. Biologic agents in osteoarthritis: hopes and disappointments. Nat Rev Rheumatol. 2013;9(7):400–10.
36. Husa M, Liu-Bryan R, Terkeltaub R. Shifting HIFs in osteoarthritis. Nat Med. 2010;16(6):641–4.
37. Liu-Bryan R, Terkeltaub R. Emerging regulators of the inflammatory process in osteoarthritis. Nat Rev Rheumatol. 2015;11(1):35–44.
38. Marcu KB, Otero M, Olivotto E, Borzi RM, Goldring MB. NF-kappaB signaling: multiple angles to target OA. Curr Drug Targets. 2010;11(5):599–613.
39. Olivotto E, Otero M, Marcu KB, Goldring MB. Pathophysiology of osteoarthritis: canonical NF-kappaB/IKKbeta-dependent and kinase-independent effects of IKKalpha in cartilage degradation and chondrocyte differentiation. RMD Open. 2015;1 Suppl 1:e000061.
40. Olivotto E, Otero M, Astolfi A, Platano D, Facchini A, Pagani S, Flamigni F, Facchini A, Goldring MB, Borzi RM, et al. IKKalpha/CHUK regulates extracellular matrix remodeling independent of its kinase activity to facilitate articular chondrocyte differentiation. PLoS One. 2013;8(9):e73024.
41. Rigoglou S, Papavassiliou AG. The NF-kappaB signalling pathway in osteoarthritis. Int J Biochem Cell Biol. 2013;45(11):2580–4.
42. Zhen G, Wen C, Jia X, Li Y, Crane JL, Mears SC, Askin FB, Frassica FJ, Chang W, Yao J, et al. Inhibition of TGF-beta signaling in mesenchymal stem cells of subchondral bone attenuates osteoarthritis. Nat Med. 2013;19(6):704–12.
43. Long E, Motwani R, Reece D, Pettit N, Hepworth J, Wong P, Reynolds P, Seegmiller R. The role of TGF-ss1 in osteoarthritis of the temporomandibular joint in two genetic mouse models. Arch Oral Biol. 2016;67:68–73.
44. Blaney Davidson EN, van der Kraan PM, van den Berg WB. TGF-beta and osteoarthritis. Osteoarthr Cartil. 2007;15(6):597–604.
45. Atsawasuwan P, Mochida Y, Katafuchi M, Kaku M, Fong KS, Csiszar K, Yamauchi M. Lysyl oxidase binds transforming growth factor-beta and regulates its signaling via amine oxidase activity. J Biol Chem. 2008; 283(49):34229–40.
46. Bonnans C, Chou J, Werb Z. Remodelling the extracellular matrix in development and disease. Nat Rev Mol Cell Biol. 2014;15(12):786–801.
47. Barker HE, Cox TR, Erler JT. The rationale for targeting the LOX family in cancer. Nat Rev Cancer. 2012;12(8):540–52.
48. Akiri G, Sabo E, Dafni H, Vadasz Z, Kartvelishvily Y, Gan N, Kessler O, Cohen T, Resnick M, Neeman M, et al. Lysyl oxidase-related protein-1 promotes tumor fibrosis and tumor progression in vivo. Cancer Res. 2003;63(7):1657–66.
49. Torres S, Garcia-Palmero I, Herrera M, Bartolome RA, Pena C, Fernandez-Acenero MJ, Padilla G, Pelaez-Garcia A, Lopez-Lucendo M, Rodriguez-Merlo R, et al. LOXL2 is highly expressed in cancer-associated fibroblasts and associates to poor colon cancer survival. Clin Cancer Res. 2015;21(21):4892–902.
50. Johnson K, Zhu S, Tremblay MS, Payette JN, Wang J, Bouchez LC, Meeusen S, Althage A, Cho CY, Wu X, et al. A stem cell-based approach to cartilage repair. Science. 2012;336(6082):717–21.
51. Hinton RJ. Genes that regulate morphogenesis and growth of the temporomandibular joint: a review. Dev Dyn. 2014;243(7):864–74.
52. Iturbide A, Garcia de Herreros A, Peiro S. A new role for LOX and LOXL2 proteins in transcription regulation. FEBS J. 2015;282(9):1768–73.
53. Iturbide A, Pascual-Reguant L, Fargas L, Cebria JP, Alsina B, Garcia de Herreros A, Peiro S. LOXL2 oxidizes methylated TAF10 and controls TFIID-dependent genes during neural progenitor differentiation. Mol Cell. 2015; 58(5):755–66.
54. Peinado H, Portillo F, Cano A. Switching on-off Snail: LOXL2 versus GSK3beta. Cell Cycle. 2005;4(12):1749–52.
55. Peinado H, Del Carmen Iglesias-de la Cruz M, Olmeda D, Csiszar K, Fong KS, Vega S, Nieto MA, Cano A, Portillo F. A molecular role for lysyl oxidase-like 2 enzyme in snail regulation and tumor progression. EMBO J. 2005;24(19): 3446–58.
56. Canesin G, Cuevas EP, Santos V, Lopez-Menendez C, Moreno-Bueno G, Huang Y, Csiszar K, Portillo F, Peinado H, Lyden D, et al. Lysyl oxidase-like 2 (LOXL2) and E47 EMT factor: novel partners in E-cadherin repression and early metastasis colonization. Oncogene. 2015;34(8):951–64.
57. Moreno-Bueno G, Salvador F, Martin A, Floristan A, Cuevas EP, Santos V, Montes A, Morales S, Castilla MA, Rojo-Sebastian A, et al. Lysyl oxidase-like 2 (LOXL2), a new regulator of cell polarity required for metastatic dissemination of basal-like breast carcinomas. EMBO Mol Med. 2011;3(9): 528–44.
58. Moon HJ, Finney J, Xu L, Moore D, Welch DR, Mure M. MCF-7 cells expressing nuclear associated lysyl oxidase-like 2 (LOXL2) exhibit an epithelial-to-mesenchymal transition (EMT) phenotype and are highly invasive in vitro. J Biol Chem. 2013;288(42):30000–8.

5

Do early life factors affect the development of knee osteoarthritis in later life

Benny Antony[1*], Graeme Jones[1], Xingzhong Jin[1] and Changhai Ding[1,2]

Abstract

Osteoarthritis (OA) mainly affects older populations; however, it is possible that early life factors contribute to the development of OA in later life. The aim of this review is to describe the association between childhood or early adulthood risk factors and knee pain, structural imaging markers and development of knee OA in later life. A narrative overview of the literature synthesising the findings of literature retrieved from searches of computerised databases and manual searches was conducted. We found that only a few studies have explored the long-term effect of childhood or early adulthood risk factors on the markers of joint health that predispose people to OA or joint symptoms. High body mass index (BMI) and/or overweight status from childhood to adulthood were independently related to knee pain and OA in later life. The findings regarding the association between strenuous physical activity and knee structures in young adults are still conflicting. However, a favourable effect of moderate physical activity and fitness on knee structures is reported. Childhood physical activity and performance measures had independent beneficial effects on knee structures including knee cartilage in children and young adults. Anterior knee pain syndrome in adolescence could lead to the development of patellofemoral knee OA in the late 40s. Furthermore, weak evidence suggests that childhood malalignment, socioeconomic status and physical abuse are associated with OA in later life. The available evidence suggests that early life intervention may prevent OA in later life.

Keywords: Childhood, BMI, Overweight, Exercise, Fitness, Physical activity, Adulthood, Knee pain, Osteoarthritis

Background

Osteoarthritis (OA) is characterised by pain, gradual loss of articular cartilage and other structural changes. OA is a disease of the whole joint, eventually leading to total joint replacement. It is the most common joint disorder in adults around the world and it is one of the most frequent causes of pain, loss of function and disability [1]. The global prevalence of radiographically confirmed symptomatic knee and hip OA in 2010 was estimated to be 3.8 % and 0.85 %, respectively [2]. OA is ranked 13th in the top 25 causes of global years lived with disability (DALYs) and the fourth leading cause that showed an increase in DALYs from 1990 to 2013 [3].

Knee OA is the most common form of OA and, currently, there are no registered disease-modifying OA drugs. There is an urgent need for research that investigates innovative and cost-effective approaches to prevent or slow down the progression of knee OA. One of the approaches is to identify and intervene in the early life risk factors that cause this major, but poorly understood, public health problem. The major risk factors associated with this disease are age, female sex, genetic factors, increased body mass index (BMI) and injury. Lifestyle factors such as physical activity and exercise have been associated with knee OA, although the evidence is inconsistent [4–6]. Low socioeconomic position and other co-morbidities, such as cardiovascular diseases, have been considered as risk factors.

OA mainly affects older populations; however, it is possible that early life factors contribute to the development of OA in later life. Considering the mechanical aspect (imbalance in the movement and physical force transmission through the joint) of knee OA, childhood risk factors such as obesity and malalignment could be

* Correspondence: Benny.EathakkattuAntony@utas.edu.au
[1]Menzies Institute for Medical Research, University of Tasmania, Private Bag 23, Hobart, Tasmania 7000, Australia
Full list of author information is available at the end of the article

of great importance in the development of this disease. However, it is difficult to identify the early life risk factors that have a life-course influence on the development of OA due to the difficulties of conducting long-term follow-up from childhood to adulthood. Therefore, only a few studies have reported the childhood risk factors for OA. The aim of this review is to describe the association between childhood or early adulthood risk factors and knee pain, structural imaging markers and the development of knee OA in later life.

Methods

The literature search involved searching relevant electronic databases (Medline, EMBASE and Google scholar), reference checking, manual searching of relevant journals and recommendations from experts. Due to the low number and diversity of studies and the diversity in outcome measures, a narrative review was felt to be most appropriate to review the relevant literature.

Early markers of OA

Our understanding of early joint changes associated with OA is increasing due to the use of advanced imaging techniques such as magnetic resonance imaging (MRI). Research on the development and validation of biomarkers, including imaging biomarkers, is a promising method for identifying the early risk factors. Many studies have explored the early life and childhood risk factors in osteoporosis research, which is mainly due to the identification of peak bone mass as a predictor of future osteoporosis or fracture risk [7]. Such markers of joint health are being established in OA research. Cartilage defects, bone marrow lesions (BMLs) and meniscal pathology (early markers of joint abnormalities) are known to occur before the clinical diagnosis of radiographic OA and can predict the development and progression of OA in later life [8]. Tibial cartilage volume in young adults has been proposed as a marker of knee joint health [9, 10] which protects against the development of knee OA in later life (similar to peak bone mass, which is a strong predictor of future risk of osteoporosis in older people) [7]. An ideal approach to identify the early life risk factors in OA is to apply advanced imaging techniques to already existing birth cohorts that have reached adulthood.

Pain is the most common presenting feature of OA, although pain is only weakly related to the structural damage seen in OA [11]. Age, previous knee injuries, overweight and knee-straining work were found to be the risk factors contributing to the incidence of knee pain. These risk factors for self-reported knee pain are similar to the risk factors for knee OA [12]. Therefore, pain should be considered as an important marker, along with other OA features.

Results

Early life obesity and adulthood knee OA

Obesity is more associated with knee OA than OA of other joints [13]. Whether childhood obesity leads to later OA has largely been unexplored. The importance of childhood overweight arises from the fact that it predicts adult obesity [14]. Adolescents who were overweight were 18 times more likely than their leaner peers to become obese in early adulthood [15]. Obesity in childhood was strongly predictive of obesity in early adulthood [16]. This tracking of obesity makes it difficult to identify the independent influence of childhood obesity on OA.

Wills and colleagues [17] suggested that obesity from childhood had an accumulative effect on knee OA development. BMI in men as early as 20 years old and women as early as 15 years old was associated with increased risk of knee OA at the age of 53 years [13, 17]. This study suggested that increases in BMI from childhood in women and from adolescence in men was positively associated with knee OA. However, prolonged exposure to high BMI throughout adulthood carried the highest risk and there was no additional risk conferred from adolescence once adult BMI had been accounted for [17]. This study defined knee OA using the symptomatic criteria at 53 years of age and did not have radiographs to confirm the structural pathology. They defined prevalent symptomatic knee OA at one time point (53 years) and could not, therefore, comment on the influence of childhood or adolescent BMI on the incidence of knee OA. The same study group previously reported that hand OA in men at the age of 53 years was associated with increased weight at the age of 26, 43 and 53 years but with decreased weight at birth. The highest risk for hand OA was observed in those who had been heaviest at age 53 years and lightest at birth [18]. However, studies reported that birth weight did not appear to be a major influence on the later development of knee OA in women [19] and the general population [20] after accounting for other confounding factors, including obesity.

BMI in young adults (mean age 23 years) was strongly associated with the incidence of knee OA, but not hip OA, at 65 years of age. For BMI assessed at ages 20 to 29 years, the incidence of knee OA at age 65 years was threefold greater in the heaviest tertile category than the incidence in the leanest tertile category of BMI after adjustment for age, physical activity and knee injury [21]. BMI at ages 20 to 29 years was more predictive of future OA than at ages 30 to 39 or 40 to 49 years [21].

Using MRI, we reported that overweight children did not differ significantly from normal weight children in knee articular cartilage volume either cross-sectionally or longitudinally over 1.6 years [22]. Similarly, we did not find any significant association between overweight status in childhood and adulthood knee structures, including cartilage volume after 25 years (data not published). However, we found that lean mass in young adults was positively and fat mass was negatively associated with tibial cartilage volume in young Australian adults [23].

Early life obesity and adulthood knee joint pain

The knee joint is commonly affected by pain in both overweight paediatric [24] and adult populations [25]. A recent systematic review that studied the relationship between overweight and various musculoskeletal complaints in children suggested that there was moderate evidence for a positive association between overweight during childhood and musculoskeletal pain with a relative risk (RR) of 1.26 (95 % confidence interval (CI) = 1.09–1.97) [26]. However, there was no relationship between body composition or body mass and patellofemoral pain in young school basketball players [27] or knee pain among school children [28].

The effect of childhood obesity on the knee joint can persist into adulthood and lead to higher knee pain in later life. A study by McFarlane et al. on the 1958 British birth cohort explored the association of weight from childhood to adulthood (BMI at 7, 11, 16, 23, 33 and 45 years) with adulthood knee pain at 45 years. They found a higher risk of adulthood knee pain for the obese relative to the underweight subjects in each age group [29]. Childhood BMI was associated with adult knee pain but this association was dependent on adulthood BMI [29]. However, BMI in the early 20s was an independent predictor of knee pain at 45 years [29]. This study had some limitations, for example, adult BMI categories were used for the definition of overweight and obesity in childhood, the reference category for comparison was an underweight group rather than normal weight, men and women were not separated for analyses and they did not use a validated scale for knee pain assessment such as the Western Ontario and McMaster Universities Osteoarthritis Index (WOMAC) scale. A similar study from our group used the Australian Schools Health and Fitness Survey (ASHFS) from 1985 and reported that the childhood overweight measures were significantly associated with adulthood knee mechanical joint pain, stiffness and physical dysfunction among males (aged 31–41 years), independent of the adult overweight measures [30]. Similarly, the change in overweight status from childhood to adulthood was also associated with knee pain; subjects who were overweight in both childhood and adult life had the greatest prevalence and double the risk of knee pain compared with subjects who had normal weight at both time points [30]. Another retrospective life course study on Finnish men ($n = 1913$) who participated in the Health 2000 Study reported that BMI at the age of 20 years increased the likelihood of knee pain and functional limitations of the knee later in life [31]. BMI at the age of 20 years increased the risk of knee pain in either knee by 38 % and functional limitations by 27 % for one standard deviation increment of BMI, respectively. Development of severe obesity in adulthood increased the risk of knee pain by 80 % and functional limitations by 90 %. The effect of obesity on functional limitations was partly mediated by traumatic knee problems during military service [31].

These results support the observation that both systemic and mechanical factors underlie the link between OA and body weight and suggest that developmental influences may be important [18]. For weight-bearing joints, the combination of increased load and changed joint biomechanics is regarded as an underlying mechanism for the association between obesity and OA. Obese individuals show altered biomechanics during everyday movements and these altered biomechanics could initiate OA by changing the load-bearing regions of the articular cartilage in the weight-bearing joints [32]. Systemic factors such as adipokines and other inflammatory markers associated with obesity may also underlie the association of obesity with OA as suggested by a higher prevalence of hand OA (non-weight bearing joint) in obese patients [18, 33].

Early life joint pain and adulthood knee OA

Knee pain is not an uncommon feature in early life [34]. Studies have found that the prevalence of knee pain is 3.9 % among children and 18.5 % in adolescents [28]. Some studies have reported an even higher prevalence of pathological knee pain in adolescents, with a range from 28.5 to 31 % [35, 36]. Knee pain in early life can result from many conditions that are not related to OA in later life. The most common causes of knee pain in early life include patellar subluxation, Osgood–Schlatter lesion (localised pain at the tibial tuberosity where the quadriceps muscles insert that is mostly associated with a growth spurt), patellar tendonitis, arthritis (bacterial, viral or inflammatory), referred pain from the hip, osteochondritis dissecans, tumours and malignancies. Similarly, anterior knee pain (AKP) is a broad symptom classification which does not imply any particular diagnosis or physical condition and is likely to be multifactorial [37]. Patellofemoral pain syndrome (PFPS) accounts for almost 50 % of nonspecific knee pain in adolescents [38]. Major symptoms of PFPS are diffuse peripatellar and retropatellar localised pain, pain provoked by ascending stairs, descending stairs, squatting, cycling and sitting with flexed knees for prolonged periods of time [39].

Similar to OA in older adults, the prevalence of PFPS has been found to be higher in females, with a prevalence that is approximately 1.5–3 times higher than males in athletic populations [40]. It is possible that these knee pain symptoms persist to later life leading to OA. There is evidence to show that 90 % of AKP sufferers had ongoing problems four years later [41] and 94 % of the AKP cases continued to experience physical difficulties for an average of 8 years following diagnosis [42]. A retrospective study investigating the association between idiopathic AKP in early adulthood and patellofemoral OA found that patients with patellofemoral OA reported more preceding AKP in their adolescence and early adult years than medial unicompartmental tibiofemoral knee OA cases [43]. A systematic review concluded that there was a paucity of high-quality research evidence regarding the link between idiopathic AKP in younger adults and the subsequent development of patellofemoral OA [44]; however, the authors indicated that the evidence from the retrospective case-control study [43] was reliable as its recall bias was minimal and the choice of the control group (medial unicompartmental tibiofemoral knee OA) was suitable. Therefore, AKP can be regarded as one of the early risk factors for knee OA.

Early life physical activity and adulthood OA

There is consistent evidence that physical activity improves pain and physical function in knee OA and moderate physical activity is recommended by the guidelines for the nonsurgical management of knee OA [45]. However, the effect of physical activity and fitness on the development and progression of OA is controversial as various studies have suggested detrimental [46], beneficial [47] or no effect [48]. The reasons for this controversy are unclear but it may be due to the fact that these studies were retrospective in nature and were not able to take into account the confounding role of injury, which increases the risk of developing OA [49]. It is also possible that knee structures behave differently during different physical activities at different life stages. Weak evidence shows that healthy articular cartilage in vivo responded beneficially to physical loading and degenerated cartilage responded detrimentally [50]. Similarly, in hamsters, physical exercise at a young age had a beneficial effect via enhancing cartilage maturation but had adverse effects on cartilage at a later age with a significant increase in the incidence of OA [51].

Our studies among children aged 9–18 years reported that physical activity was associated with increased cartilage volume both cross-sectionally [52] and longitudinally [22]. In the same study, baseline leg muscle strength was positively associated with cartilage volume accrual and partially mediated the association between physical activity and cartilage volume [22]. Similarly, an interventional study in younger adults (mean age 25 years) using delayed Gadolinium Enhanced MRI of cartilage (dGEMRIC) scans (for detecting the glycosaminoglycan (GAG) content in the cartilage) showed a positive change of dGEMRIC index over 10 weeks in women who were enrolled in a moderate running programme [53]. Similarly, a randomised controlled trial evaluated the effect of moderate exercise on GAG content in knee cartilage and found that the exercise group had an increased GAG content compared with controls in subjects aged between 35 and 50 years [54]. There was a strong correlation ($r = 0.74$) between self-reported physical activity levels and the GAG content in knee cartilage [54]. In contrast, cross-sectional studies of adult triathletes and middle-aged women found no difference in cartilage volume between those who exercised and those who did not, although bone size was generally larger in triathletes than inactive controls [55, 56]. Both studies were small in sample size and cross-sectional in nature. However, in young Australian adults we reported that physical activity measured 5 years before was positively associated with total tibial cartilage volume [57].

A twin study that explored the effect of physical activity on general health found that physical activity reduced the risk of chronic diseases and helped to maintain life satisfaction; however, there was no association between being active or less active and OA in monozygotic or dizygotic twins [58]. A study in preadolescents with lower limb pain reported that 32 % of participants had persistent pain at 1-year follow-up and 31 % reported recurring pain at 4-year follow-up, and vigorous exercise was a significant predictor of lower limb pain persistence at 1-year follow-up but hypermobility was predictive of pain recurrence 4 years later [59]. There was evidence suggesting that athletes had a higher risk of having knee OA features, including osteophytes and radiographic OA, even at a younger age [60].

A recent prospective study from our group in children with a follow-up of 25 years reported that childhood physical performance measures, such as physical work capacity at 170 beats per minute (PWC_{170}), were positively associated with adulthood (31–41 years age) tibial cartilage volume independent of adult attained fitness levels [61]. In the same study cohort, we reported that adulthood performance measures, such as leg muscle strength, long jump and PWC_{170} measures, and physical activity measures, such as vigorous, moderate and total activities, were positively associated with adulthood tibial cartilage volume [57]. However, vigorous physical activity in these young adults was weakly but positively associated with BMLs and moderate physical activity was associated with reduced BMLs [62]. Both childhood and adulthood performance measures were associated with tibial bone area and the association between performance measures and cartilage volume was partially mediated by tibial bone area growth, suggesting that greater physical fitness leads to higher cartilage volume through bone development [57, 61].

Early life injury and adulthood knee OA

Injury to the joint is a major risk factor for OA. Studies have suggested a consistent association between injury and knee OA in all age groups. Only a few studies have explored the association of childhood injury with the incidence of knee OA in later life. The effect of early life injury on OA seems to be smaller than the effect of injury in late adulthood. In a retrospective study, which explored the association between AKP in early adulthood and patellofemoral OA, patients with patellofemoral arthroplasty were found to suffer significantly more patellofemoral instability and trauma in their early adulthood than patients with medial unicompartmental arthroplasty [43]. A study exploring the persistence and recurrence of knee pain in preadolescents found that traumatic lower extremity pain had a 50 % lower risk for pain recurrence compared with non-traumatic pain, indicating a favourable long-term natural course for traumatic pain [59]. Adolescents and young adults (mean age 22) who suffered knee injury were found to be at higher risk of knee OA (RR = 2.95; 95 % CI = 1.35–6.45) at 65 years of age compared with those who did not have injury [49].

There is evidence to suggest that greater BMI in childhood is associated with increased risk of lower extremity injuries and pain [63]. Similarly, increasing BMI is associated with increased risk of lower extremity fractures, such as fractures of the foot, ankle, leg and knee, among children [64]. These injuries and fractures resulting from obesity may lead to knee OA in later life.

Early life malalignment and adulthood knee OA

Some developmental conditions, such as malalignment, have been proposed as a risk factor for the progression of knee OA, but the prospective evidence is not strong enough to support a causative role of malalignment in the development of knee OA [65]. Self-reported knee malalignment (reported as bow legs) in childhood was associated with cartilage thinning (measured as joint space narrowing using X-ray) in adults over 12 years of follow-up [66]. Similarly, increased risk of isolated knee OA occurred with early adult varus (odds ratio (OR) = 5.16; 95 % CI = 2.87–9.41) and valgus knees (OR = 3.16; 95 % CI = 1.04–9.64) [67]. The authors observed a positive association between knee OA and toe-in foot in this study and this association was explained by varus knee [67]. Although the epidemiological associations are strong, the causal relationship is not established.

There is evidence for a higher prevalence of lower extremity malalignment, fractures and musculoskeletal pain among obese children than children with normal weight [24, 26]. Studies have suggested that the association of obesity with knee OA progression is largely mediated by knee malalignment [68, 69]. Therefore, obesity-related malalignment is important in the context of life-course-approach studies for knee OA. A recent study exploring the knee alignment among obese and non-obese children found that the mean alignment was similar between obese and non-obese subjects [70]; however, in the stratified analysis, there was significantly greater variability in knee alignment among females at higher BMI and greater valgus alignment in obese adolescents in late puberty [70]. A similar study using dual-energy X-ray absorptiometry (DXA) detected a greater prevalence of lower extremity malalignment, mostly valgus deformity, in overweight children [24]. The major limitation of these studies is the use of DXA for assessment of alignment, which needs validation against radiographs. It is possible that mild malalignment with excess weight loaded on the joints over time may contribute to the increased incidence of knee pain and subsequent knee OA. However, further longitudinal studies are required to determine whether childhood obesity is a risk factor for progressive malalignment which predisposes individuals to pain and risk of early OA.

Early life socioeconomic status and adulthood knee OA

Lower socioeconomic status (SES) has been associated with knee pain, knee OA and total knee replacement in adulthood [71]. Macfarlane and colleagues have identified an association between childhood social status and adulthood wide-spread musculoskeletal pain such as knee pain at 45 years; however, the magnitude of effect of childhood social status on adulthood self-reported pain was less than that of adult social status and was partly explained by poor adult mental health, psychological distress, adverse life events and lifestyle factors [72]. Similarly, there was an independent association of both childhood and current SES with self-reported arthritis [73]. Increased BMI was the most likely mechanism underlying the association between childhood SES and arthritis onset [73].

Early life abuse and adulthood OA

Childhood abuse could be physical, sexual, emotional and/or neglect. Previous research has identified an association between childhood abuse and arthritis in adulthood [74, 75] and this association was strongest and most consistent with childhood physical abuse. The evidence of a relationship between childhood sexual abuse and arthritis is conflicting; one study showed an association [76] and another did not [75]. Individuals who reported a diagnosis of OA had significantly higher odds (OR = 1.99; 95 % CI = 1.57–2.52) of reporting childhood physical abuse [77]. This association remained significant even after controlling for demographic and SES characteristics, in addition to childhood stressors, adult health behaviours and mood disorders, which were associated with childhood physical abuse and arthritis.

Conclusions

Although the evidence for associations between childhood or early life factors and OA is limited, the existing evidence suggests that obesity from early life is independently associated with knee OA and knee pain. The evidence for injury, malalignment, childhood SES and childhood abuse are mostly from retrospective studies and such associations need to be confirmed by prospective studies. Anterior knee pain syndrome in adolescence could lead to the development of patellofemoral knee OA in the late 40s. The findings regarding the association between strenuous physical activity and knee structures in young adults are still conflicting. However, a favourable effect of moderate physical activity and fitness on knee structures is reported. Childhood physical activity and fitness may have an independent beneficial effect on knee joint health. These data suggest that early life intervention may prevent OA in later life. However, further cohort studies with larger sample sizes and long-term follow-ups are required to determine if OA in later life stems from childhood or early adulthood risk factors.

Abbreviations

AKP: Anterior knee pain; BMI: Body mass index; BML: Bone marrow lesion; CI: Confidence interval; DALYs: Disability adjusted life years; dGEMRIC: Delayed gadolinium enhanced MRI of cartilage; DXA: Dual-energy X-ray absorptiometry; GAG: Glycosaminoglycan; MRI: Magnetic resonance imaging; OA: Osteoarthritis; OR: Odds ratio; PFPS: Patellofemoral pain syndrome; PWC_{170}: Physical work capacity at 170 beats per minute; RR: Relative risk; SES: Socioeconomic status

Acknowledgements

We would like to thank Prof. Alison Venn for expert advice and the fellowship support from Arthritis Australia, Farrell Family, University of Tasmania and National Health and Medical Research Council of Australia.

Funding

This review received no funding other than salary stipends for authors as described below. BA is a recipient of the Arthritis Australia Fellowship and Farrell Family Senior Research Fellowship, CD is a recipient of an ARC Future Fellowship, XJ is a recipient of International Postgraduate Research Scholarship and GJ is a recipient of a NHMRC Practitioner Fellowship.

Authors' contributions

BA was responsible for the study planning, literature search and interpretation of the studies, prepared the initial manuscript draft and completed manuscript revisions. XJ helped in the literature search and critically revised the manuscript. GJ and CD were involved in scrutinising the literature studies and critically revised the manuscript. All authors read and approved the manuscript.

Authors' information

Dr. Benny Antony PhD is a research fellow at the Menzies Institute for Medical Research. Prof. Graeme Jones MD is a practicing rheumatologist and head of the musculoskeletal department of Menzies Institute for Medical Research. Dr. Xingzhong Jin PhD is a research fellow at the Macquire University. Prof. Changhai Ding MD is a professorial research fellow and Associate Director at the Menzies Institute for Medical Research.

Competing interests

All authors have completed the Unified Competing Interest form (available on request from the corresponding author) and declare: no support from any organisation for the submitted work; no financial relationships with any organisations that might have an interest in the submitted work in the previous three years; no other relationships or activities that could appear to have influenced the submitted work.

Author details

[1]Menzies Institute for Medical Research, University of Tasmania, Private Bag 23, Hobart, Tasmania 7000, Australia. [2]Institute of Bone & Joint Translational Research, Southern Medical University, Guangzhou, Guangdong, China.

References

1. Felson DT. Clinical practice. Osteoarthritis of the knee. N Engl J Med. 2006; 354(8):841–8.
2. Cross M, Smith E, Hoy D, Nolte S, Ackerman I, Fransen M, Bridgett L, Williams S, Guillemin F, Hill CL, et al. The global burden of hip and knee osteoarthritis: estimates from the global burden of disease 2010 study. Ann Rheum Dis. 2014;73(7):1323–30.
3. Global Burden of Disease Study C. Global, regional, and national incidence, prevalence, and years lived with disability for 301 acute and chronic diseases and injuries in 188 countries, 1990–2013: a systematic analysis for the Global Burden of Disease Study 2013. Lancet. 2015; 386(9995):743–800.
4. Richmond SA, Fukuchi RK, Ezzat A, Schneider K, Schneider G, Emery CA. Are joint injury, sport activity, physical activity, obesity, or occupational activities predictors for osteoarthritis? A systematic review. J Orthop Sports Phys Ther. 2013;43(8):515–B19.
5. Fransen M, Simic M, Harmer AR. Determinants of MSK health and disability: lifestyle determinants of symptomatic osteoarthritis. Best Pract Res Clin Rheumatol. 2014;28(3):435–60.
6. Urquhart DM, Tobing JFL, Hanna FS, Berry P, Wluka AE, Ding C, Cicuttini FM. What is the effect of physical activity on the knee joint? A systematic review. Med Sci Sports Exerc. 2011;43(3):432–42.
7. Winsloe C, Earl S, Dennison EM, Cooper C, Harvey NC. Early life factors in the pathogenesis of osteoporosis. Curr Osteoporos Rep. 2009;7(4):140–4.
8. Pelletier JP, Cooper C, Peterfy C, Reginster JY, Brandi ML, Bruyere O, Chapurlat R, Cicuttini F, Conaghan PG, Doherty M, et al. What is the predictive value of MRI for the occurrence of knee replacement surgery in knee osteoarthritis? Ann Rheum Dis. 2013;72(10):1594–604.
9. Cohen ZA, Mow VC, Henry JH, Levine WN, Ateshian GA. Templates of the cartilage layers of the patellofemoral joint and their use in the assessment of osteoarthritic cartilage damage. Osteoarthritis Cartilage. 2003;11(8):569–79.
10. Burgkart R, Glaser C, Hinterwimmer S, Hudelmaier M, Englmeier KH, Reiser M, Eckstein F. Feasibility of T and Z scores from magnetic resonance imaging data for quantification of cartilage loss in osteoarthritis. Arthritis Rheum. 2003;48(10): 2829–35.
11. Hunter DJ, Guermazi A, Roemer F, Zhang Y, Neogi T. Structural correlates of pain in joints with osteoarthritis. Osteoarthritis Cartilage. 2013;21(9):1170–8.
12. Miranda H, Viikari-Juntura E, Martikainen R, Riihimaki H. A prospective study on knee pain and its risk factors. Osteoarthritis Cartilage. 2002;10(8):623–30.
13. Martin KR, Kuh D, Harris TB, Guralnik JM, Coggon D, Wills AK. Body mass index, occupational activity, and leisure-time physical activity: an exploration of risk factors and modifiers for knee osteoarthritis in the 1946 British birth cohort. BMC Musculoskelet Disord. 2013;14:219.
14. Steinberger J, Moran A, Hong CP, Jacobs Jr DR, Sinaiko AR. Adiposity in childhood predicts obesity and insulin resistance in young adulthood. J Pediatr. 2001;138(4):469–73.
15. Whitaker RC, Wright JA, Pepe MS, Seidel KD, Dietz WH. Predicting obesity in young adulthood from childhood and parental obesity. N Engl J Med. 1997; 337(13):869–73.
16. Venn AJ, Thomson RJ, Schmidt MD, Cleland VJ, Curry BA, Gennat HC, Dwyer T. Overweight and obesity from childhood to adulthood: a follow-up of participants in the 1985 Australian Schools Health and Fitness Survey. Med J Aust. 2007;186(9):458–60.
17. Wills AK, Black S, Cooper R, Coppack RJ, Hardy R, Martin KR, Cooper C, Kuh D. Life course body mass index and risk of knee osteoarthritis at the age of 53 years: evidence from the 1946 British birth cohort study. Ann Rheum Dis. 2012;71(5):655–60.
18. Sayer AA, Poole J, Cox V, Kuh D, Hardy R, Wadsworth M, Cooper C. Weight from birth to 53 years: a longitudinal study of the influence on clinical hand osteoarthritis. Arthritis Rheum. 2003;48(4):1030–3.
19. Antoniades L, MacGregor AJ, Andrew T, Spector TD. Association of birth weight with osteoporosis and osteoarthritis in adult twins. Rheumatology (Oxford). 2003;42(6):791–6.

20. Hussain SM, Wang Y, Wluka AE, Shaw JE, Magliano DJ, Graves S, Cicuttini FM. Association of low birth weight and preterm birth with the incidence of knee and hip arthroplasty for osteoarthritis. Arthritis Care Res (Hoboken). 2015;67(4):502–8.
21. Gelber AC, Hochberg MC, Mead LA, Wang NY, Wigley FM, Klag MJ. Body mass index in young men and the risk of subsequent knee and hip osteoarthritis. Am J Med. 1999;107(6):542–8.
22. Jones G, Ding C, Glisson M, Hynes K, Ma D, Cicuttini F. Knee articular cartilage development in children: a longitudinal study of the effect of sex, growth, body composition, and physical activity. Pediatr Res. 2003;54(2): 230–6.
23. Antony B, Venn A, Cicuttini F, March L, Blizzard L, Dwyer T, Cross M, Jones G, Ding C. Association of body composition and hormonal and inflammatory factors with tibial cartilage volume and sex difference in cartilage volume in young adults. Arthritis Care Res (Hoboken). 2016;68(4):517–25.
24. Taylor ED, Theim KR, Mirch MC, Ghorbani S, Tanofsky-Kraff M, Adler-Wailes DC, Brady S, Reynolds JC, Calis KA, Yanovski JA. Orthopedic complications of overweight in children and adolescents. Pediatrics. 2006;117(6):2167–74.
25. Urwin M, Symmons D, Allison T, Brammah T, Busby H, Roxby M, Simmons A, Williams G. Estimating the burden of musculoskeletal disorders in the community: the comparative prevalence of symptoms at different anatomical sites, and the relation to social deprivation. Ann Rheum Dis. 1998;57(11):649–55.
26. Paulis WD, Silva S, Koes BW, van Middelkoop M. Overweight and obesity are associated with musculoskeletal complaints as early as childhood: a systematic review. Obes Rev. 2014;15(1):52–67.
27. Barber Foss KD, Hornsby M, Edwards NM, Myer GD, Hewett TE. Is body composition associated with an increased risk of developing anterior knee pain in adolescent female athletes? Phys Sportsmed. 2012;40(1):13–9.
28. Vahasarja V. Prevalence of chronic knee pain in children and adolescents in northern Finland. Acta Paediatr. 1995;84(7):803–5.
29. Macfarlane GJ, de Silva V, Jones GT. The relationship between body mass index across the life course and knee pain in adulthood: results from the 1958 birth cohort study. Rheumatology (Oxford). 2011;50(12):2251–6.
30. Antony B, Jones G, Venn A, Cicuttini F, March L, Blizzard L, Dwyer T, Cross M, Ding C. Association between childhood overweight measures and adulthood knee pain, stiffness and dysfunction: a 25-year cohort study. Ann Rheum Dis. 2015;74(4):711–7.
31. Frilander H, Viikari-Juntura E, Heliovaara M, Mutanen P, Mattila VM, Solovieva S. Obesity in early adulthood predicts knee pain and walking difficulties among men: a life course study. Eur J Pain. 2016;20(8):1278–87.
32. Runhaar J, Koes BW, Clockaerts S, Bierma-Zeinstra SM. A systematic review on changed biomechanics of lower extremities in obese individuals: a possible role in development of osteoarthritis. Obes Rev. 2011;12(12):1071–82.
33. Cicuttini FM, Baker JR, Spector TD. The association of obesity with osteoarthritis of the hand and knee in women: a twin study. J Rheumatol. 1996;23(7):1221–6.
34. Stovitz SD, Pardee PE, Vazquez G, Duval S, Schwimmer JB. Musculoskeletal pain in obese children and adolescents. Acta Paediatr. 2008;97(4):489–93.
35. Spahn G, Schiele R, Langlotz A, Jung R. Prevalence of functional pain of the back, the hip and the knee in adolescents. Results of a cross-sectional study. Dtsch Med Wochenschr. 2004;129(43):2285–90.
36. Fairbank JC, Pynsent PB, van Poortvliet JA, Phillips H. Mechanical factors in the incidence of knee pain in adolescents and young adults. J Bone Joint Surg Br. 1984;66(5):685–93.
37. Grelsamer R, Moss G, Ee G, Donell S. The patellofemoral syndrome; the same problem as the Loch Ness Monster? Knee. 2009;16(5):301–2.
38. Molgaard C, Rathleff MS, Simonsen O. Patellofemoral pain syndrome and its association with hip, ankle, and foot function in 16- to 18-year-old high school students: a single-blind case-control study. J Am Podiatr Med Assoc. 2011;101(3):215–22.
39. Haim A, Yaniv M, Dekel S, Amir H. Patellofemoral pain syndrome: validity of clinical and radiological features. Clin Orthop Relat Res. 2006;451:223–8.
40. Taunton JE, Ryan MB, Clement DB, McKenzie DC, Lloyd-Smith DR, Zumbo BD. A retrospective case-control analysis of 2002 running injuries. Br J Sports Med. 2002;36(2):95–101.
41. Stathopulu E, Baildam E. Anterior knee pain: a long-term follow-up. Rheumatology (Oxford). 2003;42(2):380–2.
42. Sandow MJ, Goodfellow JW. The natural history of anterior knee pain in adolescents. J Bone Joint Surg Br. 1985;67(1):36–8.
43. Utting MR, Davies G, Newman JH. Is anterior knee pain a predisposing factor to patellofemoral osteoarthritis? Knee. 2005;12(5):362–5.
44. Thomas MJ, Wood L, Selfe J, Peat G. Anterior knee pain in younger adults as a precursor to subsequent patellofemoral osteoarthritis: a systematic review. BMC Musculoskelet Disord. 2010;11:201.
45. McAlindon TE, Bannuru RR, Sullivan MC, Arden NK, Berenbaum F, Bierma-Zeinstra SM, Hawker GA, Henrotin Y, Hunter DJ, Kawaguchi H, et al. OARSI guidelines for the non-surgical management of knee osteoarthritis. Osteoarthritis Cartilage. 2014;22(3):363–88.
46. Vrezas I, Elsner G, Bolm-Audorff U, Abolmaali N, Seidler A. Case-control study of knee osteoarthritis and lifestyle factors considering their interaction with physical workload. Int Arch Occup Environ Health. 2010;83(3):291–300.
47. Teichtahl AJ, Wluka AE, Forbes A, Wang Y, English DR, Giles GG, Cicuttini FM. Longitudinal effect of vigorous physical activity on patella cartilage morphology in people without clinical knee disease. Arthritis Rheum. 2009; 61(8):1095–102.
48. Felson DT, Niu J, Clancy M, Sack B, Aliabadi P, Zhang Y. Effect of recreational physical activities on the development of knee osteoarthritis in older adults of different weights: the Framingham Study. Arthritis Rheum. 2007;57(1):6–12.
49. Gelber AC, Hochberg MC, Mead LA, Wang NY, Wigley FM, Klag MJ. Joint injury in young adults and risk for subsequent knee and hip osteoarthritis. Ann Intern Med. 2000;133(5):321–8.
50. Andriacchi TP, Mundermann A, Smith RL, Alexander EJ, Dyrby CO, Koo S. A framework for the in vivo pathomechanics of osteoarthritis at the knee. Ann Biomed Eng. 2004;32(3):447–57.
51. Julkunen P, Halmesmaki EP, Iivarinen J, Rieppo L, Narhi T, Marjanen J, Rieppo J, Arokoski J, Brama PA, Jurvelin JS, et al. Effects of growth and exercise on composition, structural maturation and appearance of osteoarthritis in articular cartilage of hamsters. J Anat. 2010;217(3):262–74.
52. Jones G, Glisson M, Hynes K, Cicuttini F. Sex and site differences in cartilage development: a possible explanation for variations in knee osteoarthritis in later life. Arthritis Rheum. 2000;43(11):2543–9.
53. Van Ginckel A, Baelde N, Almqvist KF, Roosen P, McNair P, Witvrouw E. Functional adaptation of knee cartilage in asymptomatic female novice runners compared to sedentary controls. A longitudinal analysis using delayed gadolinium enhanced magnetic resonance imaging of cartilage (dGEMRIC). Osteoarthritis Cartilage. 2010;18(12):1564–9.
54. Roos EM, Dahlberg L. Positive effects of moderate exercise on glycosaminoglycan content in knee cartilage: a four-month, randomized, controlled trial in patients at risk of osteoarthritis. Arthritis Rheum. 2005;52(11):3507–14.
55. Cotofana S, Ring-Dimitriou S, Hudelmaier M, Himmer M, Wirth W, Sanger AM, Eckstein F. Effects of exercise intervention on knee morphology in middle-aged women: a longitudinal analysis using magnetic resonance imaging. Cells Tissues Organs. 2010;192(1):64–72.
56. Eckstein F, Faber S, Muhlbauer R, Hohe J, Englmeier KH, Reiser M, Putz R. Functional adaptation of human joints to mechanical stimuli. Osteoarthritis Cartilage. 2002;10(1):44–50.
57. Antony B, Venn A, Cicuttini F, March L, Blizzard L, Dwyer T, Cross M, Jones G, Ding C. Association of physical activity and physical performance with tibial cartilage volume and bone area in young adults. Arthritis Res Ther. 2015;17:298.
58. Waller K, Kujala UM, Kaprio J, Koskenvuo M, Rantanen T. Effect of physical activity on health in twins: a 30-yr longitudinal study. Med Sci Sports Exerc. 2010;42(4):658–64.
59. El-Metwally A, Salminen JJ, Auvinen A, Kautiainen H, Mikkelsson M. Lower limb pain in a preadolescent population: prognosis and risk factors for chronicity–a prospective 1- and 4-year follow-up study. Pediatrics. 2005; 116(3):673–81.
60. Roemer FW, Jarraya M, Niu J, Silva JR, Frobell R, Guermazi A. Increased risk for radiographic osteoarthritis features in young active athletes: a cross-sectional matched case-control study. Osteoarthritis Cartilage. 2015;23(2):239–43.
61. Antony B, Jones G, Venn A, Cicuttini F, March L, Blizzard L, Dwyer T, Cross M, Ding C. Childhood physical performance measures and adulthood knee cartilage volume and bone area: a 25-year cohort study. Arthritis Care Res (Hoboken). 2015;67(9):1263–71.
62. Antony B, Venn A, Cicuttini F, March L, Blizzard L, Dwyer T, Halliday A, Cross M, Jones G, Ding C. Correlates of knee bone marrow lesions in younger adults. Arthritis Res Ther. 2016;18(1):31.
63. Adams AL, Kessler JI, Deramerian K, Smith N, Black MH, Porter AH, Jacobsen SJ, Koebnick C. Associations between childhood obesity and upper and lower extremity injuries. Inj Prev. 2013;19(3):191–7.
64. Kessler J, Koebnick C, Smith N, Adams A. Childhood obesity is associated with increased risk of most lower extremity fractures. Clin Orthop Relat Res. 2013;471(4):1199–207.

65. Tanamas S, Hanna FS, Cicuttini FM, Wluka AE, Berry P, Urquhart DM. Does knee malalignment increase the risk of development and progression of knee osteoarthritis? A systematic review. Arthritis Rheum. 2009;61(4):459–67.
66. Schouten JS, van den Ouweland FA, Valkenburg HA. A 12 year follow up study in the general population on prognostic factors of cartilage loss in osteoarthritis of the knee. Ann Rheum Dis. 1992;51(8):932–7.
67. McWilliams DF, Doherty S, Maciewicz RA, Muir KR, Zhang W, Doherty M. Self-reported knee and foot alignments in early adult life and risk of osteoarthritis. Arthritis Care Res (Hoboken). 2010;62(4):489–95.
68. Niu J, Zhang YQ, Torner J, Nevitt M, Lewis CE, Aliabadi P, Sack B, Clancy M, Sharma L, Felson DT. Is obesity a risk factor for progressive radiographic knee osteoarthritis? Arthritis Rheum. 2009;61(3):329–35.
69. Felson DT, Goggins J, Niu J, Zhang Y, Hunter DJ. The effect of body weight on progression of knee osteoarthritis is dependent on alignment. Arthritis Rheum. 2004;50(12):3904–9.
70. Bout-Tabaku S, Shults J, Zemel BS, Leonard MB, Berkowitz RI, Stettler N, Burnham JM. Obesity is associated with greater valgus knee alignment in pubertal children, and higher body mass index is associated with greater variability in knee alignment in girls. J Rheumatol. 2015;42(1):126–33.
71. Brennan SL, Lane SE, Lorimer M, Buchbinder R, Wluka AE, Page RS, Osborne RH, Pasco JA, Sanders KM, Cashman K, et al. Associations between socioeconomic status and primary total knee joint replacements performed for osteoarthritis across Australia 2003–10: data from the Australian Orthopaedic Association National Joint Replacement Registry. BMC Musculoskelet Disord. 2014;15:356.
72. Macfarlane GJ, Norrie G, Atherton K, Power C, Jones GT. The influence of socioeconomic status on the reporting of regional and widespread musculoskeletal pain: results from the 1958 British Birth Cohort Study. Ann Rheum Dis. 2009;68(10):1591–5.
73. Baldassari AR, Cleveland RJ, Callahan LF. Independent associations of childhood and current socioeconomic status with risk of self-reported doctor-diagnosed arthritis in a family-medicine cohort of North-Carolinians. BMC Musculoskelet Disord. 2013;14:327.
74. Springer KW, Sheridan J, Kuo D, Carnes M. Long-term physical and mental health consequences of childhood physical abuse: results from a large population-based sample of men and women. Child Abuse Negl. 2007; 31(5):517–30.
75. Goodwin RD, Stein MB. Association between childhood trauma and physical disorders among adults in the United States. Psychol Med. 2004; 34(3):509–20.
76. Stein MB, Barrett-Connor E. Sexual assault and physical health: findings from a population-based study of older adults. Psychosom Med. 2000;62(6):838–43.
77. Fuller-Thomson E, Stefanyk M, Brennenstuhl S. The robust association between childhood physical abuse and osteoarthritis in adulthood: findings from a representative community sample. Arthritis Rheum. 2009;61(11): 1554–62.

6

H_1-antihistamines are associated with lower prevalence of radiographic knee osteoarthritis: a cross-sectional analysis of the Osteoarthritis Initiative data

Ivan Shirinsky* and Valery Shirinsky

Abstract

Background: There is growing evidence that mast cells (MCs) play a role in knee osteoarthritis (OA). H_1-antihistamines block H_1-receptors of histamine, which is an important mediator of MCs. There is a lack of data on whether H_1-antihistamines can influence OA. We hypothesized that the use of H_1-antihistamines may be linked to the reduced prevalence of knee OA.

Methods: Baseline data from the Osteoarthritis Initiative cohort were analysed cross-sectionally. Unadjusted and adjusted logistic regression models were performed to compare the prevalence of knee OA in H_1-antihistamine users and non-users. Generalized estimating equations were used to adjust for the correlation between knees. Knee OA was defined as (1) Kellgren-Lawrence (KL) grade ≥ 2 or total joint replacement or (2) KL grade ≥ 2 and joint space narrowing or total joint replacement.

Results: The analysed sample consisted of 8545 knees (664 knees of H_1-antihistamine users and 7881 knees of H_1-antihistamine non-users). The use of H_1-antihistamines was associated with reduced prevalence of knee OA in unadjusted and adjusted models using both the first (adjusted OR, 0.77; 95% CI, 0.62, 0.96; $P < 0.02$) and second (adjusted OR, 0.75; 95% CI, 0.62, 0.93; $P < 0.008$) definitions of knee OA.

Conclusions: H_1-antihistamines are associated with a reduced prevalence of knee OA. The findings indicate that this class of drugs should be further evaluated for possible structure-modifying properties in knee OA.

Keywords: Osteoarthritis, Knee osteoarthritis, Outcomes research

Background

Mast cells (MCs) have long been considered to be inflammatory cells involved primarily in parasitic infections and allergic reactions. In recent years, an emergent role has been described for MCs in various chronic inflammatory diseases, including cancers [1], rheumatoid arthritis [2], atherosclerosis, obesity and diabetes [3]. In osteoarthritis (OA), MCs are prevalent in synovial tissue, and their presence is associated with structural damage [4]. The primary action of histamine H_1-receptor blockers (H_1-antihistamines) is to block the effects of histamine on its specific receptors. In addition, many H_1-antihistamines have anti-inflammatory effects and are able to stabilize the membranes of MC, leading to decreased release of multiple mediators of MC [5].

Therefore, H_1-antihistamines might be a candidate class of drugs to prevent and treat OA. Currently, there is a lack of data on the effects of H_1-antihistamines in knee OA in humans. In one exploratory study, H_1-antihistamines were linked to decreased progression and less pain in knee OA [6].

We hypothesized that H_1-antihistamine use may be linked to reduced prevalence of knee OA. To test this hypothesis, we evaluated the cross-sectional association between the use of oral H_1-antihistamines and radiographic

* Correspondence: ivan.shirinsky@gmail.com
Laboratory of Clinical Immunopharmacology, Federal State Budgetary Scientific Institution, Research Institute of Fundamental and Clinical Immunology, 6 Zalesskogo Street, 630047 Novosibirsk, Russia

knee OA using the data from the publicly available Osteoarthritis Initiative (OAI) cohort.

Methods

In these cross-sectional analyses we compared the knees of OAI participants taking H_1-antihistamines at baseline with the knees of control participants. For the present study, we used longitudinal data obtained from the OAI, which is publicly available at http://oai.epi-ucsf.org. Specific datasets used were "MIF00" (version 0.2.2), "AllClinical00" (version 0.2.2), "Enrollees00 (version 17)", "kXR_SQ_BU00" (version 0.6), and "Outcomes99" (version 8). The detailed information about the OAI protocol can be found elsewhere [7]. The OAI cohort consists of a progression subcohort (patients with symptomatic tibiofemoral knee OA, $n = 1390$), an incidence subcohort (subjects with increased risk of OA, $n = 3284$) and a reference control subcohort ($n = 122$). In this analysis we used the cross-sectional baseline data from both the progression and incidence subcohorts. The main inclusion criteria were the following: age between 45 and 79 years for both subcohorts, symptomatic tibiofemoral knee OA for the progression subcohort, and the presence of established or putative risk factors for incident knee OA for the incidence subcohort. The OAI subjects were recruited and enrolled between February 2004 and May 2006 at four recruitment centres in the United States. This study received ethical approval from each recruitment centre. All participants provided written informed consent. The prespecified sample size was 5000 women and men (4000 in the incidence subcohort, 800 in the progression subcohort). The sample size was expected to provide an adequate number of knees with incident and worsening OA-related structural and clinical changes to achieve the primary aims of the OAI study.

Clinical measures

Height was measured in millimetres using a calibrated, wall-mounted stadiometer. The measurement was performed twice with the subject in light clothing, without shoes, and during inspiration. Body weight was measured in kilograms with a calibrated, standard balance beam scale. The measurement was performed twice with the subject in light clothing without shoes, heavy jewellery or wallets. Body mass index (BMI) was calculated based on weight (in kg) divided by height (in cm) squared. Smoking history and education status were assessed using self-administered questionnaires. Prior knee surgery, family history of knee replacement, and Physical Activity Scale for the Elderly (PASE) were evaluated using interview.

To acquire information about the use of H_1-antihistamines, a medication inventory method was used wherein the participants brought in all of the medications they were currently taking, and the brand name, generic name or active ingredients were recorded and matched to an entry in an online medication dictionary [8]. Only participants who reported taking H_1-antihistamines for more than 1 year prior to baseline were included in the analyses.

Radiographic assessment

Posteroanterior weight-bearing knee radiographs were performed annually using a Synaflexer frame (Synarc, San Francisco, CA, USA), which allowed a fixed, standardized and reproducible knee position. X-ray interpretation was performed centrally at Boston University by three readers. In case of a disagreement about the presence of radiographic OA, the reading was adjudicated by a panel of three readers. A consensus reading was achieved when at least two of the three readers agreed.

The initial incidence and progression OAI subcohort assignments were based primarily on Kellgren-Lawrence (KL) readings at the OAI clinical centres. Because further central assessments could provide different grading results, assignment to incidence and progression subcohorts might not reflect a participant's knee OA status at baseline.

In the OAI, there were two definitions of knee OA based on central reading: (1) KL grade ≥ 2 or total joint replacement and (2) KL grade ≥ 2 and joint space narrowing (JSN) or total joint replacement. We used both definitions as outcomes of our study.

Statistical analysis

Continuous variables are presented as mean (SD), and categorical variables as number (percent). Although most of the continuous variables were not normally distributed, we used mean (SD) as the preferred statistic even in the setting of non-normally distributed data [9]. Unadjusted and adjusted logistic regression models were used to assess the association between the use of H_1-antihistamines and radiographic knee OA. Generalized estimating equations (GEEs) were used to adjust for the correlation between knees. GEE allows for not using imputation methods for the missing data, because the participants with missing data are not excluded from the analysis [10]. The models were adjusted for BMI, age, race, sex, smoking history, education status, history of prior knee surgery, family history of knee replacement, PASE and subcohort assignment. These potential confounders were selected on the basis of literature and clinical plausibility. The adjustment for the subcohort assignment was carried out because the inclusion criteria for both subcohorts were different.

Sensitivity analyses

We performed sensitivity analyses using the definition of knee OA as a KL score ≥ 2 (not including knee replacement in the definition).

Results

A sample of 4273 OAI participants (8545 knees) was analysed, and 332 of them (664 knees) used histamine H_1-receptor blockers at baseline (Fig. 1). The vast majority of H_1-antihistamine users were taking second-generation H_1-antihistamines. The compared groups consisted of middle-aged, overweight participants. There were 1518 (25%) knees with radiographic OA in the incidence subcohort and 1537 (61.4%) knees with radiographic OA in the progression subcohort using the first definition of knee OA. According to the second definition of knee OA, there were 2028 (33.6%) and 1834 (73.3%) knees with radiographic OA in the incidence and progression subcohorts, respectively.

In relative terms, the prevalence of radiographic knee OA was 15.5% and 10.8% lower in the H_1-antihistamine users group using the first and second definitions of radiographic knee OA, respectively. This difference was due to a lower proportion of patients with bilateral knee OA in the H_1-antihistamine users group (26.5% and 17% less patients with bilateral knee OA using first and second definitions of knee OA, respectively) (Table 1).

In the regression analyses, the use of H_1-antihistamines was associated with lower prevalence of radiographic knee OA using both definitions in either crude or adjusted analyses (Table 2). The sensitivity analysis did not change the direction and significance of our results shown in Table 2.

Discussion

In cross-sectional analyses of OAI data, H_1-antihistamines were associated with decreased prevalence of radiographic knee OA. Our study had the following important limitations: a cross-sectional design and a lack of precise information about the duration and dose of antihistamine use. The presence of inclusion criteria may limit the generalizability of the results.

Our data are in line with an exploratory, hypothesis-generating study performed on longitudinal OAI data. In this study, antihistamine users, defined as those using antihistamines at the first four annual visits, showed a signal for reduced changes in joint space width during 36-month follow-up. The authors did not evaluate statistical significance and did not perform adjustment for possible confounders [6]. In contrast, our analysis was cross-sectional, we used a dichotomous outcome measure of radiographic knee OA, and our models were adjusted for multiple confounders. Thus, our data may be considered as an initial line of evidence that antihistamines may influence knee OA.

The demonstrated association between H_1-antihistamine use and the decreased prevalence of knee OA may be explained in several ways. First, it is tempting to speculate that H_1-antihistamines prevent knee OA by stabilizing the membranes of MC and blocking the effects of histamine, which is their major mediator.

The role of MCs in OA was suggested more than 20 years ago by several studies showing elevation of MCs and histamine levels in synovial fluids and synovial tissues from patients with OA [11, 12]. These findings were confirmed recently, and a trend towards an association between the number of MCs and increased KL grade was also found [4].

MCs are capable to produce a plethora of mediators which are released upon different stimuli via degranulation, secretion and exocytosis. Mediators stored in MC granules are represented by amines, proteoglycans, proteases, lysosomal enzymes, and cytokines [13]. Most of these compounds may be involved in the pathogenesis of OA. Thus, histamine induced an increase in the proliferation of human articular chondrocytes [14] and upregulated production of matrix metalloproteinase (MMP)-13 and MMP-3 by these cells via H_1-receptors [15]. MC-derived

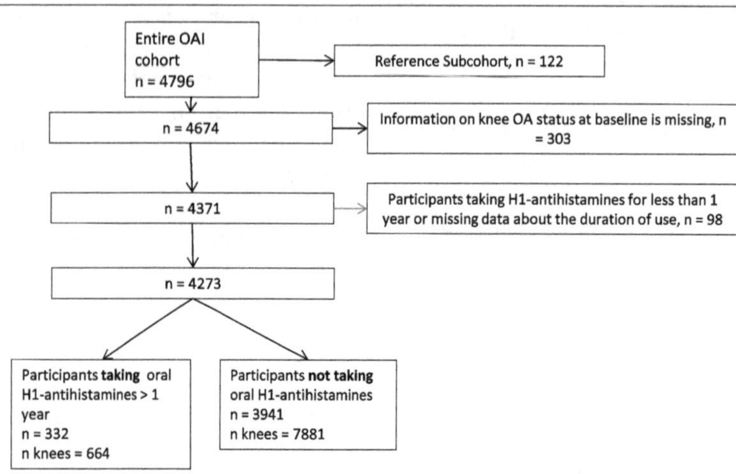

Fig. 1 Flowchart of participants selected for the analyses

Table 1 Characteristics of participants taking and not taking histamine H_1-receptor antagonists

	Participants taking H_1-antihistamines	Participants not taking H_1-antihistamines
No. of participants	332	3941
No. of knees	664	7881
Age, yr	59.84 (8.17)	61.45 (9.23)
Sex		
Female	94 (28.3)	1712 (43.4)
Male	238 (71.7)	2229 (56.6)
BMI, kg/m^2	29.18 (4.86)	28.64 (4.79)
Race		
Other non-white	3 (0.9)	64 (1.6)
White or Caucasian	261 (78.6)	3156 (80.1)
Black or African American	64 (19.3)	685 (17.4)
Asian	4 (1.2)	32 (0.8)
History of knee surgery	73 (22.0)	936 (23.8)
Family history of knee OA	60 (18.1)	611 (15.5)
PASE	160.38 (82.74)	161.68 (82.23)
Education		
Less than high school graduate	6 (1.8)	136 (3.5)
High school graduate	38 (11.4)	489 (12.4)
Some college	79 (23.8)	939 (23.8)
College graduate	63 (19.0)	846 (21.5)
Some graduate school	28 (8.4)	319 (8.1)
Graduate degree	116 (34.9)	1183 (30.0)
Smoking history		
Never	180 (54.2)	2056 (52.2)
Current	19 (5.7)	242 (6.1)
Former	129 (38.9)	1585 (40.2)
Current but never regular	2 (0.6)	6 (0.2)
WOMAC subscales		
WOMAC pain, right knee	2.93 (3.45)	2.42 (3.12)
WOMAC pain, left knee	2.70 (3.65)	2.28 (3.33)
WOMAC function, right knee	9.75 (11.28)	7.75 (10.19)
WOMAC function, left knee	9.92 (12.52)	7.92 (11.02)
KL, knees (%)		
0	256 (38.6)	2904 (36.8)
1	138 (20.8)	1386 (17.6)
2	176 (26.5)	2129 (27.0)
3	71 (10.7)	1135 (14.4)
4	18 (2.7)	272 (3.5)
Patients with knee OA, defined as KL ≥ 2 with JSN, or knee replacement (%)	145 (43.67)	1913 (48.54)
Unilateral, no. of patients (%)	87 (26.2)	974 (24.7)
Bilateral, no. of patients (%)	58 (17.5)	939 (23.8)
Patients with knee OA, defined as KL ≥ 2, or knee replacement (%)	181 (54.52)	2318 (58.84)

Table 1 Characteristics of participants taking and not taking histamine H_1-receptor antagonists *(Continued)*

	Participants taking H_1-antihistamines	Participants not taking H_1-antihistamines
Unilateral, patients (%)	92 (27.7)	1044 (26.5)
Bilateral, patients (%)	89 (26.8)	1274 (32.3)
JSN, medial compartment, knees (%)		
0	441 (66.4)	4985 (63.3)
1	154 (23.2)	1734 (22.0)
2	58 (8.7)	912 (11.6)
3	6 (0.9)	195 (2.5)
JSN, lateral compartment, knees (%)		
0	608 (91.6)	7162 (90.9)
1	26 (3.9)	340 (4.3)
2	13 (2.0)	245 (3.1)
3	12 (1.8)	79 (1.0)
Knee replacement	5 (0.8)	53 (0.7)
H_1-antihistamines		
Second-generation		
Fexofenadine	177 (53.31)	–
Cetirizine	85 (25.6)	–
Desloratadine	39 (11.75)	–
Loratadine	23 (6.93)	–
First-generation		
Diphenhydramine	7 (2.11)	–
Chlorpheniramine	4 (1.2)	–
Promethazine	5 (1.51)	–
Brompheniramine	1 (0.3)	–
Cyproheptadine	1 (0.3)	–
Dexbrompheniramine	1 (0.3)	–
Phenyltoloxamine	1 (0.3)	–
Pyrilamine	1 (0.3)	–
Duration of H_1-antihistamine use		
1–3 yr	136 (40.96)	
3–5 yr	92 (27.71)	
More than 5 yr	104 (31.33)	
Study endpoints		
Radiographic knee OA, defined as KL ≥ 2 with JSN, or knee replacement, knees (%)	203 (30.6)	2852 (36.2)
Radiographic knee OA, defined as KL ≥ 2, or knee replacement, knees (%)	270 (40.7)	3592 (45.6)

Abbreviations: OA Osteoarthritis, *BMI* Body mass index, *KL* Kellgren-Lawrence grade, *PASE* Physical Activity Scale for the Elderly, *WOMAC* Western Ontario and McMaster Universities Osteoarthritis Index, *JSN* Joint space narrowing (grades 0–3)

Data are presented as the mean (SD) or number (%). Possible ranges for WOMAC pain score are 0–20. Possible ranges for WOMAC function score are 0–68

Table 2 Association between the use of histamine H_1-receptor antagonists and prevalence of radiographic knee OA

	Non-adjusted models			Adjusted models		
	OR	95% CI	*P* value	OR	95% CI	*P* value
Radiographic knee OA, defined as KL ≥ 2 with JSN	0.78	0.63 to 0.95	0.014	0.77	0.62 to 0.96	0.02
Radiographic knee OA, defined as KL ≥ 2	0.81	0.67 to 0.99	0.041	0.75	0.62 to 0.93	0.008

Note. The models were adjusted for BMI, race, age, gender, Physical Activity scale for the elderly (PASE), history of knee surgery, family history of knee OA, smoking status, education, and Subcohort assignment. OR – odds ratio, CI – confidence interval

polyamines, which are naturally occurring, positively charged polycations, are able to promote chondrocyte differentiation, which may result in OA [16]. MC-produced chymase has potent pro-inflammatory properties and plays a key role in MMP-9 and MMP-2 activation [17]. A recent meta-analysis showed a significant link between serum levels of MMP-9, MMP-2 and OA, suggesting a contribution of these MMPs to the pathogenesis of OA [18]. MCs have also been shown to synthesize, store and release nerve growth factor (NGF) [19], which is a promising new target for the treatment of pain in OA [20]. A recent study showed that NGF-induced production of prostaglandin D_2 in joint MCs is critical for developing pain in OA [21]. One pilot observational study showed improvement of pain in patients with OA receiving therapy with anti-immunoglobulin E treatment, whose main effect is MC stabilization [22]. In addition, H_1-antihistamines have been demonstrated to exert anti-inflammatory properties via down-regulation of nuclear factor-κB and suppression of secretion of various pro-inflammatory cytokines, including tumour necrosis factor-α, interleukin (IL)-6, IL-8 and granulocyte-macrophage colony-stimulating factor, by different cell types [23–25]. Thus, a growing body of data indicates that MCs and their mediators contribute to the pathogenesis of OA. Another way of suppressing MCs may be the use of peroxisome proliferator-activated receptor-α (PPARα) agonists [26]. Clinical improvement in erosive hand OA treated with the PPARα agonist fenofibrate in a small study [27] may in part be explained by the reduced activation of MCs.

Second, the findings may be due to inherent limitations of cross-sectional studies and the presence of unidentified confounders. There is a need of prospective studies evaluating the effects of H_1-antihistamines on knee OA. Longitudinal observational studies may provide initial evidence that should be tested further in randomized controlled studies. It is agreed that to prevent several kinds of biases in the longitudinal analyses of observational cohort studies, one needs to employ a 'new-user' design that evaluates persons who were treatment-naïve at baseline and started the treatment of interest only after enrolment [28]. We were not able to perform this kind of analysis, because it would require a significantly larger sample size than that of the OAI dataset to gain sufficient statistical power using the selected knee OA outcomes. The strengths of this analysis are that it is based on a large population with a well-defined cohort, and we used standardised and reproducible procedures for knee radiograph acquisition, as well as an extensive adjudication process to determine KL and JSN grades.

Conclusions

H_1-antihistamines are associated with decreased prevalence of knee OA. In view of the absence of effective structure-modifying drugs for OA and the emerging role of MCs in OA, our findings provide an impetus for further studies evaluating H_1-antihistamines in OA.

Abbreviations

GEE: Generalized estimating equation; IL: Interleukin; JSN: Joint space narrowing; KL: Kellgren-Lawrence; MC: Mast cells; MMP: Matrix metalloproteinase; NGF: Nerve growth factor; OA: Osteoarthritis; OAI: Osteoarthritis Initiative; PASE: Physical Activity Scale for the Elderly; PPARα: Peroxisome proliferator-activated receptor-α

Acknowledgements

The OAI is a public-private partnership comprising five contracts (N01-AR-2-2258, N01-AR-2-2259, N01-AR-2-2260, N01-AR-2-2261, N01-AR-2-2262) funded by the National Institutes of Health (NIH), a branch of the Department of Health and Human Services, and conducted by the OAI study investigators. Private funding partners include Merck Research Laboratories, Novartis Pharmaceuticals Corporation, GlaxoSmithKline and Pfizer, Inc. Private sector funding for the OAI is managed by the Foundation for the National Institutes of Health. This article was prepared using an OAI public use dataset and does not necessarily reflect the opinions or views of the OAI investigators, the NIH or the private funding partners. We thank Peter Mittwede, MD, PhD, from Edanz Group (www.edanzediting.com/ac) for editing a draft of the manuscript.

Authors' contributions

Both authors contributed to the conception and design of the study and to the interpretation of the findings. IS conducted the statistical analyses. Both authors assisted in drafting the manuscript, and both of them read and approved the final draft.

Competing interests

The authors declare that they have no competing interests.

References

1. Varricchi G, Galdiero MR, Loffredo S, Marone G, Iannone R, Granata F. Are mast cells MASTers in cancer? Front Immunol. 2017;8:424.
2. Kritas SK, Saggini A, Varvara G, Murmura G, Caraffa A, Antinolfi P, Toniato E, Pantalone A, Neri G, Frydas S, et al. Mast cell involvement in rheumatoid arthritis. J Biol Regul Homeost Agents. 2013;27(3):655–60.
3. Shi GP, Bot I, Kovanen PT. Mast cells in human and experimental cardiometabolic diseases. Nat Rev Cardiol. 2015;12(11):643–58.

4. de Lange-Brokaar BJ, Kloppenburg M, Andersen SN, Dorjee AL, Yusuf E, Herb-van Toorn L, Kroon HM, Zuurmond AM, Stojanovic-Susulic V, Bloem JL, et al. Characterization of synovial mast cells in knee osteoarthritis: association with clinical parameters. Osteoarthritis Cartilage. 2016;24(4):664–71.
5. Levi-Schaffer F, Eliashar R. Mast cell stabilizing properties of antihistamines. J Invest Dermatol. 2009;129(11):2549–51.
6. Driban JB, Lo GH, Eaton CB, Lapane KL, Nevitt M, Harvey WF, McCulloch CE, McAlindon TE. Exploratory analysis of osteoarthritis progression among medication users: data from the Osteoarthritis Initiative. Ther Adv Musculoskelet Dis. 2016;8(6):207–19.
7. The osteoarthritis initiative protocol for the cohort study. http://oai.epi-csf.org/datarelease/docs/StudyDesignProtocol.pdf. Accessed 24 May 2018.
8. Pahor M, Chrischilles EA, Guralnik JM, Brown SL, Wallace RB, Carbonin P. Drug data coding and analysis in epidemiologic studies. Eur J Epidemiol. 1994;10(4):405–11.
9. Lydersen S. Statistical review: frequently given comments. Ann Rheum Dis. 2015;74(2):323–5.
10. Twisk J, de Vente W. Attrition in longitudinal studies: how to deal with missing data. J Clin Epidemiol. 2002;55(4):329–37.
11. Dean G, Hoyland JA, Denton J, Donn RP, Freemont AJ. Mast cells in the synovium and synovial fluid in osteoarthritis. Br J Rheumatol. 1993; 32(8):671–5.
12. Renoux M, Hilliquin P, Galoppin L, Florentin I, Menkes CJ. Release of mast cell mediators and nitrites into knee joint fluid in osteoarthritis–comparison with articular chondrocalcinosis and rheumatoid arthritis. Osteoarthritis Cartilage. 1996;4(3):175–9.
13. Moon TC, Befus AD, Kulka M. Mast cell mediators: their differential release and the secretory pathways involved. Front Immunol. 2014;5:569.
14. Tetlow LC, Woolley DE. Histamine stimulates the proliferation of human articular chondrocytes in vitro and is expressed by chondrocytes in osteoarthritic cartilage. Ann Rheum Dis. 2003;62(10):991–4.
15. Tetlow LC, Woolley DE. Histamine stimulates matrix metalloproteinase-3 and -13 production by human articular chondrocytes in vitro. Ann Rheum Dis. 2002;61(8):737–40.
16. Facchini A, Borzi RM, Olivotto E, Platano D, Pagani S, Cetrullo S, Flamigni F. Role of polyamines in hypertrophy and terminal differentiation of osteoarthritic chondrocytes. Amino Acids. 2012;42(2–3):667–78.
17. Tchougounova E, Lundequist A, Fajardo I, Winberg JO, Abrink M, Pejler G. A key role for mast cell chymase in the activation of pro-matrix metalloprotease-9 and pro-matrix metalloprotease-2. J Biol Chem. 2005; 280(10):9291–6.
18. Zeng GQ, Chen AB, Li W, Song JH, Gao CY. High MMP-1, MMP-2, and MMP-9 protein levels in osteoarthritis. Genet Mol Res. 2015;14(4):14811–22.
19. Leon A, Buriani A, Dal Toso R, Fabris M, Romanello S, Aloe L, Levi-Montalcini R. Mast cells synthesize, store, and release nerve growth factor. Proc Natl Acad Sci U S A. 1994;91(9):3739–43.
20. Schnitzer TJ, Marks JA. A systematic review of the efficacy and general safety of antibodies to NGF in the treatment of OA of the hip or knee. Osteoarthritis Cartilage. 2015;23(Suppl 1):S8–17.
21. Sousa-Valente J, Calvo L, Vacca V, Simeoli R, Arevalo JC, Malcangio M. Role of TrkA signalling and mast cells in the initiation of osteoarthritis pain in the monoiodoacetate model. Osteoarthritis Cartilage. 2018;26(1):84–94.
22. Aquili A, Farinelli L, Bottegoni C, Antonicelli L, Gigante A. The effect of anti-IgE therapy in knee osteoarthritis: a pilot observational study. J Biol Regul Homeost Agents. 2017;31(4 Suppl 1):1–5.
23. Carayol N, Crampette L, Mainprice B, Ben-Soussen P, Verrecchia M, Bousquet J, Lebel B. Inhibition of mediator and cytokine release from dispersed nasal polyp cells by mizolastine. Allergy. 2002;57(11):1067–70.
24. Matsubara M, Tamura T, Ohmori K, Hasegawa K. Histamine H_1 receptor antagonist blocks histamine-induced proinflammatory cytokine production through inhibition of Ca^{2+}–dependent protein kinase C, Raf/MEK/ERK and IKK/IκB/NF-κB signal cascades. Biochem Pharmacol. 2005;69(3):433–49.
25. Lippert U, Moller A, Welker P, Artuc M, Henz BM. Inhibition of cytokine secretion from human leukemic mast cells and basophils by H_1- and H_2-receptor antagonists. Exp Dermatol. 2000;9(2):118–24.
26. Sugiyama H, Nonaka T, Kishimoto T, Komoriya K, Tsuji K, Nakahata T. Peroxisome proliferator-activated receptors are expressed in human cultured mast cells: a possible role of these receptors in negative regulation of mast cell activation. Eur J Immunol. 2000;30(12):3363–70.
27. Shirinsky IV, Shirinsky VS. Treatment of erosive osteoarthritis with peroxisome proliferator-activated receptor alpha agonist fenofibrate: a pilot study. Rheumatol Int. 2014;34(5):613–6.
28. Ray WA. Evaluating medication effects outside of clinical trials: new-user designs. Am J Epidemiol. 2003;158(9):915–20.

7

The complement system is activated in synovial fluid from subjects with knee injury and from patients with osteoarthritis

André Struglics[1*†], Marcin Okroj[2,3†], Per Swärd[1], Richard Frobell[1], Tore Saxne[4], L. Stefan Lohmander[1] and Anna M. Blom[2]

Abstract

Background: The complement system is suggested to be involved in the pathogenesis of osteoarthritis (OA), and proinflammatory cytokines may play a role in OA development by inducing proteases. The association between complement factors, cytokines and OA has not been investigated. The aim of the present study was to explore the involvement of the complement system after knee trauma and in OA.

Methods: C4d, C3bBbP and soluble terminal complement complex (sTCC) resulting from complement activation were immunoassayed in synovial fluid from subjects with healthy knees (reference), OA, rheumatoid arthritis (RA; positive control), pyrophosphate arthritis (PPA; positive control) and knee injury; other biomarkers were previously assessed. Magnetic resonance imaging was used to assess joint injuries.

Results: Compared with levels in the reference group, the median concentrations of C4d, C3bBbP and sTCC in the OA, RA, PPA and knee injury groups were 2- to 34-fold increased ($p < 0.001$ to $p = 0.044$). For the knee injury group, the median concentrations of C4d, C3bBbP and sTCC were 5- to 12-fold increased ($p < 0.001$) at the day of injury; after 3–12 weeks, C3bBbP and sTCC concentrations were similar to reference levels; and C4d was still increased several years after injury. In the 0–12 weeks period after injury, the concentrations of C4d, C3bBbP and sTCC correlated positively with levels of interleukin (IL)-1β, IL-6 and tumour necrosis factor α (r_s range 0.232–0.547); none of the measured complement factors correlated with proteolytic fragments of aggrecan or cartilage oligomeric matrix protein. Knees with osteochondral fracture, with or without disrupted cortical bone, had higher concentrations of C4d ($p = 0.014$, $p = 0.004$) and sTCC ($p = 0.004$, $p < 0.001$) compared with knees without fractures.

Conclusions: The complement system is activated in OA and after knee injury. Following knee injury, this activation is instant and associated with inflammation as well as with the presence of osteochondral fractures.

Keywords: Complement, Knee injury, Osteoarthritis, Synovial fluid

Background

The complement system as a part of innate immunity is one of the first lines of defence against invading pathogens. Apart from this basic, evolutionarily conserved function, it also plays a role in scavenging of cellular debris and immune complexes, opsonisation and guidance of adaptive immunity by anaphylatoxins and stimulation of B and T lymphocytes [1]. Importantly, complement is an aggressive system capable of targeting even its own cells and tissues when improperly regulated by endogenous inhibitors and/or autoantibodies, or because of gain-of-function mutations in complement components [1, 2]. Such autoreactivity was shown to be an important constituent of pathological mechanisms of inflammatory and autoimmune diseases, including rheumatoid arthritis (RA) [3]. Cartilage degradation products released in the course of joint degenerative diseases form a separate class of potent complement modulators [4–7].

* Correspondence: andre.struglics@med.lu.se
†Equal contributors
[1]Department of Clinical Sciences Lund, Orthopaedics, Lund University, Faculty of Medicine, BMC C12, SE-221 84 Lund, Sweden
Full list of author information is available at the end of the article

Joint injury is a major risk factor for the development of post-traumatic osteoarthritis (OA) [8]. Mechanical injury to the joint leads to haemarthrosis, death of chondrocytes and bone cells [9, 10], as well as damage to the tissue extracellular matrix (ECM) directly or mediated by chondrocytes and synoviocytes via increased expression and activation of matrix-degrading enzymes stimulated by proinflammatory cytokines [11]. Furthermore, complement activation has been implicated in the connective tissue repair and inflammatory response initiated by trauma [12, 13]. These observations led us to hypothesize that mechanical joint injury may be an initial trigger of local inflammation, including activation of complement, and that subsequent ECM erosion of injured joints may reinforce complement activation in a positive feedback manner. Monitoring of the complement activation profile after injury could give information potentially important for the design of therapeutic strategies.

We therefore investigated complement activation in OA and the time-dependent activation after knee injuries. RA and pyrophosphate arthritis (PPA) samples were used as positive controls for complement activation. We measured complement activation products characteristic of classical and/or lectin (C4d) and alternative (C3bBP) pathways, as well as the soluble terminal complement complex (sTCC), in the synovial fluid from different patient diagnostic groups (Fig. 1).

Methods

Subjects

In our cross-sectional convenience cohort, 294 patients with knee injury had synovial fluid aspirated once from their knees without lavage; of those, 112 subjects did not fulfil the inclusion criteria of a randomized controlled trial [14], and the remaining 182 subjects had been studied in previous cross-sectional investigations [15–18] (Table 1).

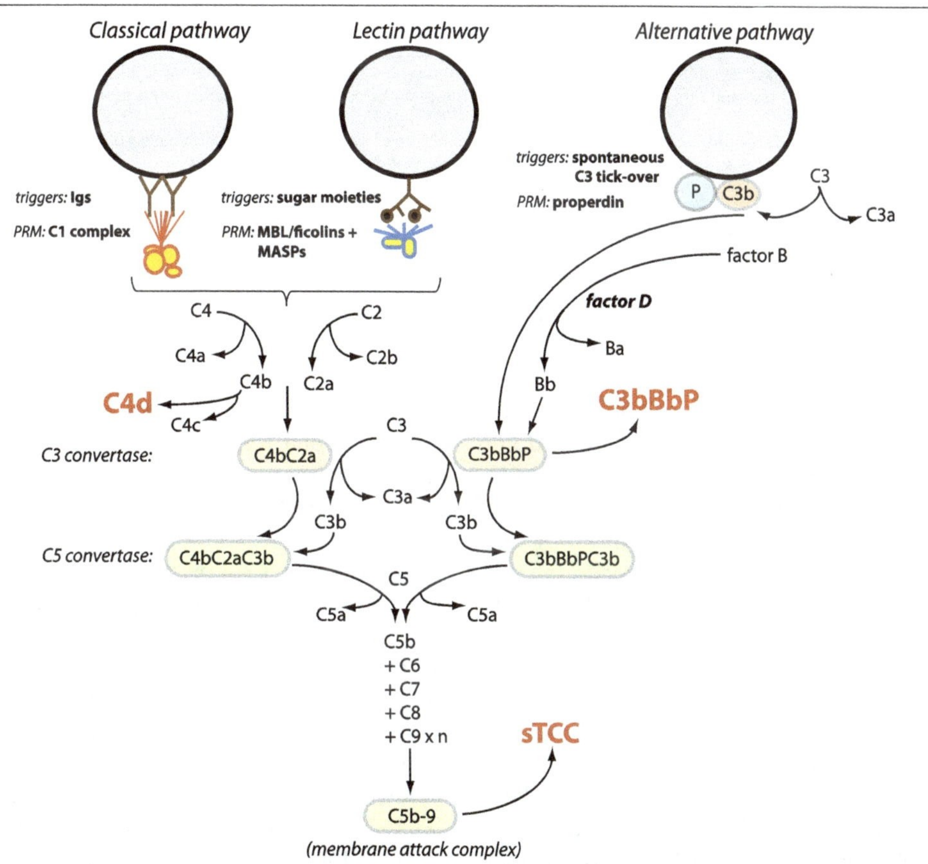

Fig. 1 A scheme of the complement system. Complement can be activated via three different routes. The classical and lectin pathways have their own specific pattern recognition molecules (PRMs), whereas the alternative pathway is activated by a spontaneous tick-over of C3 and deposition of C3b molecules onto permissive surfaces, which is facilitated by properdin (P). All pathways converge at the stage of C3 convertases, which catalyse breakdown of C3 into C3a and C3b molecules. When C3b molecules bind to the convertase complex, it gives rise to the C5 convertase. Except for the triggers indicated for each pathway in the scheme, apoptotic and necrotic cellular debris as well as degradative protein fragments from the extracellular matrix can also trigger all three pathways [4, 32]. In *red* and *boldface type* are the markers of complement activation analysed in our study: C4d, the end degradation product of C4b; C3bBbP, a soluble form of alternative C3 convertase including properdin; and sTCC, soluble terminal complement complex (a soluble form of C5b-9). *Factor D* Serine protease that cleaves factor B, *Igs* Immunoglobulins, *MASP* Mannose-binding lectin-associated serine protease, *MBL* Mannose-binding lectin

Table 1 Characteristics of the study subjects

Main diagnostic groups	Subgroups of injury	Duration, range (median)	*n* (% women)	Age in years, median (range)	Differences in age, *p* value
Reference subjects	–	NA	23 (22)	26 (15–58)	–
Osteoarthritis[a]	–	0–14.8 years (2.7)	24 (42)	64 (36–86)	**<0.001**
Rheumatoid arthritis[b]	–	0–43.0 years (10)	32 (63)	64 (32–83)	**<0.001**
Pyrophosphate arthritis	–	0–9.8 years (0.01)	25 (40)	75 (41–92)	**<0.001**
Knee injury[c]	–	0–36.9 years (0.02)	294 (27)	29 (13–65)	0.842
	Recent injury	0–83 days (4)	219 (25)	26 (13–64)	0.705
	Recent injury, substratification	0 days (0)	35 (23)	30 (14–47)	0.991
		1 day (1)	39 (21)	24 (13–57)	0.211
		2–3 days (3)	31 (29)	26 (16–54)	0.914
		4–7 days (5)	46 (28)	25 (14–64)	0.492
		8–22 days (11)	44 (30)	23 (14–57)	0.151
		23–83 days (32)	24 (13)	38 (21–59)	**0.033**
	Old injury[d]	1–36.9 years (3.3)	75 (33)	32 (18–65)	0.090
	Old injury, substratification	1–3 years (2.0)	35 (40)	33 (18–61)	0.149
		3.01–36.9 years (5.1)	40 (28)	30 (18–65)	0.121

The injury groups are presented with stratification based on time between injury and synovial fluid aspiration. Differences in age between patients and reference groups were analysed using Student's *t* test, and significant values ($p < 0.05$) are indicated by boldface type. *Duration* refers to time between injury or onset of disease and sampling. *NA* Not applicable

[a]Symptomatic and/or radiographically diagnosed idiopathic osteoarthritis (with no history of knee trauma), with information of disease duration from 17 of 24 patients. The OA score for the OA group was as follows: median = 7, range = 3–9 (information from 15 of 24 patients)

[b]Rheumatoid arthritis, with information of disease duration from 29 of 32 patients, taking the following medications: no information ($n = 1$), no medication ($n = 3$), non-steroidal anti-inflammatory and/or disease-modifying drugs ($n = 28$)

[c]The clinical diagnosis of the subjects with knee injury was as follows: isolated anterior cruciate ligament (ACL) or posterior cruciate ligament (PCL) injuries (ACL $n = 39$, PCL $n = 4$), ACL injury with meniscal tear ($n = 69$), ACL injury with meniscal tear and other ligament injuries ($n = 37$), ACL injury with other ligament injuries ($n = 47$), isolated meniscal tear ($n = 58$), meniscal tear with other (not ACL) ligament injuries ($n = 7$), patellar dislocation with or without soft tissue injuries ($n = 13$), other types of injuries (medial or lateral collateral ligament tears $n = 7$, give-way $n = 2$), no signs of soft tissue injury ($n = 10$)

[d]Six patients in the old injury group had post-traumatic OA (based on OA score ≥5 [20]), and the group had the following OA score: median = 2, range = 1–8 (information from 63 of 75 patients)

On the basis of time between injury and synovial fluid aspiration, the subjects with knee injury were stratified into a recent injury group (sampling 0–83 days, or 0–12 weeks, after injury) and an old injury group (sampling 1–37 years after injury), and these groups were substratified by time after injury into groups of 24–46 subjects each (Table 1). From another convenience cohort, we used 23 reference subjects (without a history of knee symptoms or knee injury, or with normal findings in clinical, radiographic and arthroscopic examinations), and 24 patients with OA, 32 with RA and 25 with PPA (RA and PPA, positive controls for complement activation) who had synovial fluid aspirated from their knees (Table 1). These samples have been used in previous investigations [14–19]. For the patients in the OA and old injury groups, an OA score (ranging from 1 to 10) for their affected joints was assessed by arthroscopy and radiography, with a score of 1 representing a normal joint by arthroscopy and radiography, scores of 2–5 representing an increasing extent and severity of fibrillation and clefts by arthroscopy and appearing normal on a radiograph, and scores of 6–10 representing increasing degrees of radiographic joint space narrowing [20].

Synovial fluid was aspirated (without lavage) from each subject at one time point only, centrifuged at $3000 \times g$ for 10 minutes at 4 °C, and the supernatants were then stored at −80 °C.

Analysis of C4d, C3bBbP and sTCC in synovial fluid

Concentrations of C4d [21], C3bBbP and sTCC (C5b-9) [22] in synovial fluid were measured by performing sandwich enzyme-linked immunosorbent assays (ELISAs). Briefly, for the C4d assay, a capture antibody against a C4d neoepitope, together with a mouse anti-C4d detection antibody (A253; Quidel, San Diego, CA, USA), followed by peroxidase-conjugated goat anti-mouse (P0447; Dako, Carpinteria, CA, USA) were used. For the C3bBbP assay, a capture antibody against properdin (A235; Quidel), together with a rabbit anti-C3c detection antibody (P0062; Dako), followed by peroxidase-conjugated goat anti-rabbit (P0448; Dako) were used. For the sTCC assay, we used a monoclonal capture antibody against a C9 neoepitope (clone ae11, HM2167; Hycult Biotech, Uden, the Netherlands), together with an in-house biotinylated monoclonal anti-C6 antibody (A219; Quidel), followed by a streptavidin-

HRP reagent. The read-out of each of these assays was given in complement activation units (CAU), a defined arbitrary unit set for the International Complement Standard #2 sample, which is serum pooled from approximately 1000 healthy individuals and incubated with activators of all three complement pathways [22].

Other biomarkers and cytokines

A subset of synovial fluid samples from the recent injury group ($n = 111–181$) were previously assayed for the following biomarkers: sulfated glycosaminoglycan (sGAG, a marker for total aggrecan); ARGS neoepitope of aggrecan (ARGS-aggrecan from aggrecanase cleavage at the $TEGE^{392}\downarrow^{393}ARGS$ site of aggrecan); osteocalcin, secreted protein acidic and rich in cysteine (SPARC), also known as osteonectin, osteopontin, cartilage oligomeric matrix protein (COMP); type II collagen epitope (C2C); osteopontin; and the proinflammatory cytokines interleukin (IL)-1β, IL-6, IL-8 and tumour necrosis factor α (TNF-α) [14, 17, 19, 23].

Image acquisition and analysis

Magnetic resonance imaging (MRI) using a 1.5-Tesla scanner was conducted in a subfraction of the recent injury group as described elsewhere [19]. Briefly, synovial fluid was aspirated 0–23 days after injury, and MRI scans were acquired within a median of 8 days (range 1–38) after injury in 98 of the 219 subjects of the recent injury group. MRI studies were assessed by an experienced musculoskeletal radiologist for anterior cruciate ligament (ACL) tears, meniscal tears, post-traumatic bone marrow lesions (BMLs), apparent cartilage defects (evident irregularity of cartilage) and osteochondral (OC) fractures with or without disrupted cortical bone. Such fractures were considered a proxy for the strength of impact forces applied over the articular surface at the time of injury [19, 24]. These factors were classified as present or absent for the entire knee.

Statistics and calculations

According to Shapiro-Wilk tests, synovial fluid C4d, C3bBbP and sTCC concentrations were not normally distributed in all diagnostic groups; therefore, when all groups were compared, non-parametric analysis was conducted. Between-groups comparisons were made using Mann-Whitney rank-sum tests, and for correlation analysis, Spearman's rank correlation (r_s) analysis was used. Student's t test was used for comparison of age between subject groups. All of these tests were two-tailed. For a subset ($n = 98$) of the recent injury group, one-way analysis of covariance (ANCOVA) was used to investigate differences in synovial fluid C4d, C3bBbP and sTCC concentrations with regard to structural joint damage as visualized by MRI. After $\log_{10}$ transformation, the data were normally distributed according to the Shapiro-Wilks test, and ANCOVA was done with adjustments for days between injury and synovial fluid aspiration, age and sex. The mean and 95 % CI were calculated using $\log_{10}$-transformed data, but they are presented as linear data.

Samples with concentrations below the lower limit of detection (LLOD) were imputed and given a value equal to half the value of the LLOD. The synovial fluid concentrations of C4d, C3bBbP and sTCC, as well as the amount of samples with imputed values (between 0 and 17 % depending on groups) in the different subject groups, are provided in Additional file: Table S1. In the group-level analysis, the imputed values were included. In the correlation analysis, samples with and without (measured values only) imputed values were analysed, but significance was considered only when both analyses showed correlation, and the presented data (r_s and p values) include imputed values. IBM SPSS version 21 software (IBM, Armonk, NY, USA) was used for statistical analysis, and p values less than 0.05 were considered significant. Expressions such as "higher" and "increase" in the text are based on statistically significant differences.

Results

Technical performance of the C4d, C3bBbP and sTCC ELISAs with synovial fluid

The LLOD and upper limit of detection (ULOD) for the C4d ELISA were 0.05 and 25 CAU, respectively (Additional file 2: Table S2). Within this range, good dilution linearity was observed for synovial fluid control samples diluted 1:5 to 1:40, mean recoveries between 97 % and 104 %, and reference and patient synovial fluid samples were used at the same dilutions. The LLOD and ULOD for the C3bBbP and sTCC assays were 0.05 and 50, respectively, and 0.02 and 10 CAU, respectively (Additional file 2: Table S2). The control synovial fluid samples showed poor dilution linearity in the C3bBbP and sTCC assays, mean recoveries were 54–150 % for C3bBbP and 60–141 % for sTCC; therefore, all analysis of the reference and patient synovial fluid samples were done at the same dilution of 1:20. Spiking the synovial fluid control samples with different amounts of standards showed good recovery for the C4d and C3bBbP assays (mean recoveries between 79 % and 99 % and between 96 % and 107 %, respectively), while the sTCC assay showed lower recovery of 68–77 %. As also shown for measurements in serum and plasma samples [21, 22], the C4d, C3bBbP and sTCC concentrations in synovial fluid were not affected by repeated freeze-thaw cycles, tested for up to

15 cycles (Additional file 2: Table S2). The intra-assay coefficient of variation (CV, within plates) for the synovial fluid control samples was approximately similar between the C4d, C3bBbP and sTCC assays (between 9 % and 10 %), while the inter-assay CV (between plates) was higher for the C3bBbP and sTCC assays (both 23 %) compared with the C4d assay (16 %) (Additional file 2: Table S2).

Concentrations of C4d, C3bBbP and sTCC in synovial fluid were higher in the arthritis groups than in the reference group

The concentrations of C4d, C3bBbP and sTCC were higher in the OA, RA and PPA groups than in the reference group. Median levels increased between 4- and 34-fold (C4d), 2- and 5-fold (C3bBbP), and 4- and 12-fold (sTCC) (Fig. 2a, Additional file 1: Table S1). The highest

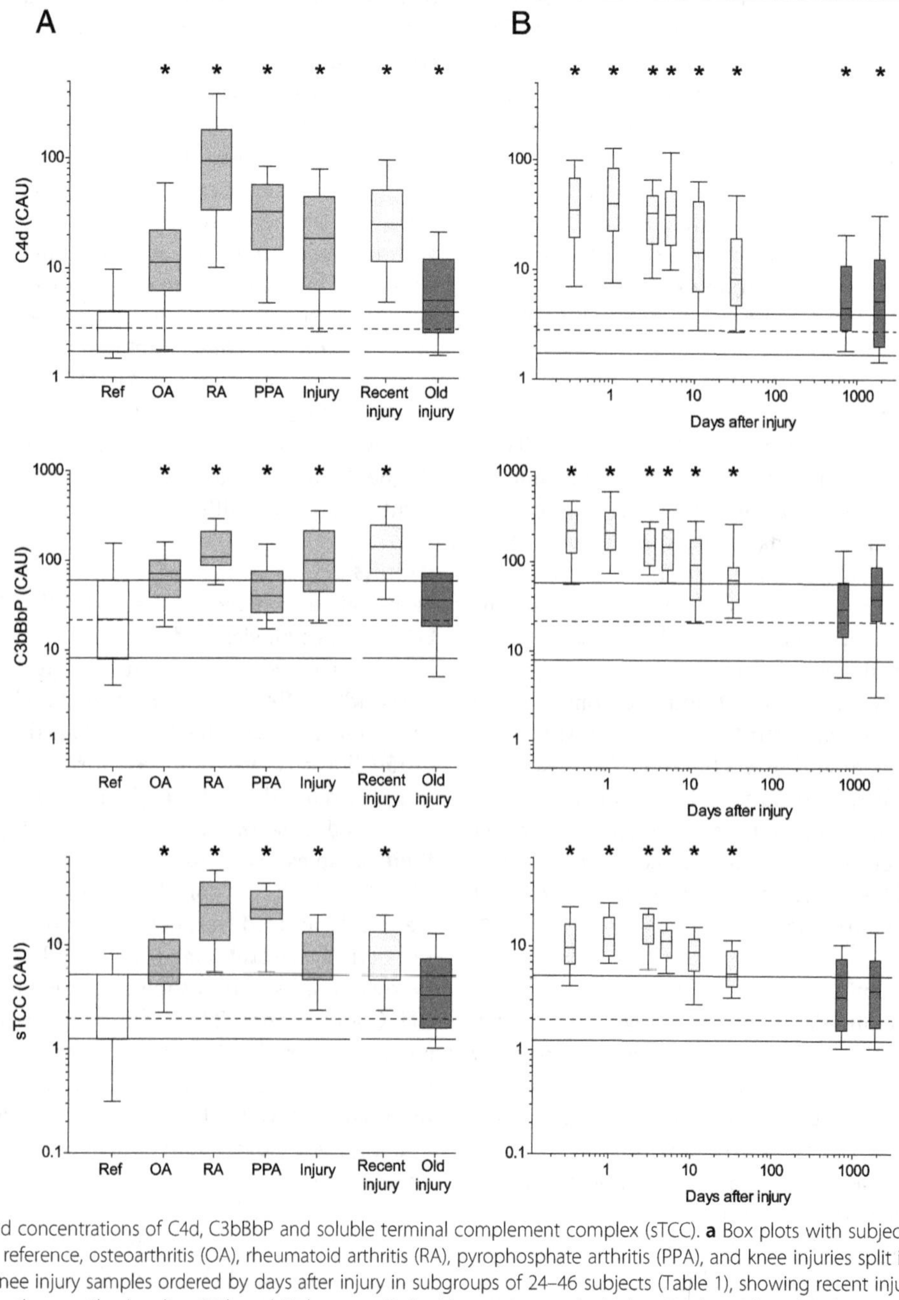

Fig. 2 Synovial fluid concentrations of C4d, C3bBbP and soluble terminal complement complex (sTCC). **a** Box plots with subjects ordered by the diagnostic groups: reference, osteoarthritis (OA), rheumatoid arthritis (RA), pyrophosphate arthritis (PPA), and knee injuries split into recent injury and old injury. **b** Knee injury samples ordered by days after injury in subgroups of 24–46 subjects (Table 1), showing recent injury and old injury groups. Boxes show the quartiles (median, 25th and 75th percentiles) with error bars and whiskers for the 10th and 90th percentiles. The quartiles of the reference group are extended as *thin horizontal lines* in both panels for comparison. Statistically significant group differences, determined by Mann-Whitney *U* test, versus the reference group are indicated by *asterisks (*)* and are presented in Additional file 1: Table S1. *CAU* Complement activation units

synovial fluid concentrations of C4d, C3bBbP and sTCC were found in the RA group (Fig. 2a, Additional file 1: Table S1).

The synovial fluid concentrations of C4d, C3bBbP and sTCC did not differ between men and women in the different subject groups (Additional file 3: Table S3). The subjects in the OA, RA and PPA groups were older than the subjects in the reference group (Table 1). Also, there was a positive correlation in the OA and PPA groups between age and concentrations of sTCC, and in the reference group for C4d; no other correlation between age and concentration of complement products was found in the subject groups (Additional file 3: Table S3). On one hand, this suggests that, compared with the reference group, the increased levels of C3bBbP in the OA, RA and PPA groups, as well as the increased levels of sTCC in the RA group, were due to disease mechanisms and not to differences in age. On the other hand, the increased levels of C4d in the OA, RA and PPA groups, as well as the increased levels of sTCC in the OA and PPA groups, could also be due partially to differences in age between the disease and reference groups.

Concentrations of C4d, C3bBbP and sTCC in synovial fluid were higher in the knee injury group than in the reference group

The concentrations of C4d, C3bBbP and sTCC were higher in the knee injury group than in the reference group, with median increases of 7-, 5- and 4-fold, respectively (Fig. 2a, Additional file 1: Table S1). The synovial fluid concentrations of C4d, C3bBbP and sTCC did not differ between men and women in the knee injury group (Additional file 3: Table S3). There was no difference in mean age between the reference group and the knee injury group (0–37 years after injury), or between the reference group and the recent injury (0–83 days after injury) and old injury (1–37 years after injury) subgroups (Table 1). This suggests that the increased levels of activated complement products in the synovial fluid of injured knees compared with reference knees were due to the knee trauma.

The elevated concentrations of C4d, C3bBbP and sTCC were seen immediately after injury (day 0, the day of injury) as 12-, 10- and 12-fold increases of median levels compared with the reference group, with a lower still significantly elevated level in knees aspirated over the first 12 weeks after injury (Fig. 2b, Additional file 1: Table S1). As seen by using correlation analysis, the synovial fluid concentrations of C4d, C3bBbP and sTCC in the recent injury group (0–83 days after injury) decreased with time after injury (Fig. 2b, Additional file 3: Table S3), while no lower levels were observed over later times in the old injury group (1–37 years after injury) (Additional file 3: Table S3). Many years after injury, the synovial fluid concentration of C4d was still elevated 2-fold compared with levels in the reference group (Fig. 2b, Additional file 1: Table S1), although this increase could be due in part to the fact that some patients in the old injury group had post-traumatic OA (Table 1).

Correlation between activated complement products

In all the subject groups, the synovial fluid concentrations of C4d and sTCC showed a moderate to strong positive correlation (Table 2). In the reference, RA and knee injury groups, there was a moderate to strong positive correlation between C4d and C3bBbP, and in the RA and knee injury groups, there was also a moderate positive correlation between C3bBbP and sTCC (Table 2).

Correlation between activated complement products and other biomarkers in the recent injury group

For the recent injury group (0–83 days after injury), we performed a correlation analysis between synovial fluid concentrations of the activated complement factors and the levels of proinflammatory cytokines and biomarkers of cartilage (sGAG, ARGS-aggrecan, COMP and C2C) and bone (osteocalcin, SPARC and osteonectin). A weak to moderate positive correlation was found for the C4d, C3bBbP and sTCC concentrations and the levels of cytokines, where C4d and TNF showed the strongest correlation ($r_s = 0.547$). No correlation was found between the concentrations of activated complement products and the levels of aggrecan markers sGAG and ARGS-aggrecan or between activated complement products and COMP (Table 3). A weak negative correlation was found between the concentrations of type II collagen epitope C2C and the level of C4d. Also, C4d, C3bBbP and sTCC concentrations showed weak to moderate positive correlations with the levels of SPARC, and concentrations of C4d and C3bBbP had a weak positive correlation with the levels of osteocalcin (Table 3).

Association between activated complement products and MRI findings in the recent injury group

For a subset of the recent injury group, we compared MRI features with synovial fluid concentrations of the complement factors. Knees with any OC fracture (with or without disrupted cortical bone) had higher concentrations of C4d and sTCC than knees without an OC fracture (Table 4). Knees with an OC fracture with disrupted cortical bone had higher concentrations of C4d and sTCC than knees without an OC fracture, and they also higher concentrations of C4d than knees with an OC fracture without disrupted cortical bone (Table 4). There were no significant differences between knees with an OC fracture without disrupted cortical bone and knees without OC fracture (data not shown). There was

Table 2 Correlation between C4d, C3bBbP and sTCC in reference and patient groups

	Reference ($n = 23$)		Osteoarthritis ($n = 24$)		Rheumatoid arthritis ($n = 32$)	
	C4d	C3bBbP	C4d	C3bBbP	C4d	C3bBbP
C3bBbP	**0.428 (0.041)**	–	0.080 (0.710)	–	**0.536 (0.002)**	–
sTCC	**0.625 (0.001)**	0.409 (0.053)	**0.754 (<0.001)**	−0.298 (0.157)	**0.752 (<0.001)**	**0.509 (0.003)**
	Pyrophosphate arthritis ($n = 25$)		Knee injury ($n = 294$)			
	C4d	C3bBbP	C4d	C3bBbP		
C3bBbP	−0.085 (0.685)	–	**0.674 (<0.001)**	–		
sTCC	**0.496 (0.012)**	0.345 (0.091)	**0.643 (<0.001)**	**0.494 (<0.001)**		

sTCC Soluble terminal complement complex
Correlation using Spearman's rho (r_s) between synovial fluid biomarkers of complement system analysed in different subject groups. Significant correlations ($p < 0.05$) are indicated by boldface type. The table shows r_s with p values in brackets

no difference in the synovial fluid concentrations of the complement factors between knees that acquired an ACL injury and knees without an ACL injury, although knees with a meniscal tear had lower concentrations of sTCC than knees without a meniscal tear (Table 4).

Discussion

Using synovial fluid from subjects in different diagnostic groups, we show that C4d, C3bBbP and sTCC concentrations were elevated not only in our positive controls RA and PPA but also in OA knees and in knee injury compared with levels in the healthy reference group knees. In injured knees, this increase was immediate, seen in knees aspirated on the day of injury, compared with lower levels in knees aspirated up to weeks after injury. Compared with levels of reference knees, knees aspirated several years after injury only showed elevated levels of C4d.

Table 3 Correlation between C4d, C3bBbP, sTCC and other biomarkers in the recent injury group

Biomarkers	n	C4d	C3bBbP	sTCC
IL-1β	112	**0.397 (<0.001)**	**0.232 (0.014)**	**0.297 (0.001)**
IL-6	112	**0.364 (<0.001)**	**0.235 (0.013)**	**0.268 (0.004)**
IL-8	112	**0.355 (<0.001)**	0.183 (0.054)	**0.372 (<0.001)**
TNF-α	112	**0.547 (<0.001)**	**0.317 (0.001)**	**0.391 (<0.001)**
sGAG	181	0.108 (0.148)	0.092 (0.218)	0.132 (0.077)
ARGS	111	−0.023 (0.811)	−0.113 (0.238)	0.176 (0.065)
COMP	112	−0.019 (0.845)	−0.149 (0.116)	−0.057(0.549)
C2C	164	**−0.181 (0.020)**	−0.101 (0.197)	−0.085 (0.279)
Osteocalcin	112	**0.265 (0.005)**	**0.192 (0.043)**	0.016 (0.871)
SPARC	112	**0.476 (<0.001)**	**0.221 (0.019)**	**0.401 (<0.001)**
Osteopontin	112	0.167 (0.079)	0.098 (0.302)	0.165 (0.083)

Abbreviations: IL Interleukin, *TNF-α* Tumour necrosis factor α, *sGAG* Sulfated glycosaminoglycan, *ARGS* ARGS-aggrecan, *COMP* Cartilage oligomeric matrix protein, *C2C* Type II collagen epitope, *SPARC* Secreted protein acidic and rich in cysteine, *sTCC* Soluble terminal complement complex
Correlation using Spearman rho (r_s), between synovial fluid biomarkers was analysed in samples from the recent injury group (0–83 days after injury). Significant correlations ($p < 0.05$) are shown in boldface type. The table shows r_s with p values in brackets. References to biomarkers: cytokines, ARGS, sGAG, osteocalcin, SPARC, osteopontin [14], COMP [19], C2C [23]

Complement C4d fragment (a proteolytic fragment of C4 with unknown biological function) is an early-stage marker for the classical and lectin pathways, C3bBbP (a C3 convertase) is an early stage marker for the alternative pathway, and sTCC (also known as *membrane attack complex* [MAC]) is a late-stage marker for all three pathways [1]. In autoimmune diseases such as RA, all three pathways are activated [3]. Analysis of synovial fluid by mass spectrometry and ELISA has shown that levels of complement components are elevated in patients with OA compared with levels found in healthy individuals [25–27]. Further, patients with OA had increased synovial fluid concentrations of C3a, an anaphylatoxin (i.e., stimulator of inflammation) that can be generated from all three pathways, and of sTCC compared with levels in healthy control subjects [27]. Our results confirm that patients with OA have increased concentrations of sTCC, and they extend previous findings by showing that the alternative pathway, together with the classical and/or lectin complement pathways, was activated in the synovial fluid of patients with OA and after knee injury.

Complement factors present in the synovial fluid after knee trauma may originate from intra-articular bleeding (i.e., haemarthrosis from the ligaments and/or from the synovium) or may be produced by synovial cells (leucocytes and synoviocytes) and/or chondrocytes [27–31]. Joint bleeding is very common after acute knee injury, and 96 of the 98 recent injury samples with available MRI data had haemarthrosis in our study. At the moment of knee trauma, impact forces can also result in BMLs and OC fractures visualized by MRI. On the basis of previous evidence [24], we anticipated that the presence of OC fractures could be used as a proxy for a strong impact trauma and that disruption of the cortical bone may be an indicator of more severe joint trauma. Complement is involved in fracture healing, where it

Table 4 C4d, C3bBbP, sTCC concentrations in the recent injury group in relation to structural features

	Any OC fracture ($n = 67$)	vs.	No OC fracture ($n = 31$)	vs.	OC fracture with disrupted cortical bone ($n = 38$)	vs.	OC fracture without disrupted cortical bone ($n = 29$)
	Mean (95 % CI)	*p* value	Mean (95 % CI)	*p* value	Mean (95 % CI)	*p* value	Mean (95 % CI)
C4d	38.90 (32.01–47.29)	**0.014**	23.92 (15.17–37.70)	**0.004**	45.42 (33.95–60.79)	**0.025**	31.76 (25.00–40.35)
C3bBbP	235.61 (203.19–273.15)	0.478	213.60 (162.33–281.06)	0.612	237.30 (195.79–287.61)	0.637	233.35 (182.64–298.19)
sTCC	12.81 (11.35–14.47)	**0.004**	9.27 (7.20–11.94)	**<0.001**	14.26 (12.20–16.68)	0.056	11.13 (9.20–13.46)
	ACL injury ($n = 60$)	vs.	No ACL injury ($n = 38$)				
	Mean (95 % CI)	*p* value	Mean (95 % CI)				
C4d	34.34 (28.39–41.52)	0.418	31.86 (20.87–48.66)				
C3bBbP	231.42 (198.93–269.28)	0.417	223.67 (174.62–286.48)				
sTCC	11.53 (10.26–12.97)	0.885	11.61 (9.08–14.85)				
	Meniscal tear ($n = 43$)	vs.	No meniscal tear ($n = 55$)				
	Mean (95 % CI)	*p* value	Mean (95 % CI)				
C4d	29.36 (21.57–39.98)	0.565	36.86 (28.42–47.80)				
C3bBbP	204.27 (172.78–241.49)	0.399	249.23 (205.21–302.69)				
sTCC	9.91 (8.46–11.62)	**0.013**	13.05 (11.08–15.37)				

Abbreviations: ACL Anterior cruciate ligament, *OC* Osteochondral, *sTCC* Soluble terminal complement complex

Magnetic resonance imaging results were available for a subfraction of the recent injury group ($n = 98$). Between-groups statistical testing was performed using analysis of covariance of log_{10}-transformed concentrations with adjustment for days between the injury and synovial fluid aspiration, age at injury, and sex. Significant differences ($p < 0.05$) are shown in boldface type. Concentrations in complement activation units are presented as linear data as means with 95 % CI in brackets

affects osteoblasts and osteoclasts. These bone cells also produce C3 and C5, and type I collagen is capable of activating platelets, forming sTCC and upregulating receptors for C3a and C5a [32, 33]. At the fracture edge of matrix cracks, the chondrocyte death rate is very high, and damage-associated molecular patterns released from dying cells (i.e., cellular debris such as mitochondria, histones, DNA) contributes to an activation of the innate system [10, 32, 34] and directly triggers C1q [35]. Further, factor VII-acting serine protease, an activator of the coagulation system that is activated by DNA and histones, together with plasmin and clotting factors (e.g., thrombin and factor Xa) can generate C3a/C3b and C5a/C5b [32, 36]. Together, this might explain why patients with knee injury with OC fractures who have major cell osteocyte and chondrocyte death and intra-articular bleeding also have increased complement factor activation of C4d and sTCC compared with patients without such fractures, as shown in our present study.

Previously, we showed that patients with recent knee injury have signs of cartilage degradation, as reflected by an increased release into synovial fluid over several weeks of proteolytic products of aggrecan, type II collagen and COMP [14–17, 19, 23, 37, 38]. Many of the ECM proteins and their fragments, such as aggrecan, chondroadherin, fibromodulin and osteoadherin, activate the classical complement pathway [6, 7, 27, 39], while others, such as COMP and type II collagen, activate the alternative pathway [5, 40]. However, several ECM proteins also inhibit complement: Proline/arginine-rich end leucine-rich repeat protein (PRELP) and the NC4 domain of type IX collagen directly inhibit formation of MAC [41, 42]; biglycan, decorin and COMP inhibit the classical pathway via binding of C1q [5, 43]; and PRELP inhibits the alternative pathway [41]. The ECM proteins and their fragments thus seem to have dual effects on complement, either activating or inhibiting it. This duality could in part explain why in the synovial fluid from the recent injury group no correlations were found between the cartilage protein fragments and the components of the different complement pathways.

Compared with individuals with healthy knees, TNF-α concentrations in synovial fluid are increased in patients with OA and also in patients with recent (weeks) as well as old (years) knee injuries [14, 38, 44–46]. Interestingly, in this study, the strongest correlation for the recent injury group samples (0–83 days after injury) was between synovial fluid concentrations of C4d and TNF-α ($r_s = 0.547$), and the levels of C4d were also found to be elevated many years after injury. This resembles what was found for patients with ACL injury, who had elevated synovial fluid levels of TNF-α 5 years after injury [38].

In injured knee joints, proinflammatory cytokines are produced by chondrocytes and synoviocytes and by infiltrated leucocytes, resulting in the production and activation of matrix metalloproteases (MMPs) and aggrecanases [11, 47, 48]. As a parallel route, complement components such as sublytic concentrations of MAC stimulate chondrocytes to produce MMPs and aggrecanases [27], and complement anaphylatoxins (C3a and C5a) stimulate granulocytes, macrophages, and B and T cells to produce proinflammatory cytokines [3]. Further, it has been shown that C1s (a protease of the classical pathway) can activate proMMP-9, and C1s can also cleave types I, II and IV collagens [49, 50]. This indicates that there are several possible routes for the induction of extracellular proteases in these patients.

In patients with a recent knee injury (0–5 weeks), the release into the synovial fluid of proinflammatory cytokines IL-1β, IL-6 and TNF-α precedes the release of cartilage degradation products of aggrecan, COMP and type II collagen [14, 19, 23, 38]. In the same patients in the present study, we found no correlation between the complement factors C4d, C3bBbP and sTCC and cartilage degradation products of aggrecan, type II collagen and COMP; however, the complement factor concentrations correlated positively with proinflammatory cytokine levels of IL-1β, IL-6 and TNF-α. This supports the concept that complement together with coagulation represents an alternative route to activation of cytokine pathways, and together these routes drive the catabolic process seen as cartilage degradation after joint injury and most likely later in OA.

This study has certain limitations. First, the lack of dilution linearity for the C3bBbP and sTCC assays using synovial fluid samples complicated the assessments, and only relative comparison could be made by using the same dilution (1:20) for all samples. Second, because the subjects in the OA, RA and PPA groups were older than the subjects in the reference group, we cannot exclude the possibility that the increased levels of the complement factors found in these patient groups could be due partly to differences in age. Third, the knee injury group was cross-sectional, so the design precludes drawing firm conclusions of trends in time because no repeated sampling was done within individual patients. Hence, our suggestions regarding differences in complement activation over time need to be confirmed in longitudinal studies. Finally, we measured only the soluble components of C4d, C3bBbP and sTCC found in synovial fluid, and these also ought to be analysed as cell-bound (e.g., chondrocytes, synoviocytes) components for the different diagnostic groups.

Conclusions

We show that alternative and classical and/or lectin complement pathways are activated in the synovial fluid of subjects with knee injury and in patients with OA. After an injury to the knee, the complement factors C4d, C3bBbP and sTCC are instantly activated and are associated with proinflammatory cytokines, while C4d and sTCC are associated with OC fractures.

This and previous reports have suggested that complement is activated in OA [27]. Knee injury is a well-known and strong risk factor for rapid knee OA development, but the driving mechanisms are not well understood. The sudden activation of complement after knee injury found in this study, especially among those with more severe trauma, most likely represents one of several important pathways involved in the onset of this complex disease. Therefore, more clinical studies using longitudinal cohorts are needed to elucidate these pathological pathways to determine if or when to use complement inhibitors as a treatment strategy for OA.

Abbreviations

ACL: Anterior cruciate ligament; ANCOVA: Analysis of covariance; BML: Bone marrow lesion; CAU: Complement activation units; COMP: Cartilage oligomeric matrix protein; CV: Coefficient of variation; ECM: Extracellular matrix; ELISA: Enzyme-linked immunosorbent assay; Ig: Immunoglobulin; IL: Interleukin; LLOD: Lower limit of detection; MAC: Membrane attack complex; MASP: Mannose-binding lectin-associated serine protease; MBL: Mannose-binding lectin; MMP: Matrix metalloprotease; MRI: Magnetic resonance imaging; NA: Not applicable; OA: Osteoarthritis; OC: Osteochondral; P: Properdin; PCL: Posterior cruciate ligament, PPA, Pyrophosphate arthritis; PRELP: Proline/arginine-rich end leucine-rich repeat protein; PRM: Pattern recognition molecule; RA: Rheumatoid arthritis; sGAG: Sulfated glycosaminoglycan; SPARC: Secreted protein acidic and rich in cysteine; sTCC: Soluble terminal complement complex; TNF: Tumour necrosis factor; ULOD: Upper limit of detection; ARGS: ARGS-aggrecan, C2C, type II collagen epitope C2C

Acknowledgements

We thank Tom Eirik Mollnes (Oslo University Hospital) for his kind gift of the complement standard, and Torsten Boegård (Lund University) for assessing the MRI scans.

Funding

Funding for this work was provided as project grants from the Swedish Research Council (to AMB, RF, LSL), the Lund University Faculty of Medicine (to RF, AS), the King Gustaf V 80th Birthday Fund (to AMB, AS), the Kock Foundation (to AMB, AS), the Swedish Rheumatism Association (to AS), the Alfred Österlunds Foundation (to AMB, AS), the Medical Training and Research Agreement (ALF) and Skåne University Hospital (to AMB, RF, AS), the Thelma Zoega Foundation (to RF), the Crafoord Foundation (RF) and the National Science Centre Poland (2014/14/E/NZ6/00182; to MO).

Authors' contributions

AS designed the study, performed the statistical calculations and drafted the manuscript. MO participated in the design of the study, carried out the immunoassays and drafted the manuscript. PS carried out the immunoassays and helped with the statistical calculations. RF collected the cohorts and analysed the MRI data. TS collected the cohorts and drafted the manuscript. LSL participated in the design of the study, collected the cohorts and drafted the manuscript. AMB participated in the design of the study and drafted the manuscript. All authors read and approved the final manuscript. AS takes responsibility for the integrity of the work.

Competing interests

The authors declare that they have no competing interests.

Author details
[1]Department of Clinical Sciences Lund, Orthopaedics, Lund University, Faculty of Medicine, BMC C12, SE-221 84 Lund, Sweden. [2]Department of Translational Medicine, Division of Medical Protein Chemistry, Lund University, Faculty of Medicine, Lund, Sweden. [3]Department of Medical Biotechnology, Intercollegiate Faculty of Biotechnology UG-MUG, Medical University of Gdańsk, Gdańsk, Poland. [4]Department of Clinical Sciences Lund, Rheumatology, Lund University, Faculty of Medicine, Lund, Sweden.

References

1. Ricklin D, Hajishengallis G, Yang K, Lambris JD. Complement: a key system for immune surveillance and homeostasis. Nat Immunol. 2010;11(9):785–97.
2. Merle NS, Church SE, Fremeaux-Bacchi V, Roumenina LT. Complement system part I –molecular mechanisms of activation and regulation. Front Immunol. 2015;6:262.
3. Okroj M, Heinegård D, Holmdahl R, Blom AM. Rheumatoid arthritis and the complement system. Ann Med. 2007;39(7):517–30.
4. Happonen KE, Heinegård D, Saxne T, Blom AM. Interactions of the complement system with molecules of extracellular matrix: relevance for joint diseases. Immunobiology. 2012;217(11):1088–96.
5. Happonen KE, Saxne T, Aspberg A, Mörgelin M, Heinegård D, Blom AM. Regulation of complement by cartilage oligomeric matrix protein allows for a novel molecular diagnostic principle in rheumatoid arthritis. Arthritis Rheum. 2010;62(12):3574–83.
6. Melin Fürst C, Mörgelin M, Vadstrup K, Heinegård D, Aspberg A, Blom AM. The C-type lectin of the aggrecan G3 domain activates complement. PLoS One. 2013;8(4):e61407.
7. Sjöberg A, Onnerfjord P, Mörgelin M, Heinegård D, Blom AM. The extracellular matrix and inflammation: fibromodulin activates the classical pathway of complement by directly binding C1q. J Biol Chem. 2005;280(37):32301–8.
8. Lohmander LS, Englund PM, Dahl LL, Roos EM. The long-term consequence of anterior cruciate ligament and meniscus injuries: osteoarthritis. Am J Sports Med. 2007;35(10):1756–69.
9. Johnson DL, Urban Jr WP, Caborn DN, Vanarthos WJ, Carlson CS. Articular cartilage changes seen with magnetic resonance imaging-detected bone bruises associated with acute anterior cruciate ligament rupture. Am J Sports Med. 1998;26(3):409–14.
10. Tochigi Y, Zhang P, Rudert MJ, Baer TE, Martin JA, Hillis SL, et al. A novel impaction technique to create experimental articular fractures in large animal joints. Osteoarthritis Cartilage. 2013;21(1):200–8.
11. Goldring MB. The role of the chondrocyte in osteoarthritis. Arthritis Rheum. 2000;43(9):1916–26.
12. Huber-Lang M, Kovtun A, Ignatius A. The role of complement in trauma and fracture healing. Semin Immunol. 2013;25(1):73–8.
13. Schmal H, Salzmann GM, Niemeyer P, Langenmair E, Guo R, Schneider C, et al. Early intra-articular complement activation in ankle fractures. Biomed Res Int. 2014;2014:426893.
14. Swärd P, Frobell R, Englund M, Roos H, Struglics A. Cartilage and bone markers and inflammatory cytokines are increased in synovial fluid in the acute phase of knee injury (hemarthrosis) – a cross-sectional analysis. Osteoarthritis Cartilage. 2012;20(11):1302–8.
15. Larsson S, Lohmander LS, Struglics A. Synovial fluid level of aggrecan ARGS fragments is a more sensitive marker of joint disease than glycosaminoglycan or aggrecan levels: a cross-sectional study. Arthritis Res Ther. 2009;11(3):R92.
16. Lohmander LS, Atley LM, Pietka TA, Eyre DR. The release of crosslinked peptides from type II collagen into human synovial fluid is increased soon after joint injury and in osteoarthritis. Arthritis Rheum. 2003;48(11):3130–9.
17. Lohmander LS, Ionescu M, Jugessur H, Poole AR. Changes in joint cartilage aggrecan after knee injury and in osteoarthritis. Arthritis Rheum. 1999;42(3):534–44.
18. Struglics A, Hansson M, Lohmander LS. Human aggrecanase generated synovial fluid fragment levels are elevated directly after knee injuries due to proteolysis both in the inter globular and chondroitin sulfate domains. Osteoarthritis Cartilage. 2011;19(8):1047_57.
19. Swärd P, Struglics A, Englund M, Roos HP, Frobell RB. Soft tissue knee injury with concomitant osteochondral fracture is associated with higher degree of acute joint inflammation. Am J Sports Med. 2014;42(5):1096–102.
20. Dahlberg L, Ryd L, Heinegård D, Lohmander LS. Proteoglycan fragments in joint fluid: influence of arthrosis and inflammation. Acta Orthop Scand. 1992;63(4):417–23.
21. Blom AM, Osterborg A, Mollnes TE, Okroj M. Antibodies reactive to cleaved sites in complement proteins enable highly specific measurement of soluble markers of complement activation. Mol Immunol. 2015;66(2):164–70.
22. Bergseth G, Ludviksen JK, Kirschfink M, Giclas PC, Nilsson B, Mollnes TE. An international serum standard for application in assays to detect human complement activation products. Mol Immunol. 2013;56(3):232–9.
23. Kumahashi N, Sward P, Larsson S, Lohmander LS, Frobell R, Struglics A. Type II collagen C2C epitope in human synovial fluid and serum after knee injury – associations with molecular and structural markers of injury. Osteoarthritis Cartilage. 2015;23(9):1506–12.
24. Frobell RB, Roos HP, Roos EM, Hellio Le Graverand MP, Buck R, Tamez-Pena J, et al. The acutely ACL injured knee assessed by MRI: are large volume traumatic bone marrow lesions a sign of severe compression injury? Osteoarthritis Cartilage. 2008;16(7):829–36.
25. Gobezie R, Kho A, Krastins B, Sarracino DA, Thornhill TS, Chase M, et al. High abundance synovial fluid proteome: distinct profiles in health and osteoarthritis. Arthritis Res Ther. 2007;9(2):R36.
26. Ritter SY, Subbaiah R, Bebek G, Crish J, Scanzello CR, Krastins B, et al. Proteomic analysis of synovial fluid from the osteoarthritic knee: comparison with transcriptome analyses of joint tissues. Arthritis Rheum. 2013;65(4):981–92.
27. Wang Q, Rozelle AL, Lepus CM, Scanzello CR, Song JJ, Larsen DM, et al. Identification of a central role for complement in osteoarthritis. Nat Med. 2011;17(12):1674–9.
28. Bradley K, North J, Saunders D, Schwaeble W, Jeziorska M, Woolley DE, et al. Synthesis of classical pathway complement components by chondrocytes. Immunology. 1996;88(4):648–56.
29. Corvetta A, Pomponio G, Rinaldi N, Luchetti MM, Di Loreto C, Stramazzotti D. Terminal complement complex in synovial tissue from patients affected by rheumatoid arthritis, osteoarthritis and acute joint trauma. Clin Exp Rheumatol. 1992;10(5):433–8.
30. John T, Stahel PF, Morgan SJ, Schulze-Tanzil G. Impact of the complement cascade on posttraumatic cartilage inflammation and degradation. Histol Histopathol. 2007;22(7):781–90.
31. Sjöberg AP, Trouw LA, Blom AM. Complement activation and inhibition: a delicate balance. Trends Immunol. 2009;30(2):83–90.
32. Huber-Lang M, Ignatius A, Brenner RE. Role of complement on broken surfaces after trauma. Adv Exp Med Biol. 2015;865:43–55.
33. Ignatius A, Schoengraf P, Kreja L, Liedert A, Recknagel S, Kandert S, et al. Complement C3a and C5a modulate osteoclast formation and inflammatory response of osteoblasts in synergism with IL-1β. J Cell Biochem. 2011;112(9):2594–605.
34. Martin JA, Buckwalter JA. Post-traumatic osteoarthritis: the role of stress induced chondrocyte damage. Biorheology. 2006;43(3-4):517–21.
35. Martin M, Leffler J, Blom AM. Annexin A2 and A5 serve as new ligands for C1q on apoptotic cells. J Biol Chem. 2012;287(40):33733–44.
36. Amara U, Flierl MA, Rittirsch D, Klos A, Chen H, Acker B, et al. Molecular intercommunication between the complement and coagulation systems. J Immunol. 2010;185(9):5628–36.
37. Lohmander LS, Saxne T, Heinegård DK. Release of cartilage oligomeric matrix protein (COMP) into joint fluid after knee injury and in osteoarthritis. Ann Rheum Dis. 1994;53(1):8–13.
38. Struglics A, Larsson S, Kumahashi N, Frobell R, Lohmander LS. Changes in cytokines and aggrecan ARGS neoepitope in synovial fluid and serum and in C-terminal crosslinking telopeptide of type II collagen and N-terminal crosslinking telopeptide of type I Collagen in urine over five years after anterior cruciate ligament rupture: an exploratory analysis in the knee anterior cruciate ligament, nonsurgical versus surgical treatment trial. Arthritis Rheumatol. 2015;67(7):1816–25.
39. Sjöberg AP, Manderson GA, Mörgelin M, Day AJ, Heinegård D, Blom AM. Short leucine-rich glycoproteins of the extracellular matrix display diverse patterns of complement interaction and activation. Mol Immunol. 2009;46(5):830–9.
40. Hanauske-Abel HM, Pontz BF, Schorlemmer HU. Cartilage specific collagen activates macrophages and the alternative pathway of complement: evidence for an immunopathogenic concept of rheumatoid arthritis. Ann Rheum Dis. 1982;41(2):168–76.

41. Happonen KE, Furst CM, Saxne T, Heinegård D, Blom AM. PRELP protein inhibits the formation of the complement membrane attack complex. J Biol Chem. 2012;287(11):8092–100.
42. Kalchishkova N, Furst CM, Heinegård D, Blom AM. NC4 domain of cartilage-specific collagen IX inhibits complement directly due to attenuation of membrane attack formation and indirectly through binding and enhancing activity of complement inhibitors C4B-binding protein and factor H. J Biol Chem. 2011;286(32):27915–26.
43. Groeneveld TW, Oroszlan M, Owens RT, Faber-Krol MC, Bakker AC, Arlaud GJ, et al. Interactions of the extracellular matrix proteoglycans decorin and biglycan with C1q and collectins. J Immunol. 2005;175(7):4715–23.
44. Higuchi H, Shirakura K, Kimura M, Terauchi M, Shinozaki T, Watanabe H, et al. Changes in biochemical parameters after anterior cruciate ligament injury. Int Orthop. 2006;30(1):43–7.
45. Kapoor M, Martel-Pelletier J, Lajeunesse D, Pelletier JP, Fahmi H. Role of proinflammatory cytokines in the pathophysiology of osteoarthritis. Nat Rev Rheumatol. 2011;7(1):33–42.
46. Sohn DH, Sokolove J, Sharpe O, Erhart JC, Chandra PE, Lahey LJ, et al. Plasma proteins present in osteoarthritic synovial fluid can stimulate cytokine production via Toll-like receptor 4. Arthritis Res Ther. 2012;14(1):R7.
47. Bondeson J, Wainwright SD, Lauder S, Amos N, Hughes CE. The role of synovial macrophages and macrophage-produced cytokines in driving aggrecanases, matrix metalloproteinases, and other destructive and inflammatory responses in osteoarthritis. Arthritis Res Ther. 2006;8(6):R187.
48. Moradi B, Rosshirt N, Tripel E, Kirsch J, Barie A, Zeifang F, et al. Unicompartmental and bicompartmental knee osteoarthritis show different patterns of mononuclear cell infiltration and cytokine release in the affected joints. Clin Exp Immunol. 2015;180(1):143–54.
49. Sakiyama H, Inaba N, Toyoguchi T, Okada Y, Matsumoto M, Moriya H, et al. Immunolocalization of complement C1s and matrix metalloproteinase 9 (92 kDa gelatinase/type IV collagenase) in the primary ossification center of the human femur. Cell Tissue Res. 1994;277(2):239–45.
50. Yamaguchi K, Sakiyama H, Matsumoto M, Moriya H, Sakiyama S. Degradation of type I and II collagen by human activated C1-s. FEBS Lett. 1990;268(1):206–8.

8

Exploring determinants predicting response to intra-articular hyaluronic acid treatment in symptomatic knee osteoarthritis: 9-year follow-up data from the Osteoarthritis Initiative

Jean-Pierre Pelletier[1*], Jean-Pierre Raynauld[1], François Abram[2], Marc Dorais[3], Philippe Delorme[4] and Johanne Martel-Pelletier[1]

Abstract

Background: The weight of recommendation for intra-articular therapies such as hyaluronic acid injections varies from one set of guidelines to another, and they have not yet reached unanimity with respect to the usefulness of intra-articular hyaluronic acid (IAHA) injections for the symptomatic treatment of knee osteoarthritis (OA). Among the reasons for the controversy is that the current literature provides inconsistent results and conclusions about such treatment. This study aimed at identifying determinants associated with a better response to IAHA treatment in knee OA.

Methods: Subjects were selected from the Osteoarthritis Initiative database. Participants were subjects who had radiographic OA, received one IAHA treatment, and had data on demographics and Western Ontario and McMaster Universities Osteoarthritis Index (WOMAC) scores at visits before (T0) and after (T1; within 6 months) treatment. Pain was analyzed for demographic, clinical, and imaging characteristics at T0 and change over time (T0 to T1). Subjects with WOMAC pain > 0 at T0 were subdivided into Low, Moderate, and High pain groups based on tertile analysis. Further analyses were done with the High pain group (score ≥ 8), which was divided into responders (improvement in pain ≥ 20%) and nonresponders (unchanged or worsening of pain).

Results: Participants (n = 310) received a total of 404 treatments (one per knee). In the Low and Moderate pain groups vs the High pain group, participants had significantly lower score at T0 ($p < 0.001$), and the Low vs High pain group had significantly lower BMI ($p = 0.002$), greater joint space width (JSW) ($p = 0.010$) and knee cartilage volume ($p \leq 0.009$), and smaller synovial effusion ($p = 0.033$). In the High pain group, responders vs nonresponders were usually younger ($p = 0.014$), with greater cartilage volume in the medial compartment ($p = 0.046$), a trend toward greater JSW, and a significant improvement in all WOMAC scores ($p < 0.001$), while nonresponders showed worsening of symptoms.

Conclusions: This study identified reliable predictive determinants that can distinguish patients who could best benefit from IAHA treatment: high levels of knee pain, younger, and less severe structural damage. These could be implemented in clinical practice as a useful guide for physicians.

Keywords: Osteoarthritis, Hyaluronic acid injection, Knee pain, Treatment responders

* Correspondence: dr@jppelletier.ca
[1]Osteoarthritis Research Unit, University of Montreal Hospital Research Centre (CRCHUM), 900 Saint-Denis, Suite R11.412, Montreal, QC H2X 0A9, Canada
Full list of author information is available at the end of the article

Background

Treatment of knee osteoarthritis (OA) focuses on symptom relief and improvement of function. In addition to nonpharmacological measures, if needed, a number of oral, topical, and intra-articular therapies including acetaminophen, nonsteroidal anti-inflammatory drugs (NSAIDs) and symptomatic slow-acting drugs are used as first-line treatment for OA [1–4].

The weight of recommendation for intra-articular therapies, such as steroids and hyaluronic acid (IAHA) injections, which are the most commonly listed [1–7], varies from one set of guidelines to another, and they have not yet reached unanimity with respect to the usefulness of IAHA injections for the symptomatic treatment of knee OA [8, 9]. Among the reasons for the controversy is that the current literature provides inconsistent results and conclusions about such treatment [10–12].

The Osteoarthritis Initiative (OAI) cohort provides a unique opportunity for the prospective follow-up of subjects with knee OA over an extended period of time, up to nine years so far. This cohort has been used to follow the natural history of the disease and to evaluate the efficacy of some OA treatments on disease progression and symptoms [13–15]. It provides a real-life scenario to extend our understanding of the effects of potential treatments on disease outcome.

This study aimed at identifying determinants that best correlate with the level of response to IAHA in participants with symptomatic knee OA.

Methods

Study patients

Data used for this study were from the OAI database, which is publicly available online (https://oai.epi-ucsf.org/datarelease/). The individuals were from the Incidence and Progression subcohorts (Fig. 1). The selection of subjects for the evaluation of the effects of IAHA injections was based on the following question that participants in the OAI cohort were asked at each visit: "During the past 6 months, have you had a treatment with injections of hyaluronic acid in either of your knees (right, left, both) for your arthritis?" Treatment was given as one injection per week for 3–5 weeks. Selected patients had radiographic OA (Kellgren–Lawrence (KL) grade ≥ 1) and had received one treatment with IAHA in one or both knees during the course of follow-up. In addition, to be included in the present study, data had to be available regarding the disease symptoms on the yearly visit that took place before (T0) and after (T1) the IAHA treatment. Data on OA patient demographics, symptoms (Western Ontario and McMaster Universities Osteoarthritis Index (WOMAC)), imaging (radiography, magnetic resonance imaging (MRI)), and concomitant arthritis drug treatments were obtained from the OAI website and the MR images were assessed by our imaging group. Of note, patients with secondary causes of knee OA were excluded. A total of 310 participants provided data for 404 knees that received IAHA injections.

Symptoms as predictors of treatment response

The study design allowed the assessment of the symptomatic effect of one treatment with IAHA explored up to a maximum period of 6 months after administration of the treatment. All participants who had one IAHA treatment in one or both knees and for whom data were available from the visits before and after the treatment were studied.

The WOMAC questionnaire is self-administered and scores are built upon three domains (pain (0–20), stiffness (0–8), and function (0–68)), and their summation yields a total score (0–96). Data on symptoms were also evaluated with regard to the use of other drugs, including arthritis drug treatment, taken by the patients at T0. The participant population was subdivided based on the level of the WOMAC pain scores using tertile analysis. Only those with WOMAC pain scores > 0 at T0 were used for the analysis. In participants with WOMAC pain score = 8, the symptomatic responders were defined as having experienced an improvement in WOMAC pain score ≥ 20% from T0 to T1. WOMAC pain score data were analyzed with regard to the demographic and clinical data at T0 and change in WOMAC pain score over time (from T0 to T1).

Imaging characteristics at T0 as predictors of disease response

Participants who had one IAHA treatment in one or both knees for whom data were available at T0 and T1 were studied.

The KL score and the joint space width (JSW) data were obtained from the OAI database (central reading). The MR images were acquired using a double-echo steady-state imaging protocol from 3.0 T apparatus (Magnetom Trio, Siemens) at the four OAI clinical centers. Fully automated and validated quantitative MRI technology was used to assess the cartilage volume [15, 16], incidence and severity of bone marrow lesions (BMLs) [17], and synovial fluid effusion size [18], and a validated scoring method was used to assess meniscal extrusion [19]. For the cartilage volume and BML assessments, the global knee comprises the condyles plus tibial plateaus, and for cartilage the subregions include medial and lateral compartments (condyle plus tibial plateau).

Statistical analysis

Participants with WOMAC pain score = 0 at T0 were excluded. The cohort was divided into three groups based on tertile analysis of the WOMAC pain scores:

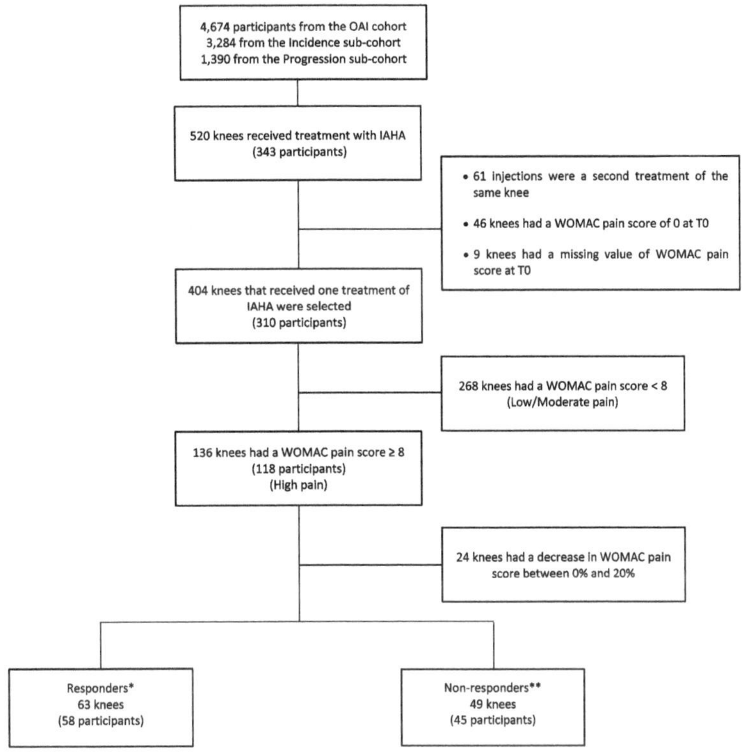

Fig. 1 Participant disposition. *Responders had a decrease in WOMAC pain score of at least 20% between T0 and T1 (WOMAC ≥ 20%). **Nonresponders had the same WOMAC pain score or an increase in WOMAC pain score between T0 and T1 (WOMAC ≤ 0%). T0 visit before intra-articular hyaluronic acid (IAHA) treatment, T1 visit after IAHA treatment, OAI Osteoarthritis Initiative, WOMAC Western Ontario and McMaster Universities Osteoarthritis Index

Low, 0 < WOMAC pain < 4; Moderate, 4 ≤ WOMAC pain ≤ 7; High, WOMAC pain ≥ 8. Responders were defined as participants in the High pain group who showed an improvement, measured from the preinjection status (T0 to T1), in symptom variables (WOMAC pain) of ≥ 20%. Nonresponders were those in the High pain group who had no improvement (stable) or worsening (increase > 0) of pain.

Comparisons between the groups were analyzed using Student's *t* test (Wilcoxon Mann–Whitney/Kruskal Wallis if nonnormal distribution) for continuous variables and Pearson's chi-squared test (Fisher's exact test if sample size was too small) for categorical variables. Multivariate linear analyses were performed adjusting for the potential confounding factors (age, sex, and body mass index (BMI)) at T0. All tests were two-sided and $p \leq 0.050$ was considered statistically significant. All statistical analyses were performed using SAS software, version 9.3 (SAS Institute, Cary, NC, USA).

Results

Demographic, symptom and imaging characteristics at T0 and change in symptoms based on WOMAC scores

The distribution and characteristics information of the study participants (n = 310) are presented in Tables 1 and 2. Participants received a total of 404 treatments (one per knee) in the right and/or left knee (Fig. 1).

Demographics and imaging were balanced at T0 with the exception that those in the Low pain group were predominantly from the Incidence subcohort, male, and with lower BMI compared to the participants in the High pain group (WOMAC pain ≥ 8). Compared to the High pain group, the Moderate pain group also had more participants in the Incidence cohort. With regard to knee structure, the Low pain group vs the High pain group showed a greater JSW and cartilage volume, smaller effusion size, and numerical trends for lower KL grade and BML score. These findings indicate that participants in the High pain group also had more severe disease.

As expected, the average WOMAC pain and other WOMAC scores at T0 progressively and significantly increased from the Low pain group to the High pain group (Table 2). The change in WOMAC pain score showed, for the total population studied, that the level of pain had slightly increased over time. When data were analyzed by group, an increase in WOMAC score was found in the Low and Moderate pain groups while a reduction in the score (less symptoms) was observed in the High pain group.

Table 1 Demographics and imaging characteristics at T0

	Total ($n = 404$)[a]	Low,[b] $0 <$ WOMAC pain[c] < 4 ($n = 118$)	Moderate, $4 \leq$ WOMAC pain[c] ≤ 7 ($n = 150$)	High, WOMAC pain[c] ≥ 8 ($n = 136$)	Low vs High p value[d]	Moderate vs High p value[d]
Subcohort						
Incidence	47% (189)	54% (64)	50% (75)	37% (50)		
Progression	53% (215)	46% (54)	50% (75)	63% (86)	**0.005**[e]	**0.024**[e]
Injected knee						
Right	50% (204)	51% (60)	51% (76)	50% (68)		
Left	50% (200)	49% (58)	49% (74)	50% (68)	0.893[e]	0.910[e]
Sex, male	41% (165)	46% (54)	43% (65)	34% (46)	0.052[e]	0.099[e]
Age (years)	66 ± 9	66 ± 9	66 ± 9	64 ± 9	0.140	0.190
	($n = 364$)	($n = 110$)	($n = 134$)	($n = 120$)		
Body mass index	30.39 ± 5.30	28.98 ± 4.48	30.74 ± 4.99	31.30 ± 6.07	**0.002**	0.353
Kellgren–Lawrence	($n = 208$)	($n = 62$)	($n = 78$)	($n = 68$)		
Grade 0, 1	15% (31)	23% (14)	14% (11)	9% (6)		
Grade 2	26% (55)	29% (18)	26% (20)	25% (17)		
Grade 3	35% (72)	32% (20)	33% (26)	38% (26)		
Grade 4	24% (50)	16% (10)	27% (21)	28% (19)	0.088[e]	0.769[e]
	($n = 226$)	($n = 67$)	($n = 86$)	($n = 73$)		
Joint space width (mm)	3.34 ± 1.62	3.78 ± 1.79	3.23 ± 1.57	3.06 ± 1.45	**0.010**	0.430
Magnetic resonance imaging						
Cartilage volume (mm^3)	($n = 239$)	($n = 69$)	($n = 92$)	($n = 78$)		
Global knee	9371 ± 2788	10,196 ± 2356	9060 ± 2959	9009 ± 2813	**0.002**	0.917
Medial compartment	4351 ± 1615	4861 ± 1515	4093 ± 1644	4205 ± 1582	**0.008**	0.670
Lateral compartment	5020 ± 1490	5335 ± 1209	4967 ± 1627	4805 ± 1519	**0.009**	0.760
Bone marrow lesion (global knee)	($n = 246$)	($n = 73$)	($n = 92$)	($n = 81$)		
Presence	42% (104)	44% (32)	36% (33)	48% (39)	0.592[e]	0.102[e]
Score	1.97 ± 3.37	1.54 ± 2.54	1.86 ± 3.95	2.49 ± 3.28	0.090	0.058
Medial meniscus	($n = 248$)	($n = 74$)	($n = 95$)	($n = 79$)		
No extrusion	64% (159)	68% (50)	67% (64)	57% (45)		
Extrusion	36% (89)	32% (24)	33% (31)	43% (34)	0.177[e]	0.158[e]
	($n = 231$)	($n = 67$)	($n = 87$)	($n = 77$)		
Synovial fluid volume (ml)	20.12 ± 13.59	17.43 ± 11.46	19.77 ± 13.25	22.86 ± 15.22	**0.033**	0.203

Results are shown as mean ± standard deviation or % and number (n) of participants' IAHA injected knees. Bold data are significant at $p < 0.05$
T0 visit before IAHA treatment, *IAHA* intra-articular hyaluronic acid, *WOMAC* Western Ontario and McMaster Universities Osteoarthritis Index
[a]Number of injected knees based on 310 participants
[b]The level of pain on the WOMAC score was divided into three groups (Low, Moderate, and High) based on tertile analysis
[c]WOMAC Likert 3.1 (scale 0–20) pain scores at T0. Participants with WOMAC pain score = 0 were excluded from analysis
[d]Continuous variables were compared using Student's t test/Mann–Whitney test
[e]Proportions compared using the chi-squared test/Fisher's exact test

There were significant differences between the Low and High pain groups, and between the Moderate and High pain groups.

Data analyzed based on whether participants had an increased, stable, or decreased level of pain (% change in WOMAC pain) (Table 2) revealed that the proportion of participants with a decrease in pain level ≥ 20% was greatest in the High pain group and that this group also had a significantly smaller proportion of participants with an increase in pain. The WOMAC function and total scores yielded results very similar to those of the pain. With regard to the use of concomitant arthritis medication (Table 3), the number of participants taking glucosamine and chondroitin sulfate was significantly lower in the High pain group than in the other two groups; however, the number receiving steroid injections

Table 2 Symptoms (WOMAC scores) at T0

	Total ($n = 404$)[a]	Low,[b] $0 <$ WOMAC pain[c] < 4 ($n = 118$)	Moderate, $4 \leq$ WOMAC pain[c] ≤ 7 ($n = 150$)	High, WOMAC pain[c] ≥ 8 ($n = 136$)	Low vs High p value[d]	Moderate vs High p value[d]
WOMAC at T0						
	($n = 404$)	($n = 118$)	($n = 150$)	($n = 136$)		
Pain (0–20)	6.13 ± 3.69	2.07 ± 0.80	5.37 ± 1.10	10.48 ± 2.19	**< 0.001**	**< 0.001**
	($n = 390$)	($n = 116$)	($n = 146$)	($n = 128$)		
Function (0–68)	19.27 ± 11.63	8.61 ± 5.53	18.46 ± 8.23	29.87 ± 9.55	**< 0.001**	**< 0.001**
	($n = 404$)	($n = 118$)	($n = 150$)	($n = 136$)		
Stiffness (0–8)	2.85 ± 1.68	1.84 ± 1.53	2.73 ± 1.38	3.85 ± 1.54	**< 0.001**	**< 0.001**
	($n = 390$)	($n = 116$)	($n = 146$)	($n = 128$)		
Total (0–96)	28.17 ± 15.80	12.49 ± 6.76	26.56 ± 9.32	44.23 ± 11.71	**< 0.001**	**< 0.001**
WOMAC change (T0 to T1)	($n = 404$)	($n = 118$)	($n = 150$)	($n = 136$)		
Pain	0.28 ± 3.90	1.90 ± 2.81	1.25 ± 3.72	−2.21 ± 3.71	**< 0.001**	**< 0.001**
Decrease ≥ 20% (responders)	31% (125)	19% (22)	27% (40)	46% (63)		
0% < decrease < 20%	8% (31)	0% (0)	5% (7)	18% (24)		
Stable = 0% (nonresponders)	14% (55)	14% (17)	14% (21)	13% (17)		
Increase > 0% (nonresponders)	48% (193)	67% (79)	55% (82)	24% (32)	**< 0.001**[e]	**< 0.001**[e]
	($n = 390$)	($n = 116$)	($n = 146$)	($n = 128$)		
Function	0.95 ± 12.50	5.35 ± 9.84	2.56 ± 11.60	−4.89 ± 13.50	**< 0.001**	**< 0.001**
	($n = 404$)	($n = 118$)	($n = 150$)	($n = 136$)		
Stiffness	0.18 ± 1.84	0.43 ± 1.53	0.29 ± 1.77	−0.16 ± 2.10	**0.010**	**0.032**
	($n = 390$)	($n = 116$)	($n = 146$)	($n = 128$)		
Total	1.35 ± 16.71	7.62 ± 13.02	4.12 ± 15.43	−7.50 ± 17.51	**< 0.001**	**< 0.001**

Results are shown as mean ± standard deviation or % and number (n) of participants' IAHA injected knees. Bold data are significant at $p < 0.05$
T0 visit before IAHA treatment, *T1* visit after IAHA treatment, *IAHA* intra-articular hyaluronic acid, *WOMAC* Western Ontario and McMaster Universities Osteoarthritis Index
[a]Number of injected knees based on 310 participants
[b]The level of pain on WOMAC score was divided into three groups (Low, Moderate, and High) based on tertile analysis
[c]WOMAC Likert 3.1 (scale 0–20) pain scores at T0. Participants with WOMAC pain score = 0 were excluded from analysis. A higher score indicates more pain/symptoms and greater function impairment
[d]Continuous variables were compared using Student's t test/Mann–Whitney test
[e]Proportions compared using the chi-squared test/Fisher's exact test

was significantly higher than in the Low pain group. No differences were observed for NSAIDs with or without analgesics or bone anti-remodeling agents.

Responders and nonresponders

The participants with a WOMAC pain score ≥ 8 at T0 (High pain group) were identified as the population of most interest for at least two reasons. First, the level of pain is clinically meaningful and experienced by the majority of knee OA patients seen in consultation who are subject to therapeutic intervention including the use of IAHA injections. Secondly, this is the group of participants in which a greater number were found to experience an improvement in symptoms with IAHA treatment (Table 2). These participants' data (WOMAC pain score ≥ 8 at T0) were further divided into responders and nonresponders (Tables 4 and 5) based on the level of change in the WOMAC score following treatment: responders had a WOMAC pain score decrease ≥ 20%; and nonresponders had a stable or increased WOMAC pain score. Those with a decrease in WOMAC pain < 20% were excluded from the analysis because this level of change (improvement) is generally regarded as not really clinically meaningful.

As shown by the participant characteristics at T0 (Table 4), the majority were responders to IAHA treatment (63 vs 49). The responders were usually younger ($p = 0.014$), with greater cartilage volume in the medial compartment ($p = 0.046$), and a tendency to have greater JSW. No differences were found between responders and nonresponders with regard to BML incidence or score, incidence of medial meniscal extrusion, or synovial effusion size.

Table 3 Concomitant arthritis medication at T0

	Total ($n = 404$)[a]	Low,[b] $0 <$ WOMAC pain[c] < 4 ($n = 118$)	Moderate, $4 \leq$ WOMAC pain[c] ≤ 7 ($n = 150$)	High, WOMAC pain[c] ≥ 8 ($n = 136$)	Low vs High p value[d]	Moderate vs High p value[d]
	($n = 311$)	($n = 89$)	($n = 119$)	($n = 103$)		
NSAIDs ± analgesics	74% (230)	74% (66)	69% (82)	80% (82)	0.370	0.070
	($n = 311$)	($n = 89$)	($n = 119$)	($n = 103$)		
Anti-bone remodeling	17% (52)	18% (16)	18% (22)	14% (14)	0.404	0.324
	($n = 404$)	($n = 118$)	($n = 150$)	($n = 136$)		
Steroid injections	18% (72)	12% (14)	17% (26)	24% (32)	**0.016**	0.193
	($n = 400$)	($n = 117$)	($n = 148$)	($n = 135$)		
Glucosamine ± chondroitin sulfate	49% (194)	56% (65)	52% (77)	39% (52)	**0.007**	**0.023**

Results are shown as % and number (n) of participants' IAHA injected knees. Bold data are significant at $p < 0.05$

T0 visit before IAHA treatment, *NSAID* nonsteroidal anti-inflammatory drug, *IAHA* intra-articular hyaluronic acid, *WOMAC* Western Ontario and McMaster Universities Osteoarthritis Index

[a]Number of injected knees based on 310 participants

[b]The level of pain on WOMAC score was divided into three groups (Low, Moderate, and High) based on tertile analysis

[c]WOMAC Likert 3.1 (scale 0–20) pain scores at T0. Participants with WOMAC pain score = 0 were excluded from analysis

[d]Proportions compared using the chi-squared test/Fisher's exact test

Moreover, the participant characteristics at T0 with regard to symptoms (WOMAC scores; Table 5) were found not to be significantly different between responders and nonresponders when adjusted for age, sex, and BMI. With regard to the WOMAC score change, the differences between responders and nonresponders in all WOMAC scores were found highly significant (Table 5). The mean reduction in WOMAC pain score was almost 50% in responders, with 41% of participants having a reduction > 40% (Table 5). The reductions in WOMAC function, stiffness, and total scores were less pronounced than the WOMAC pain, with a similar proportion experiencing a reduction > 40% (Table 5). The changes in the WOMAC scores in the nonresponder group were positive, indicating, as expected, a worsening of symptoms (Table 5). Overall, there were no significant differences in the use of concomitant arthritis medication (as described in Table 3) between the Low, Moderate and High pain groups, and no significant differences in such use were observed between responders and nonresponders (data not shown).

Discussion

This study demonstrated for the first time, in a large longitudinal database analysis, that injections of IAHA can be effective for the symptomatic treatment of knee OA. The results showed that the treatment was not only useful for the relief of knee pain but that it also improved joint function, especially in patients with certain demographic and clinical characteristics. Data clearly suggested that IAHA injections could be effective for a subset of OA patients: those with greater knee pain at the time of the injections (WOMAC pain ≥ 8), younger age, higher BMI, greater radiographic JSW, and, as assessed by MRI, greater cartilage volume, which indicates less structural damage. Among this subset, the responders were those of younger age, with greater cartilage volume in the medial compartment, and a tendency for a greater JSW. To our knowledge, this is the first time that a subset of predictive variables for good response to IAHA injection therapy has been identified in a longitudinal assessment.

Another key finding was the need to select the responders to IAHA therapy using a cutoff point of at least 20% improvement in WOMAC pain in a population that had a pain score of at least 8 out of 20. T0 pain score ≥ 8 was chosen as it corresponds to a level of symptoms that is perceived as clinically meaningful for patients and, accordingly, was part of the inclusion criteria for many previous clinical trials. Here, such participants demonstrated clinically meaningful results of identifying predictors of response and optimizing patient stratification based on a relatively small population. Although the pain improvement cutoff point of 20% might seem somewhat arbitrary, it is well in accordance with the OMERACT group definition [20] of what minimal pain improvement should be in a responder. Interestingly, this subgroup representing 41% of the responders had > 40% pain improvement, a clear landmark that yielded even more clinical importance. This subgroup, however, was too small to further identify predictors of such excellent response to IAHA therapy.

This study has limitations. Because of the OAI questionnaire design, it was impossible to differentiate between the many different IAHA preparations based on molecular weight (MW), reticulation process, or treatment regimen. Hence, all preparations were considered as a single group. Some studies have demonstrated that IAHA preparations

Table 4 Demographics and imaging characteristics at T0—responders and nonresponders

	Total	High,[a] WOMAC pain[b] ≥ 8			
	Responders and nonresponders (n = 112)[c]	Responders[d] (n = 63)	Nonresponders[e] (n = 49)	p value[f]	p value[g]
Subcohort					
Incidence	34% (38)	35% (22)	33% (16)		
Progression	66% (74)	65% (41)	67% (33)	0.802[h]	-
Injected knee					
Right	50% (56)	46% (29)	55% (27)		
Left	50% (56)	54% (34)	45% (22)	0.341[h]	–
Sex, male	33% (37)	35% (22)	31% (15)	0.631[h]	–
Age (years)	64 ± 9	62 ± 8	67 ± 9	**0.014**	–
	(n = 101)	(n = 58)	(n = 43)		
Body mass index	31.23 ± 6.29	32.09 ± 6.04	30.06 ± 6.50	0.163	–
Kellgren–Lawrence	(n = 60)	(n = 34)	(n = 26)		
Grade 0, 1	10% (6)	9% (3)	12% (3)		
Grade 2	25% (15)	26% (9)	23% (6)		
Grade 3	37% (22)	32% (11)	42% (11)		
Grade 4	28% (17)	32% (11)	23% (6)	0.812[h]	–
	(n = 61)	(n = 33)	(n = 29)		
Joint space width (mm)	3.07 ± 1.46	3.37 ± 1.46	2.74 ± 1.42	0.102	0.150
Magnetic resonance imaging					
Cartilage volume (mm^3)	(n = 71)	(n = 42)	(n = 29)		
Global knee	8746 ± 2554	9016 ± 2707	8354 ± 2306	0.196	0.263
Medial compartment	4065 ± 1472	4334 ± 1455	3675 ± 1434	0.054	**0.046**
Lateral compartment	4680 ± 1417	4682 ± 1517	4679 ± 1286	0.695	0.809
Bone marrow lesion (global knee)	(n = 72)	(n = 43)	(n = 29)		
Presence	49% (35)	51% (22)	45% (13)	0.598[h]	–
Score	2.47 ± 3.16	2.47 ± 3.25	2.47 ± 3.08	0.899	0.901
Medial meniscus	(n = 71)	(n = 41)	(n = 30)		
No extrusion	58% (41)	56% (23)	60% (18)		
Extrusion	42% (30)	44% (18)	40% (12)	0.742[h]	–
	(n = 69)	(n = 40)	(n = 29)		
Synovial fluid volume (ml)	22.95 ± 15.79	22.90 ± 16.63	23.01 ± 14.84	0.766	0.982

Results are shown as mean ± standard deviation or % and number (n) of participants' IAHA injected knees. Bold data are significant at $p < 0.05$

T0 visit before IAHA treatment, *T1* visit after IAHA treatment, *IAHA* intra-articular hyaluronic acid, *WOMAC* Western Ontario and McMaster Universities Osteoarthritis Index

[a]The level of pain on WOMAC score was divided into three groups (Low, Moderate, and High) based on tertile analysis: High represents patients in the highest tertile

[b]WOMAC Likert 3.1 (scale 0–20) pain scores at T0

[c]Number of injected knees based on 99 participants

[d]Responders had a decrease in WOMAC pain score of at least 20% between T0 and T1

[e]Nonresponders had the same WOMAC pain score or an increase in WOMAC pain score between T0 and T1

[f]Continuous variables were compared using Student's t test/Mann–Whitney test

[g]Continuous variables were analyzed using a linear mixed model adjusted for age, sex, and body mass index

[h]Proportions compared using the chi-squared test/Fisher's exact test

of higher MW (> 3000 kDa) have a tendency to offer better long-term knee pain relief [10, 21], and many meta-analyses, including those that do not recommend IAHA, acknowledge more favorable outcomes with high-MW HA preparations.

We also recognize that this study does not include a control group and that IAHA responders may also relate to a "placebo/regression to the mean" effect. However, the aim of the present study was not to determine whether IAHA is effective per se, but to determine

Table 5 WOMAC scores and changes—participants with WOMAC pain score[a] ≥ 8 at T0

	Total	High,[b] WOMAC pain[a] ≥ 8			
	Responders and nonresponders (n = 112)[c]	Responders[d] (n = 63)	Nonresponders[e] (n = 49)	p value[f]	p value[g]
WOMAC at T0					
	(n = 112)	(n = 63)	(n = 49)		
Pain (0–20)	10.44 ± 2.28	10.87 ± 2.37	9.88 ± 2.05	**0.008**	0.112
	(n = 104)	(n = 62)	(n = 42)		
Function (0–68)	29.93 ± 9.43	30.95 ± 8.93	28.41 ± 10.04	0.229	0.223
	(n = 112)	(n = 63)	(n = 49)		
Stiffness (0–8)	3.85 ± 1.50	3.87 ± 1.40	3.82 ± 1.64	0.966	0.364
	(n = 104)	(n = 62)	(n = 42)		
Total (0–96)	44.24 ± 11.67	45.63 ± 11.07	42.20 ± 12.36	0.146	0.163
WOMAC change (T0 to T1)					
	(n = 112)	(n = 63)	(n = 49)		
Pain	−2.41 ± 4.06	−5.31 ± 2.84	1.33 ± 1.52	**< 0.001**	**< 0.001**
20% ≤ decrease < 40%		59% (37)			
Decrease > 40%		41% (26)			
	(n = 104)	(n = 62)	(n = 42)		
Function	−5.30 ± 14.52	−11.88 ± 10.99	4.42 ± 13.69	**< 0.001**	**< 0.001**
20% ≤ decrease < 40%		44% (27)			
Decrease > 40%		21% (13)			
	(n = 112)	(n = 63)	(n = 49)		
Stiffness	−0.16 ± 2.16	−0.75 ± 2.03	0.59 ± 2.10	**< 0.010**	**< 0.001**
20% ≤ decrease < 40%		30% (19)			
Decrease > 40%		25% (16)			
	(n = 104)	(n = 62)	(n = 42)		
Total	−8.17 ± 18.97	−17.95 ± 14.13	6.27 ± 15.76	**< 0.001**	**< 0.001**
20% ≤ decrease < 40%		44% (27)			
Decrease > 40%		27% (17)			

Results are shown as mean ± standard deviation or % and number (n) of participants' IAHA injected knees. Bold data are significant at $p < 0.05$
T0 visit before IAHA treatment, *TI* visit after IAHA treatment, *IAHA* intra-articular hyaluronic acid, *WOMAC* Western Ontario and McMaster Universities Osteoarthritis Index
[a]The level of pain on WOMAC score was divided into three groups (Low, Moderate, and High) based on tertile analysis: High represents patients in the highest tertile
[b]WOMAC Likert 3.1 (scale 0–20) pain scores at T0
[c]Number of injected knees based on 99 participants
[d]Responders had a decrease in WOMAC pain score of at least 20% between T0 and T1
[e]Nonresponders had the same WOMAC pain score or an increase in WOMAC pain score between T0 and T1
[f]Continuous variables were compared using Student's t test/Mann–Whitney test
[g]Continuous variables were analyzed using a linear mixed model adjusted for age, sex, and body mass index

which baseline characteristics may predict responders to such injections vs those who do not respond.

The database information on concomitant therapies including analgesics, NSAIDs, and steroid injections did not identify any difference in the use of such medication between the responders and the nonresponders to IAHA treatment. Furthermore, study power issues precluded the use of these pain treatments as combination therapies with the IAHA administration at T0 to probe a multiplicative effect. One might have expected a better response to IAHA treatment in participants in whom preexisting analgesic usage was present and expect a decrease in the analgesic usage over time if IAHA had been effective. However, the design of the present study and the 12-month interval administration of the OAI questionnaire made it impossible to detect important analgesic use interaction. This problem may be better addressed by comparing those treated with IAHA with a separate control group that was not exposed to analgesics. Moreover, the important issue of compliance and usage frequency of the concomitant therapies, as they could impact upon pain improvement independent of

IAHA usage, could not be fully addressed using information provided by the OAI self-administered questionnaires, contrary to a pill count commonly performed in randomized controlled trials.

Another limitation relates to the participants' characteristics of the population from the OAI cohort which may differ from those in IAHA clinical trials. For instance, 24% of our study population had a KL grading of 4, which would be considered by many as a suboptimal group for response to IAHA treatment. However, despite this uncommon use of IAHA for end-stage radiographic OA, the response to therapy was numerically better (32% vs 23%). These results are in line with previous observations [22].

Surprisingly, 118 out of the 404 IAHA injected knees had a T0 WOMAC pain score of less than 4 out of 20. This could indicate that IAHA was potentially used for knee OA pain prevention and/or joint protection, rather than for treatment of actual pain. Previous studies using the OAI cohort [14, 15] revealed that the participants are overall relatively young compared to those included in most OA clinical trials and have less severe symptoms or are symptom free. Another possible explanation for a low pain score at T0 could be the administration of a 12-month interval questionnaire as per the OAI design, which may not be optimal to timely match symptom assessments for the IAHA treatment.

Statistical power may also be an issue since, by selecting subjects that had received one IAHA treatment but also had all demographic, clinical, and MRI information, the patient number was reduced from 4674 subjects to a mere 404 participants' knees, of which only 136 had WOMAC pain > 8 pre treatment, which is somewhat limited for multivariate analyses.

Importantly, information about the IAHA safety, especially the local injection site reactions reported by patients, was not available from the OAI questionnaires and data sets. Clinical trials have determined that IAHA injections are occasionally accompanied by pain, swelling, or effusion of the treated knee, most of these being self-limited [11, 12]. The effect of repetitive IAHA injections over time with regard to efficacy and safety was also not evaluated in our study.

Further work is needed to assess the structural impact (i.e., knee cartilage protection) of such IAHA injections using the unique opportunity offered by the OAI cohort of analyzing cartilage volume, bone marrow lesions, and meniscal integrity assessed by MRI. A small and unique 2-year randomized controlled trial [23] has already suggested a beneficial effect of Hylan GF-20, a high-MW HA, on cartilage volume and defect scores. Since the present study probed MRI acquisitions only for a maximum of 12 months, it is very likely that the time span may be too narrow to demonstrate such an effect.

This study provides new information about the efficacy and usefulness of IAHA treatment that could assist clinicians' decision-making in treating patients with knee OA, especially with regard to the controversy in recent years surrounding IAHA injections [5, 8, 9]. While some question its efficacy, the reality is that IAHA is approved for knee OA treatment worldwide and has been used for decades [5, 7–9]. A number of guidelines based on systematic review of the randomized controlled trial data on IAHA concluded that, despite mixed results, the overall data support the efficacy of IAHA injections and recommend such therapy [1, 3] or are uncertain [2], while others are strongly against it [6].

Conclusions

This study adds evidence of the usefulness of IAHA therapy, especially for a subset of knee OA patients with high levels of knee pain, younger age, higher BMI, and less severe structural damage. In an era of OA therapeutic choice paucity, this will help in selecting patients for whom IAHA can be an effective way to locally treat knee OA symptoms. However, longer term and controlled studies, as well as safety assessments, should be conducted in the same context of longitudinal follow-up to further probe these initial findings.

Abbreviations

BMI: Body mass index; BML: Bone marrow lesion; IAHA: Intra-articular hyaluronic acid; JSW: Joint space width; KL: Kellgren–Lawrence; MRI: Magnetic resonance imaging; MW: Molecular weight; NSAID: Nonsteroidal anti-inflammatory drug; OA: Osteoarthritis; OAI: Osteoarthritis Initiative; OMERACT: Outcome Measures in Rheumatology; T0: Yearly visit that took place before the IAHA treatment; T1: Yearly visit that took place after the IAHA treatment; WOMAC: Western Ontario and McMaster Universities Osteoarthritis Index

Acknowledgements

The authors would like to thank the OAI participants and Coordinating Center for their work in generating the clinical and radiological data of the OAI cohort and for making them publicly available. They also thank Virginia Wallis for her assistance with the manuscript preparation.

Funding

This initiative was funded by Sanofi Canada through an unrestricted educational grant. Sanofi Canada had no role in the design of the study, the collection, analysis, and interpretation of data, or the writing of the manuscript. The OAI is a public–private partnership comprised of five contracts (NO1-AR-2-2258; NO1-AR-2-2259; NO1-AR-2-2260; NO1-AR-2-2261; NO1-AR-2-2262) funded by the National Institutes of Health, a branch of the Department of Health and Human Services, in four clinical sites (University of Maryland School of Medicine and Johns Hopkins University, Baltimore, MD, USA; Ohio State University, Columbus, OH, USA; University of Pittsburgh, PA, USA; Memorial Hospital of Rhode Island, Pawtucket, RI, USA) and conducted by the OAI study investigators. Private funding partners include Merck Research Laboratories, Novartis Pharmaceuticals Corporation, GlaxoSmithKline, and Pfizer Inc. Private-sector funding for the OAI is managed by the Foundation for the National Institutes of Health.

Authors' contributions

J-PP, J-PR, MD, and JM-P contributed to study conception and design. J-PP, J-PR, FA, PD, and JM-P contributed to acquisition, analysis and interpretation of data. J-PP, J-PR, and JM-P contributed to drafting of the manuscript. J-PP, J-PR, FA, MD, PD, and JM-P contributed to critical revision and approval of the final manuscript.

Competing interests

J-PP is a shareholder in ArthroLab and consultant for Sanofi Canada. J-PR is a consultant for ArthroLab and Sanofi Canada. FA is an employee of ArthroLab. MD is a consultant for ArthroLab. PD is an employee of ArthroLab. JM-P is a shareholder in ArthroLab and consultant for Sanofi Canada.

Author details

[1]Osteoarthritis Research Unit, University of Montreal Hospital Research Centre (CRCHUM), 900 Saint-Denis, Suite R11.412, Montreal, QC H2X 0A9, Canada. [2]Medical Imaging Research & Development, ArthroLab Inc, Montreal, QC, Canada. [3]StatSciences Inc, Notre-Dame-de-l'Île-Perrot, QC, Canada. [4]ArthroLab Inc, Montreal, QC, Canada.

References

1. Bruyere O, Cooper C, Pelletier JP, Maheu E, Rannou F, Branco J, Luisa Brandi M, Kanis JA, Altman RD, Hochberg MC, et al. A consensus statement on the European Society for Clinical and Economic Aspects of Osteoporosis and Osteoarthritis (ESCEO) algorithm for the management of knee osteoarthritis—from evidence-based medicine to the real-life setting. Semin Arthritis Rheum. 2016;45(4 Suppl):S3–11.
2. McAlindon TE, Bannuru RR, Sullivan MC, Arden NK, Berenbaum F, Bierma-Zeinstra SM, Hawker GA, Henrotin Y, Hunter DJ, Kawaguchi H, et al. OARSI guidelines for the non-surgical management of knee osteoarthritis. Osteoarthr Cartil. 2014;22(3):363–88.
3. Hochberg MC, Altman RD, April KT, Benkhalti M, Guyatt G, McGowan J, Towheed T, Welch V, Wells G, Tugwell P. American College of Rheumatology 2012 recommendations for the use of nonpharmacologic and pharmacologic therapies in osteoarthritis of the hand, hip, and knee. Arthritis Care Res (Hoboken). 2012;64(4):465–74.
4. Jordan KM, Arden NK, Doherty M, Bannwarth B, Bijlsma JW, Dieppe P, Gunther K, Hauselmann H, Herrero-Beaumont G, Kaklamanis P, et al. EULAR Recommendations 2003: an evidence based approach to the management of knee osteoarthritis: Report of a Task Force of the Standing Committee for International Clinical Studies Including Therapeutic Trials (ESCISIT). Ann Rheum Dis. 2003;62(12):1145–55.
5. Bhandari M, Bannuru RR, Babins EM, Martel-Pelletier J, Khan M, Raynauld JP, Frankovich R, McLeod D, Devji T, Phillips M, et al. Intra-articular hyaluronic acid in the treatment of knee osteoarthritis: a Canadian evidence-based perspective. Ther Adv Musculoskel Dis. 2017;9(9):231–46.
6. Jevsevar DS. Treatment of osteoarthritis of the knee: evidence-based guideline, 2nd edition. J Am Acad Orthop Surg. 2013;21(9):571–6.
7. Cooper C, Rannou F, Richette P, Bruyere O, Al-Daghri N, Altman RD, Luisa Brandi M, Collaud Basset S, Herrero-Beaumont G, Migliore A, et al. Use of intra-articular hyaluronic acid in the management of knee osteoarthritis in clinical practice. Arthritis Care Res (Hoboken). 2017;69(9):1287–96.
8. Migliore A, Bizzi E, Herrero-Beaumont J, Petrella RJ, Raman R, Chevalier X. The discrepancy between recommendations and clinical practice for viscosupplementation in osteoarthritis: mind the gap. Eur Rev Med Pharmacol Sci. 2015;19(7):1124–9.
9. Altman RD, Schemitsch E, Bedi A. Assessment of clinical practice guideline methodology for the treatment of knee osteoarthritis with intra-articular hyaluronic acid. Semin Arthritis Rheum. 2015;45(2):132–9.
10. Bellamy N, Campbell J, Robinson V, Gee T, Bourne R, Wells G. Viscosupplementation for the treatment of osteoarthritis of the knee. Cochrane Database Syst Rev. 2006;2:CD005321.
11. Bannuru RR, Schmid CH, Kent DM, Vaysbrot EE, Wong JB, McAlindon TE. Comparative effectiveness of pharmacologic interventions for knee osteoarthritis: a systematic review and network meta-analysis. Ann Intern Med. 2015;162(1):46–54.
12. Rutjes AW, Juni P, da Costa BR, Trelle S, Nuesch E, Reichenbach S. Viscosupplementation for osteoarthritis of the knee: a systematic review and meta-analysis. Ann Intern Med. 2012;157(3):180–91.
13. Raynauld JP, Pelletier JP, Abram F, Dodin P, Delorme P, Martel-Pelletier J. Long-term effects of glucosamine and chondroitin sulfate on the progression of structural changes in knee osteoarthritis: six-year followup data from the Osteoarthritis Initiative. Arthritis Care Res (Hoboken). 2016; 68(10):1560–6.
14. Roubille C, Martel-Pelletier J, Abram F, Dorais M, Delorme P, Raynauld JP, Pelletier JP. Impact of disease treatments on the progression of knee osteoarthritis structural changes related to meniscal extrusion: data from the OAI progression cohort. Semin Arthritis Rheum. 2015;45(3):257–67.
15. Martel-Pelletier J, Roubille C, Abram F, Hochberg MC, Dorais M, Delorme P, Raynauld JP, Pelletier JP. First-line analysis of the effects of treatment on progression of structural changes in knee osteoarthritis over 24 months: data from the osteoarthritis initiative progression cohort. Ann Rheum Dis. 2015;74(3):547–56.
16. Dodin P, Pelletier JP, Martel-Pelletier J, Abram F. Automatic human knee cartilage segmentation from 3D magnetic resonance images. IEEE Trans Biomed Eng. 2010;57:2699–711.
17. Dodin P, Abram F, Pelletier J-P, Martel-Pelletier J. A fully automated system for quantification of knee bone marrow lesions using MRI and the osteoarthritis initiative cohort. J Biomed Graph Comput. 2013;3(1):51–65.
18. Li W, Abram F, Pelletier JP, Raynauld JP, Dorais M, d'Anjou MA, Martel-Pelletier J. Fully automated system for the quantification of human osteoarthritic knee joint effusion volume using magnetic resonance imaging. Arthritis Res Ther. 2010;12(5):R173.
19. Berthiaume MJ, Raynauld JP, Martel-Pelletier J, Labonté F, Beaudoin G, Bloch DA, Choquette D, Haraoui B, Altman RD, Hochberg M, et al. Meniscal tear and extrusion are strongly associated with the progression of knee osteoarthritis as assessed by quantitative magnetic resonance imaging. Ann Rheum Dis. 2005;64:556–63.
20. Pham T, van der Heijde D, Altman RD, Anderson JJ, Bellamy N, Hochberg M, Simon L, Strand V, Woodworth T, Dougados M. OMERACT-OARSI initiative: Osteoarthritis Research Society International set of responder criteria for osteoarthritis clinical trials revisited. Osteoarthr Cartil. 2004;12(5):389–99.
21. Altman RD, Devji T, Bhandari M, Fierlinger A, Niazi F, Christensen R. Clinical benefit of intra-articular saline as a comparator in clinical trials of knee osteoarthritis treatments: a systematic review and meta-analysis of randomized trials. Semin Arthritis Rheum. 2016;46(2):151–9.
22. Altman R, Lim S, Steen RG, Dasa V. Hyaluronic acid injections are associated with delay of total knee replacement surgery in patients with knee osteoarthritis: evidence from a large U.S. health claims database. PLoS One. 2015;10(12):e0145776.
23. Wang Y, Hall S, Hanna F, Wluka AE, Grant G, Marks P, Feletar M, Cicuttini FM. Effects of Hylan G-F 20 supplementation on cartilage preservation detected by magnetic resonance imaging in osteoarthritis of the knee: a two-year single-blind clinical trial. BMC Musculoskelet Disord. 2011;12:195.

9

Development of a clinical prediction algorithm for knee osteoarthritis structural progression in a cohort study: value of adding measurement of subchondral bone density

Michael P. LaValley[1], Grace H. Lo[2,3], Lori Lyn Price[4], Jeffrey B. Driban[5], Charles B. Eaton[6] and Timothy E. McAlindon[5*]

Abstract

Background: Risk prediction algorithms increase understanding of which patients are at greatest risk of a harmful outcome. Our goal was to create a clinically useful prediction algorithm for structural progression of knee osteoarthritis (OA), using medial joint space loss as a proxy; and to quantify the benefit of including periarticular bone mineral density (BMD) in the algorithm.

Methods: Participants were from the Osteoarthritis Initiative (OAI) Progression Cohort, with X-ray readings of medial joint space at 36- and 48-month visits, and a 30- or 36-month medial-to-lateral tibial BMD ratio (M:L BMD ratio) value. Loss of medial joint space was the outcome and clinically available factors associated with OA progression were employed in the base prediction algorithm, with M:L BMD ratio added to an enhanced prediction algorithm. The benefit of adding M:L BMD ratio was evaluated by change in area under the ROC curve (AUC), net reclassification improvement (NRI), and integrated discrimination improvement (IDI).

Results: Five hundred thirty-three participants were included; 51 (14%) had medial joint space loss; 47% were female; the mean (SD) age was 64.6 (9.2) years and BMI was 29.6 (4.8) kg/m^2. The base algorithm model included age, BMI, gender, recent injury, knee pain, and hand OA as predictors and had an AUC value of 0.65. The algorithm adding M:L BMD ratio had an AUC value of 0.73, and the AUC, NRI and IDI were all significantly improved ($p \leq 0.002$).

Conclusions: This clinical prediction algorithm predicts structural progression in individuals with OA using only clinically available predictors supplemented by the M:L BMD ratio, a biomarker that could be made available at clinical sites.

Keywords: Arthritis, Calibration, Discrimination, Joint space loss, Logistic regression, ROC curve, X-ray

Background

Osteoarthritis (OA) is the most common type of arthritis and is a substantial public health problem [1, 2]. Treatments for OA include nonsteroidal anti-inflammatory drugs (NSAIDs), physical therapy, and ultimately arthroplasty. A challenge in the clinical management of patients with OA is the variable pace of disease progression and prediction of which patients are in need of intervention [3]. Therefore, there is an important need for an algorithm that can stratify OA patients by their level of risk for progression over a short period of time. In addition, such an algorithm could be used to stratify subjects for inclusion in clinical trials for development of additional therapies [4].

There have been statistical models developed to predict the incidence [5–7] and progression [7–9] of structural changes in knee OA progression in the OA literature, however, their use may be difficult due to inclusion of

* Correspondence: tmcalindon@tuftsmedicalcenter.org
[5]Division of Rheumatology Tufts Medical Center, Box #406, 800 Washington Street, Boston, MA 02111, USA
Full list of author information is available at the end of the article

radiographic or genetic biomarkers that require specialized equipment or personnel for assessment.

A different potential biomarker for knee OA structural progression is the medial-to-lateral tibial plateau bone mineral density ratio (M:L BMD ratio). This ratio can be acquired from dual-energy X-ray absorptiometry (DXA) scanners which are currently available for clinical imaging at many sites. The M:L BMD ratio may serve as a useful component of a prediction tool as it provides a measure of the bone underlying the knee, and the measurement can be semi-automated. DXA studies of periarticular bone have shown that knee compartments with localized OA have greater BMD than uninvolved regions [10–13]. This difference has been commonly standardized as the calculated ratio of BMD between the two compartments [11–17]. Use of this internal reference conveniently controls for individual variations in BMD [11] and the ratio is precise, with reported coefficients of variation ranging from 1 to 7% [10–16, 18, 19]. The M:L BMD ratio is predictive of knee OA severity [11, 13] and is highly correlated with compartment-specific joint space narrowing (JSN), osteophytes and sclerosis [16]. The co-location of radiographic sclerosis and region measured for the M:L BMD ratio suggests that these two measures may both reflect a similar process [16]. However, the M:L BMD ratio appears to be a more sensitive measure of this process because removal of radiographs which exhibit sclerosis on radiographs only partly attenuates its association with OA [16]. Furthermore, the M:L BMD ratio is associated with subchondral pathologies such as bone marrow lesions (which are themselves associated with OA progression) [15, 16, 20–25]. Two small longitudinal studies showed that unloading a knee is associated with a reduction of the M:L BMD ratio, suggesting that it is also responsive to changes in knee loading [11, 17].

Study objectives

The first objective of this study was to develop and evaluate two prediction algorithms for knee OA structural progression in participants with existing knee OA. These algorithms will be (1) a base model, which includes factors that are currently readily available in a typical setting, and (2) an enhanced model that adds the M:L BMD ratio to the base model. The second objective was to quantify the improvement in prediction obtained when the M:L BMD ratio is added to the base model.

Methods

Source of study participants: the Osteoarthritis Initiative (OAI) progression cohort

The OAI is a multicenter cohort study that collected longitudinal clinical and image data in participants with, or at high risk of, knee OA over a 9-year period [26]. OAI progression cohort participants were 45–79 years of age at recruitment in the clinical sites of Baltimore, MD, Pawtucket, RI, Columbus, OH and Pittsburgh, PA, and had symptomatic knee OA in at least one knee.

So that the study sample mirrored subjects in clinical care for knee OA, we included participants from the progression cohort of the OAI. At the OAI baseline visit, these participants had knee pain, aching or stiffness on most days of 1 month of the preceding year and radiographic tibiofemoral knee OA (Osteoarthritis Research Society International (OARSI) atlas grades 1–3) on a fixed-flexion radiograph at recruitment in at least one knee, but not necessarily in their study knee. Most subjects had radiographic OA in their study knee, but we also chose to include the participants without OA in their study knee in our analyses to reflect clinical care of patients with contralateral OA. More information on the inclusion and exclusion criteria for the OAI progression cohort is available at http://oai.epi-ucsf.org. This study was approved by the Institutional Review Boards at the four clinical sites, Baylor College of Medicine, and Tufts Medical Center.

The goal of the Bone Ancillary Study was to investigate the influence of bone on structural progression in knee OA. Participants in this ancillary study were recruited from the four OAI clinical sites at the 30- or 36-month visit at which visit knee DXA scans were acquired (August 2007 to April 2009). While 600 participants was the ancillary study enrollment target for the progression cohort, 629 were ultimately enrolled. For this analysis we used progression cohort participants who were included in the Bone Ancillary Study who also had radiographic readings from the 36- and 48-month OAI examinations.

Outcome: progression measures

At the 24-, 36- and 48-month examinations, posterior-anterior radiographs were taken with a fixed flexion in weight-bearing position using a positioning frame to provide optimal assessment of change in joint space. All radiographs were read for medial and lateral joint space using the OARSI 0–3 scale [27] by trained readers and within grade scores (e.g., 2.2, 2.4, etc.) were allowed. The reliability for these readings (read-reread) was high (weighted kappa [intra-rater reliability] = 0.88 [95% CI 0.80–0.95]). The 24-month radiographs were further evaluated for the Kellgren and Lawrence grade [28], and we use the knees with grades of 2 or more in subset analyses of knees with radiographic OA. All radiographic readings were obtained from the OAI public data release (kXR_SQ_BU_03 (versions 5.5 and 6.3) and kXR_SQ_BU_06).

Our measurement for structural OA progression was loss of medial joint space within a single knee from each participant on the radiograph between the 36- and 48-month examinations. We did not include loss of lateral joint space as a progression as there were few of these and they may reflect a different process. We took any increase in the medial joint space value, including increases within an OARSI grade (such as from 2.0 to 2.4), as a progression event. In addition, any knee replacements that occurred by the 48-month visit in study knees with predominantly medial involvement at the 36-month radiograph, by consensus of the authors, were counted as progression events.

Exposure (biomarker): M:L BMD ratio

Our exposure of main interest is the M:L BMD ratio, a DXA imaging biomarker for knee OA [29]. The M:L BMD ratio measure of the study knee was acquired at recruitment of a participant into the Bone Ancillary Study, either at the OAI 30- or 36-month examination, using the techniques described below.

Tibial plateau dual-energy X-ray absorptiometry

The proximal tibiae were evaluated using one of four identical DXA systems (Lunar Prodigy Advance, GE Lunar Corp., Madison WI, USA) at each OAI clinical site with investigational knee software (enCORE 2007 Version 11.20.068). The lower extremity was positioned with the long axis of the tibia perpendicular to the X-ray beam, and neutrally rotated. A foam knee positioner, which was posterior to the popliteal fossa, placed the knee in mild flexion. The foot positioner was then applied to the ipsilateral foot using a Velcro strap around the perimeter of the foot and the positioner. This resulted in the ipsilateral toes oriented perpendicular to the scanning bed and the plantar surface of the ipsilateral foot adjacent to the perpendicular edge of the positioner, parallel to the lower border of the scanner bed. A positioning laser centered the scanner arm 5 centimeters below the inferior pole of the patella. The knee was then imaged using DXA (Fig. 1).

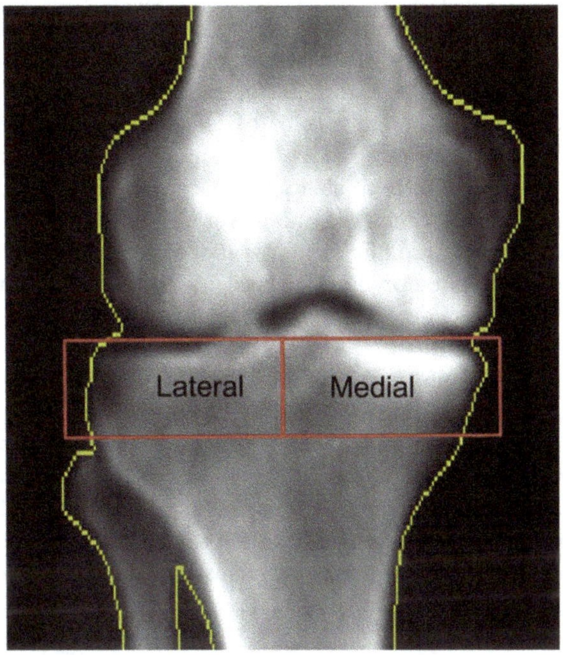

Fig. 1 DXA knee scan with regions of interest for the M:L BMD ratio

Tibial plateau dual-energy X-ray absorptiometry image analysis

Two DXA analysts determined the tibial plateau BMD measurements using a customizable region of interest. The height of the medial and lateral tibial regions of interest was fixed at 20 mm while the region of interest width in the medio-lateral direction was set as half the distance between the medial and lateral bone edges along a line midway between the far medial and lateral points of the tibial plateau (Fig. 1) [14]. The bone edges (*yellow outline*) served as the outer border of the region of interests. The regions of interest were positioned so that their top edges were just superior and parallel to the medial joint surfaces of the tibia [14]. The medial and lateral tibial bone mineral densities were divided to generate M:L BMD ratio scores. The scan-rescan (with repositioning) intra-class correlation was 0.993 (95% CI 0.982–0.997) [29]. Both the intra-rater reliability and inter-rater reliability (measurement-remeasurement) were excellent at 0.98–0.99.

Predictive factors

For our base model we evaluated readily available clinical predictors from the OAI data, based on their reported connection to knee OA structural progression in the literature, with the consideration that there should be close to ten progression events per included predictor [30]. From the literature we chose to include age, gender and body mass index (BMI), knee pain and injury regardless of statistical significance [31, 32] Other potential predictors were screened in bivariate analyses with progression in our study sample, and included if their p values were 0.2 or less. While radiographic measures, such as Kellgren and Lawrence grade, joint space width, or knee alignment, can be strong predictors of OA progression, we did not include these in the prediction models as they would require advanced radiographic assessment which is not standard in routine clinical management for OA. However, we did include the presence of Kellgren and Lawrence grade of 2 or more at the 24-month examination as a descriptive factor and to perform a subgroup analysis restricted to knees with radiographic OA.

In our base model we included gender, age, BMI, knee pain, previous injury to the knee (yes/no), and the presence of hand OA (yes/no). BMI was calculated by dividing the weight of the subject in kilograms by the height (squared) of the subject in meters, with both measures taken from the DXA examination evaluation. The knee pain assessment was from a 0–10 visual analog scale for pain in the study knee from the 36-month examination. The presence of a knee injury was taken to be a positive response to the question "Were you injured badly enough to limit ability to walk for at least 2 days, since last visit about 12 months ago?" administered at the 36-month examination. We judged hand OA to be present if three or more Heberden's nodes (from both hands) were detected in the clinical examination at recruitment to the OAI as this cutoff gave the strongest association with progression. Predictive factors and presence of radiographic OA were compared between knees which were excluded from analysis due to lack of a measure of 48-month medial joint space and those included in the prediction analysis. Logistic regression models were used to provide univariate and multivariable adjusted odds ratios for association with progression.

Statistical modeling and assessment

To evaluate the linearity of association between continuous predictors and the dichotomous outcome of OA progression (yes/no), we compared the goodness of fit of logistic regression models using either natural cubic splines that can accommodate non-linear effects or linear trends to model the association [33, 34]. The base prediction model was constructed using logistic regression and the predictive factors listed above. The BMD enhanced prediction model was constructed using logistic regression with the same predictive factors but also adding the M:L BMD ratio biomarker. The analysis used the presence of loss in medial joint space between the 36- and 48-month examinations as the outcome as the biomarker assessment strictly precedes all joint space measures used for the outcome. In a subgroup analysis, we performed the same evaluation restricted to subjects whose knees had more advanced osteoarthritis as measured by a Kellgren and Lawrence score of 2 or more at the 24-month examination.

The prediction models were evaluated on two characteristics – discrimination and calibration. Discrimination measures how well the model distinguishes between participants who experience OA progression and those who do not. Discrimination was assessed using area under the curve (AUC), with guidelines suggesting that values of at least 0.70 are needed for adequate prediction [35]. Calibration measures if the model systematically over or under-predicts OA progression. While calibration is often assessed using the Hosmer and Lemeshow test, this approach has been criticized [36] and we employ an approach which evaluates the intercept and slope from a new logistic regression model fit to the same outcome and using only the predictions from the preceding model as a predictor. If the new logistic regression intercept is close to 0 and the slope close to 1 then the initial model is well calibrated.

To evaluate whether a new biomarker is informative beyond previously established markers and predictors, the predictive ability of the model enhanced with the new biomarker is compared to the base model. Change in the AUC between models gives the change in overall discrimination; the net reclassification improvement (NRI) adds the percent of observations with OA progression that have an increased predicted value in the enhanced model and the percent of observations without progression that have a reduction in predicted value. The integrated discrimination improvement (IDI) adds the average increase in predicted values in the observations with OA progression to the average decrease in predicted values in observations without OA progression [37]. As a prediction algorithm based on a logistic regression model with few OA progression events per predictor is prone to produce overly optimistic estimates that do not generalize to other data sets, so we used an internal validation approach to reduce this bias [33]. The internal validation uses a tenfold cross-validation procedure to produce predicted values with reduced bias for use in assessing the logistic regression discrimination, calibration, and improvement measures.

Results

Description of cohort

Out of 629 Bone Ancillary Study participants from the OAI progression subcohort, 96 participants were excluded due to indeterminate medial progression values (missing the 48-month visit, or unreadable medial joint space on either the 36 or 48-month radiograph), leaving 533 participants for the primary analysis. The excluded subjects had a higher mean BMI ($p = 0.04$) and had higher percentages of females ($p < 0.01$), knee injury ($p < 0.01$), and radiographic OA ($p < 0.01$) than subjects remaining in the analysis.

There were 51 knees with medial joint space progression (9.6%), including five knees which underwent total knee replacement with predominately medial OA at 36 months. Table 1 provides the descriptive characterization of these knees both overall and by progression status.

Logistic regression modeling

Univariate and multivariate odds ratios for the associations between descriptive characteristics and OA progression are shown in Table 2. The continuous values of age, body mass index, and M:L BMD are modeled as linear terms in the regression corresponding to a one standard deviation increase in value.

Table 1 Descriptive characteristics by primary analysis outcome

Characteristic	Overall (*n* = 533)	Non-progressors (*n* = 482)	Progressors (*n* = 51)
Female (*n*, %)	252 (47%)	226 (47%)	26 (51%)
Age years (mean, SD)	64.6 (9.2)	64.2 (9.2)	68.3 (7.5)
Body mass index kg/m^2 (mean, SD)	29.6 (4.8)	29.5 (4.7)	30.4 (4.9)
Knee pain (mean, SD)	3.5 (2.8)	3.4 (2.8)	4.1 (2.7)
Recent injury (*n*, %)	11 (2%)	9 (2%)	2 (4%)
Hand OA (*n*, %)	191 (36%)	160 (33%)	31 (61%)
M:L BMD (mean, SD)	1.1 (0.2)	1.1 (0.1)	1.2 (0.2)
Radiographic knee OA (*n*, %)	369 (69%)	324 (67%)	45 (88%)

OA osteoarthritis, *M:L BMD ratio* medial-to-lateral tibial plateau bone mineral density ratio

Initial analyses indicated that the M:L BMD ratio, age and BMI had non-linear trends as predictors of medial joint space loss, and were modeled using natural cubic splines. The knee pain measure did show a linear trend with medial joint space loss and was used as a linear predictor. Figure 2 shows the form of the spline for M:L BMD ratio in the initial analysis: the risk of medial joint space loss is close to 0 for ratio values below 1, there is an upward bend for values near 1, and then a linear increase in the risk for ratio values above 1.

The base model includes age and BMI as natural cubic splines, knee pain as a linear term, and sex, recent injury, and presence of hand OA as dichotomous predictors. The BMD enhanced model has the same set of predictors plus a natural cubic spline for the M:L BMD ratio. Adding in the spline for M:L BMD increases the AUC measure of discrimination from 0.65 in the base model to 0.73 in the BMD enhanced model, for a difference of 0.08 with a 95% confidence interval from 0.03 to 0.13 ($p = 0.002$). The BMD enhanced model has an AUC value above the threshold of 0.70 which denotes acceptable discrimination [35]. Both models show good calibration with intercept estimates equal to 0 out to 5 decimal places, and slopes equal to 1 out to 4 decimal places.

Table 2 Univariate and multivariate associations with the primary analysis outcome

Characteristic	Univariate odds ratio (95% CI)	Multivariable odds ratio (95% CI)
Female	1.18 (0.66, 2.11)	1.06 (0.56, 2.01)
Age, years[a]	1.58 (1.18, 2.16)	1.45 (1.02, 2.08)
Body mass index kg/m^2 [a]	1.20 (0.90, 1.59)	1.32 (0.95, 1.84)
Knee pain[a]	1.28 (0.96, 1.70)	1.06 (0.77, 1.47)
Recent injury	2.14 (0.32, 8.60)	2.58 (0.39, 16.92)
Hand OA	3.12 (1.74, 5.72)	2.68 (1.39, 5.19)
M:L BMD[a]	1.94 (1.47, 2.58)	1.76 (1.32, 2.35)
Radiographic knee OA	3.33 (1.50, 8.87)	2.20 (0.88, 5.50)

OA osteoarthritis, *M:L BMD ratio* medial-to-lateral tibial plateau bone mineral density ratio

[a]Odds ratio estimates per 1 standard deviation change in predictor

Evaluation of improvement in prediction with M:L BMD

Figure 3 shows the cross-validated predicted probability of progression from the base model on the horizontal axis and the cross-validated predicted probability from the BMD enhanced model on the vertical axis for each participant. Improvement in prediction in the BMD enhanced model compared to the base model is shown by most participants with OA progression (*solid blue points*) appearing above the diagonal line and most participants without progression (*red circles*) below the diagonal. The results displayed in Fig. 3 are quantified using the NRI and IDI in Table 3. The percentage of the 51 subjects who did experience progression who had an increased predicted risk or progression from the BMD enhanced model compared to the base model minus those with a decrease in risk was 22%. In the 482 subjects without progression, the net percentage of subjects with decreased predicted risk was 27%. From these values, the overall NRI value is 0.49 and this is statistically significant ($p = 0.001$). In participants with joint space loss there is an average increase in predicted value of 0.04 in the BMD enhanced model compared to the base; and the average predicted value is the same in both models for participants without joint space loss. This gives an IDI value of 0.04 which is also statistically significant ($p = 0.002$).

In the subgroup analysis that was restricted to the 365 knees with Kellgren and Lawrence grade of 2 or more at the 24-month examination, 45 had medial joint space progression (12.3%). While the AUC, NRI and IDI values were as good or better than those in the full analysis, neither the base nor BMD enhanced model had adequate calibration. The intercept estimates were far from 0 (-0.99 in the base model, and -0.63 for the BMD enhanced model), and the slopes well below 1 (0.47 in the base model, 0.63 in the BMD enhanced model). The slopes below 1 indicate that the predictions were too

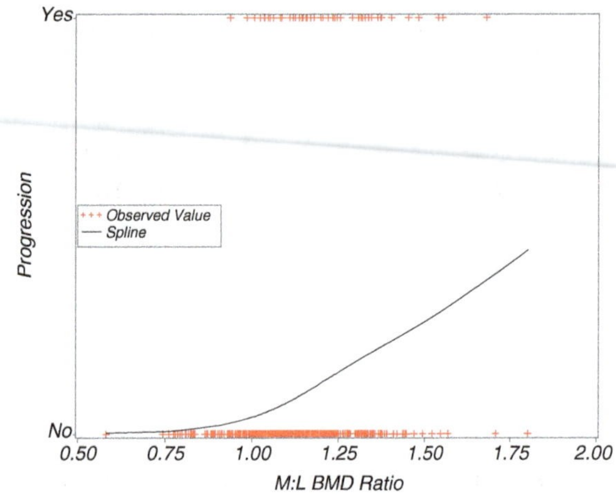

Fig. 2 Unadjusted predicted risk of medial progression from univariate logistic regression with a natural cubic spline for M:L BMD ratio. Uses the outcomes from the primary analysis. *M:L BMD ratio* medial-to-lateral tibial plateau bone mineral density ratio

extreme in these subgroup models – low predictions were exaggeratedly low, and high predictions exaggeratedly high – indicating the subgroup was too small to adequately fit the models [36].

Discussion

We found the M:L BMD ratio together with routine clinically available patient characteristics to provide acceptable prediction of loss of medial joint space over 1 year of follow-up. In addition, the M:L BMD ratio provided a significant improvement in prediction above what would be possible using only the clinically available patient characteristics, using both the net reclassification improvement and the integrated discrimination improvement measures. However, when restricted to the subgroup of knees with advanced OA (Kellgren and Lawrence grade of 2 or more), the M:L BMD ratio model was not well-calibrated, which could indicate the model having too many terms to estimate with the reduced sample size.

There have been five sets of prediction rules developed for knee OA of which we are aware: Zhang et al. used clinical factors along with radiographic information to develop two prediction rules for incidence and one for progression of knee OA [7]; Kraus et al. used clinical data along with a radiographic fractal signature analysis to develop a prediction rule for progressive OA [9]; Kerkhof et al. used clinical, radiographic and genetic information to predict incidence of knee OA [5]; Blanco et al. used clinical and genetic data to predict progression to end-stage OA (Kellgren and Lawrence grade 4 or total knee replacement) [8]; and Losina et al. used their osteoarthritis policy model to calculate lifetime risk of symptomatic knee OA using demographic, occupational, family history, and medical diagnosis of knee OA [6]. While we focused on progression of knee OA, our prediction model is different than those of Zhang, Kraus, Kerkhof, Blanco, or Losina. To maintain clinical utility for our prediction model, only easily obtainable patient and clinical factors were used except for the M:L BMD ratio biomarker, which would provide a new usage of the broadly available DXA scanners. In addition, previous efforts have based outcomes directly on changes in Kellgren and Lawrence grade, where we have focused on the medial compartment to reduce heterogeneity in the outcome.

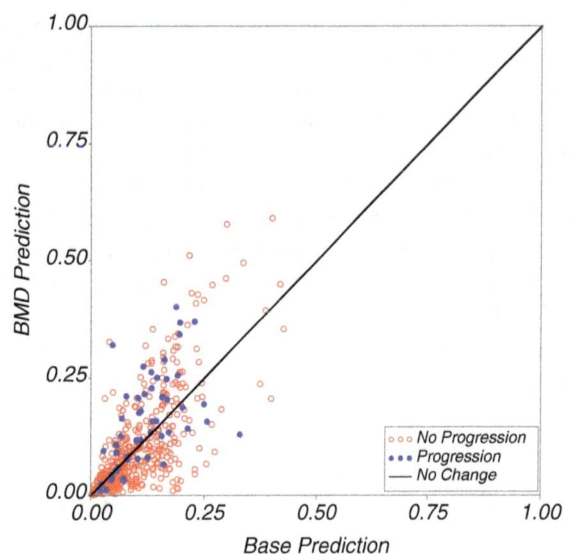

Fig. 3 Predicted risk of progression from the model including M:L BMD ratio on the Y-axis plotted against predicted probability of progression in the base model on the X-axis for the primary analysis outcome. A strong biomarker is shown by having the participants with progression *above the diagonal line* and the participants without progression *below the line*. *BMD* bone mineral density

Limitations of study

Current literature on prediction rules call for validation of rules on external datasets, as the results are generally less impressive in data not used to generate the prediction rules. However, we did not have access to another dataset with both measures of OA progression and the M:L BMD ratio biomarker. Our use of cross-validation did reduce the bias in assessment of the prediction algorithms, but ideally these should be evaluated in an independent dataset. We hope to perform this external validation in future work. In addition, even though we are using a large number of participants with symptomatic knee OA, the number of progression events was not as large as would be

Table 3 Improvement measures comparing base and BMD models in primary analysis

Improvement measure	Outcome	Base model	BMD model	Comparison
Net reclassification improvement			Net % improvement	NRI (95% CI)
	OA progression	Ref	22%	0.49 (0.20, 0.77)
	No OA progression	Ref	27%	
Integrated discrimination improvement		Base model average prediction	BMD model average prediction	IDI (95% CI)
	OA progression	0.12	0.16	0.04 (0.01, 0.06)
	No OA progression	0.09	0.09	

BMD bone mineral density, *OA* osteoarthritis

ideal for development of a prediction rule. This led us to be more sparing in the use of potential predictors in the base model than we would have preferred.

As our interest was to create prediction rules for OA progression that would be relevant for patients in clinical care for osteoarthritis we used subjects with initial findings of osteoarthritis from the OAI cohort. However, some knees still had OARSI grade 0, i.e., intact medial joint space, at the 36-month evaluation. So, our progression measure includes what might be considered incident joint space loss as well as progression of previously reduced joint space. As incident and progressive OA may have different risk factors, our progression model may mix these disparate predictors. However, these are still the predictors that would apply to patients in clinical care with a mix of incident and progressive disease at different locations with the knee. In addition, we have attempted to use the predictors that would be available in the clinical context, with the exception of our main exposure, the M:L BMD value. While this is not available in clinical care, it could provide a means of using widely available DXA scanners to better utilize the quality of bone in caring for OA patients. In addition, we have limited our evaluation to changes in the medial joint space, which excludes the less common, but still important, lateral compartment changes.

Finally, we note that there has been controversy over how to best study the progression of OA as it is challenging to provide causal interpretations for adjusted estimates in studies of subjects with established disease [38]. However, these predictive algorithms and models do not address the causality of exposures and biomarkers, just their ability to provide an early warning of future disease outcomes. So, these concerns regarding causality do not apply to this research.

Conclusions

So, in conclusion, we found that a prediction model composed of patient characteristics and the M:L BMD ratio provided adequate prediction of medial-compartment knee OA progression. The M:L ratio biomarker provided an important component of this prediction rule as it statistically significantly increased the discrimination and enhanced the predictive ability of this rule.

Abbreviations

AUC: Area under the curve; BMD: Bone mineral density; BMI: Body mass index; DXA: Dual-energy X-ray absorptiometry; IDI: Integrated discrimination improvement; JSN: Joint space narrowing; M:L BMD ratio: Medial-to-lateral tibial plateau bone mineral density ratio; NRI: Net reclassification improvement; OA: Osteoarthritis; OAI: Osteoarthritis Initiative; OARSI: Osteoarthritis Research Society International

Funding

Periarticular Bone Density as a Biomarker for Early Knee Osteoarthritis" is sponsored by National Institutes of Health/National Institute of Arthritis and Musculoskeletal and Skin Diseases (NIH/NIAMS) (McAlindon R01 AR 060718) providing support for design and conduct of the study, analysis, and interpretation of the data; and preparation and review of this work. Dr. Lo is supported by K23 AR062127, an NIH/NIAMS-funded mentored award, providing support for design and conduct of the study, analysis, and interpretation of the data; and preparation and review of this work. This work is supported in part with resources at the VA HSR&D Center for Innovations in Quality, Effectiveness and Safety (#CIN 13-413), at the Michael E. DeBakey VA Medical Center, Houston, TX, USA. The Osteoarthritis Initiative is a public-private partnership comprised of five contracts (N01-AR-2-2258; N01-AR-2-2259; N01-AR-2-2260; N01-AR-2-2261; N01-AR-2-2262) funded by the National Institutes of Health, a branch of the Department of Health and Human Services, and conducted by the Osteoarthritis Initiative Study Investigators. Private funding partners include Merck Research Laboratories; Novartis Pharmaceuticals Corporation, GlaxoSmithKline; and Pfizer, Inc. Private sector funding for the Osteoarthritis Initiative is managed by the Foundation for the National Institutes of Health.

Authors' contributions

TM and GL made substantial contributions to study conception and design, and to data acquisition, analysis, and interpretation. LLP and JD were involved in the study design, data acquisition, analysis, and interpretation. CE made substantial contributions to analysis and interpretation of data. ML performed the statistical analyses, interpreted the results, and wrote the manuscript draft while TM, GL, LLP, JD and CE revised it critically. ML, TM, GL, LLP, JD, and CE read and approved the final manuscript.

Competing interests

The authors declare that they have no competing interests.

Ethics approval and consent to participate

This study received ethical approval from each OAI clinical site (Memorial Hospital of Rhode Island Institutional Review Board, The Ohio State University's Biomedical Sciences Institutional Review Board, University of Pittsburgh Institutional Review Board, and University of Maryland Baltimore - Institutional Review Board), and the OAI coordinating center (Committee on Human Research at University of California, San Francisco), the Tufts Health Sciences Institutional Review Board, and the Baylor College of Medicine Institutional Review Board. All patients provided written informed consent for participation in the OAI.

Author details

[1]Department of Biostatistics, Boston University School of Public Health, 801 Massachusetts Avenue 3rd Floor, Boston, MA 02118, USA. [2]Medical Care Line and Research Care Line, Houston VA HSR&D Center for Innovations in Quality, Effectiveness and Safety, Michael E. DeBakey Medical Center, Houston, TX 77030, USA. [3]Section of Immunology, Allergy, and Rheumatology, Baylor College of Medicine, 1 Baylor Plaza, BCM-285, Houston, TX 77030, USA. [4]Institute for Clinical Research and Health Policy Studies at Tufts Medical Center, Tufts Clinical and Translational Science Institute, Tufts University, 800 Washington Street, Box #63, Boston, MA 02111, USA. [5]Division of Rheumatology Tufts Medical Center, Box #406, 800 Washington Street, Boston, MA 02111, USA. [6]Department of Family Medicine, Alpert Medical School of Brown University, 111 Brewster Street, Pawtucket, RI 02860, USA.

References

1. Jinks C, Jordan K, Croft P. Osteoarthritis as a public health problem: the impact of developing knee pain on physical function in adults living in the community: (KNEST 3). Rheumatology (Oxford). 2007;46(5):877–81.
2. Neogi T, Zhang Y. Epidemiology of osteoarthritis. Rheum Dis Clin North Am. 2013;39(1):1–19.
3. Arden N, Richette P, Cooper C, Bruyere O, Abadie E, Branco J, Brandi ML, Berenbaum F, Clerc C, Dennison E, et al. Can we identify patients with high risk of osteoarthritis progression who will respond to treatment? A focus on biomarkers and frailty. Drugs Aging. 2015;32(7):525–35.
4. Kent DM, Hayward RA. Limitations of applying summary results of clinical trials to individual patients: the need for risk stratification. JAMA. 2007; 298(10):1209–12.
5. Kerkhof HJ, Bierma-Zeinstra SM, Arden NK, Metrustry S, Castano-Betancourt M, Hart DJ, Hofman A, Rivadeneira F, Oei EH, Spector TD, et al. Prediction model for knee osteoarthritis incidence, including clinical, genetic and biochemical risk factors. Ann Rheum Dis. 2014;73(12):2116–21.
6. Losina E, Klara K, Michl GL, Collins JE, Katz JN. Development and feasibility of a personalized, interactive risk calculator for knee osteoarthritis. BMC Musculoskelet Disord. 2015;16(1):312.
7. Zhang W, McWilliams DF, Ingham SL, Doherty SA, Muthuri S, Muir KR, Doherty M. Nottingham knee osteoarthritis risk prediction models. Ann Rheum Dis. 2011;70(9):1599–604.
8. Blanco FJ, Moller I, Romera M, Rozadilla A, Sanchez-Lazaro JA, Rodriguez A, Galvez J, Fores J, Monfort J, Ojeda S, et al. Improved prediction of knee osteoarthritis progression by genetic polymorphisms: the Arthrotest Study. Rheumatology (Oxford). 2015;54(7):1236–43.
9. Kraus VB, Feng S, Wang S, White S, Ainslie M, Brett A, Holmes A, Charles HC. Trabecular morphometry by fractal signature analysis is a novel marker of osteoarthritis progression. Arthritis Rheum. 2009;60(12):3711–22.
10. Bohr HH, Schaadt O. Mineral content of upper tibia assessed by dual photon densitometry. Acta Orthop Scand. 1987;58(5):557–9.
11. Akamatsu Y, Koshino T, Saito T, Wada J. Changes in osteosclerosis of the osteoarthritic knee after high tibial osteotomy. Clin Orthop. 1997;334:207–14.
12. Madsen OR, Schaadt O, Bliddal H, Egmose C, Sylvest J. Bone mineral distribution of the proximal tibia in gonarthrosis assessed in vivo by photon absorption. Osteoarthritis Cartilage. 1994;2:141–7.
13. Wada M, Maezawa Y, Baba H, Shimada S, Sasaki S, Nose Y. Relationships among bone mineral densities, static alignment and dynamic load in patients with medial compartment knee osteoarthritis. Rheumatology (Oxford). 2001;40(5):499–505.
14. Hurwitz DE, Sumner DR, Andriacchi TP, Sugar DA. Dynamic knee loads during gait predict proximal tibial bone distribution. J Biomech. 1998; 31(5):423–30.
15. Lo GH, Hunter DJ, Zhang Y, McLennan CE, Lavalley MP, Kiel DP, McLean RR, Genant HK, Guermazi A, Felson DT. Bone marrow lesions in the knee are associated with increased local bone density. Arthritis Rheum. 2005;52(9): 2814–21.
16. Lo GH, Zhang Y, McLennan CE, Niu J, Kiel DP, McLean RR, Aliabadi P, Felson DT, Hunter DJ. The ratio of medial to lateral tibial plateau bone mineral density and compartment specific tibiofemoral osteoarthritis. Osteoarthritis Cartilage. 2006;14(10):984–90.
17. Katsuragawa Y, Fukui N, Nakamura K. Change of bone mineral density with valgus knee bracing. Int Orthop. 1999;23(3):164–7.
18. Clarke S, Wakeley C, Duddy J, Sharif M, Watt I, Ellingham K, Elson DJ, Nickols G, Kirwan JR. Dual-energy X-ray absorptiometry applied to the assessment of tibial subchondral bone mineral density in osteoarthritis of the knee. Skeletal Radiol. 2004;33:588–95.
19. Hulet C, Sabatier JP, Souquet D, Locker B, Marcelli C, Vielpeau C. Distribution of bone mineral density at the proximal tibia in knee osteoarthritis. Calcif Tissue Int. 2002;71(4):315–22.
20. Carbone LD, Nevitt MC, Wildy K, Barrow KD, Harris F, Felson D, Peterfy C, Visser M, Harris TB, Wang BW, et al. The relationship of antiresorptive drug use to structural findings and symptoms of knee osteoarthritis. Arthritis Rheum. 2004;50(11):3516–25.
21. Felson DT, Chaisson CE, Hill CL, Totterman SM, Gale ME, Skinner KM, Kazis L, Gale DR. The association of bone marrow lesions with pain in knee osteoarthritis. Ann Intern Med. 2001;134(7):541–9.
22. Felson DT, McLaughlin S, Goggins J, LaValley MP, Gale ME, Totterman S, Li W, Hill C, Gale D. Bone marrow edema and its relation to progression of knee osteoarthritis. Ann Intern Med. 2003;139(5 Pt 1):330–6.
23. Hunter DJ, Zhang Y, Niu J, Goggins J, Amin S, Lavalley MP, Guermazi A, Genant H, Gale D, Felson DT. Increase in bone marrow lesions associated with cartilage loss: A longitudinal magnetic resonance imaging study of knee osteoarthritis. Arthritis Rheum. 2006;54(5):1529–35.
24. Pessis E, Drape JL, Ravaud P, Chevrot A, Dougados M, Ayral X. Assessment of progression in knee osteoarthritis: results of a 1 year study comparing arthroscopy and MRI. Osteoarthritis Cartilage. 2003;11(5):361–9.
25. Sowers MF, Hayes C, Jamadar D, Capul D, Lachance L, Jannausch M, Welch G. Magnetic resonance-detected subchondral bone marrow and cartilage defect characteristics associated with pain and X-ray-defined knee osteoarthritis. Osteoarthritis Cartilage. 2003;11(6):387–93.
26. Felson DT, Nevitt MC. Epidemiologic studies for osteoarthritis: new versus conventional study design approaches. Rheum Dis Clin North Am. 2004; 30(4):783–97. vii.
27. Altman RD, Gold GE. Atlas of individual radiographic features in osteoarthritis, revised. Osteoarthritis Cartilage. 2007;15(Suppl A):A1–56.
28. Kellgren JH, Lawrence JS. Radiological assessment of osteo-arthrosis. Ann Rheum Dis. 1957;16(4):494–502.
29. Lo GH, Tassinari AM, Driban JB, Price LL, Schneider E, Majumdar S, McAlindon TE. Cross-sectional DXA and MR measures of tibial periarticular bone associate with radiographic knee osteoarthritis severity. Osteoarthritis Cartilage. 2012;20(7):686–93.
30. Peduzzi P, Concato J, Kemper E, Holford TR, Feinstein AR. A simulation study of the number of events per variable in logistic regression analysis. J Clin Epidemiol. 1996;49(12):1373–9.
31. Cooper C, Snow S, McAlindon TE, Kellingray S, Stuart B, Coggon D, Dieppe PA. Risk factors for the incidence and progression of radiographic knee osteoarthritis. Arthritis Rheum. 2000;43(5):995–1000.
32. Silverwood V, Blagojevic-Bucknall M, Jinks C, Jordan JL, Protheroe J, Jordan KP. Current evidence on risk factors for knee osteoarthritis in older adults: a systematic review and meta-analysis. Osteoarthritis Cartilage. 2015;23(4):507–15.
33. Harrell FE. Regression modeling strategies. New York: Springer-Verlag; 2001.
34. Hastie T, Tibshirani R, Friedman J. The elements of statistical learning. New York: Springer-Verlag; 2001.
35. Hosmer DW, Lemeshow S. Applied logistic regression. 2nd ed. New York: Wiley; 2000.
36. Steyerberg EW, Vergouwe Y. Towards better clinical prediction models: seven steps for development and an ABCD for validation. Eur Heart J. 2014;35(29):1925–31.

10

Chondroitin sulfate efficacy versus celecoxib on knee osteoarthritis structural changes using magnetic resonance imaging

Jean-Pierre Pelletier[1*], Jean-Pierre Raynauld[1,2], André D. Beaulieu[3], Louis Bessette[4], Frédéric Morin[5], Artur J. de Brum-Fernandes[6], Philippe Delorme[7], Marc Dorais[8], Patrice Paiement[7], François Abram[7] and Johanne Martel-Pelletier[1]

Abstract

Background: In osteoarthritis (OA) treatment, although chondroitin sulfate (CS) was found in a number of studies using radiography to have a structure-modifying effect, to date CS use is still under debate. A clinical study using quantitative magnetic resonance imaging (qMRI) is therefore of the utmost importance. Here we report data from a 24-month, randomised, double-blind, double-dummy, controlled, comparative exploratory study of knee OA. The primary endpoint was to determine the effect of CS 1200 mg/day versus celecoxib 200 mg/day on cartilage volume loss (CVL) in the lateral compartment over time as measured by qMRI. Secondary endpoints included assessment of the OA structural changes and signs and symptoms of OA.

Methods: qMRI was performed at baseline and at 12 and 24 months. CVL, bone marrow lesion size, and synovial thickness were evaluated using qMRI. The primary statistical analysis was carried out on the modified intention-to-treat (mITT) population ($n = 138$) using chi-squared, Fisher's exact, Wilcoxon Mann–Whitney, and Student's t tests and analysis of covariance. Analyses were also conducted on the according-to-protocol (ATP; $n = 120$) population.

Results: In the adjusted mITT analysis, compared with celecoxib treatment, patients treated with CS had a significant reduced CVL at 24 months in the medial compartment (celecoxib −8.1 % ± 4.2, CS −6.3 % ± 3.2; $p = 0.018$) and medial condyle (−7.7 % ± 4.7, −5.5 % ± 3.9; $p = 0.008$); no significant effect was seen in the lateral compartment. In the ATP population, CS reduced CVL in the medial compartment at 12 months (celecoxib −5.6 % ± 3.0, CS −4.5 % ± 2.6; $p = 0.049$) and 24 months (celecoxib −8.4 % ± 4.2, CS −6.6 % ± 3.3; $p = 0.021$), and in the medial condyle at 24 months (celocoxib −8.1 % ± 4.7, CS −5.7 % ± 4.0; $p = 0.010$). A trend towards a statistically reduced synovial thickness (celecoxib +17.96 ± 33.73 mm, CS −0.66 ± 22.72 mm; $p = 0.076$) in the medial suprapatellar bursa was observed in CS patients. Both groups experienced a marked reduction in the incidence of patients with joint swelling/effusion and in symptoms over time. Data showed similar good safety profiles including cardiovascular adverse events for both drugs.

Conclusion: This study demonstrated, for the first time in a 2-year randomised controlled trial using qMRI, the superiority of CS over celecoxib at reducing CVL in knee OA patients.

Keywords: Chondroitin sulfate, Symptomatic slow-acting drug in osteoarthritis, Osteoarthritis, Knee, Celecoxib

* Correspondence: dr@jppelletier.ca
[1]Osteoarthritis Research Unit, University of Montreal Hospital Research Centre (CRCHUM), 900 Saint-Denis, Suite R11.412, Montreal, Quebec H2X 0A9, Canada
Full list of author information is available at the end of the article

Background

Knee osteoarthritis (OA) is one of the most common musculoskeletal disorders, which causes joint pain, stiffness, and loss of function [1, 2]. Current treatment recommendations include a combination of non-pharmacological (e.g. education, exercise, weight loss) and pharmacological (e.g. acetaminophen, non-steroidal anti-inflammatory drugs (NSAIDs)) treatments, and some also suggest the use of symptomatic slow-acting drugs for osteoarthritis (SYSADOA) [3–5], which include chondroitin sulfate (CS) and glucosamine. However, the use of the latest line of treatment has not reached a general consensus among different guidelines [6, 7], due in part to the unavailability of prescription quality SYSADOAs indicated for use in OA that have been evaluated by the US Food and Drug Administration [6].

The goals of OA therapy are to decrease pain and maintain or improve joint function. Existing pharmacologic therapies for OA, namely NSAIDs and analgesics, help to reduce symptoms, but are only moderately effective and expose patients to potential significant toxicity (cardiovascular, hepatic, renal, and other adverse events (AEs)) and problems resulting from interactions with other medications. A recent systematic literature review suggests that paracetamol, especially at the upper end of standard analgesic doses, can also induce gastrointestinal events (i.e. gastroduodenal ulcers and complications such as upper gastrointestinal haemorrhages) and renal events (decrease in glomerular filtration rate) [8]. For this reason, attention has recently been focused on the investigation and development of new types of drugs and treatments that can improve the clinical symptoms of OA and show better safety profiles, such as symptomatic SYSADOAs. SYSADOAs such as CS are characterised by a slow onset of action and a global efficacy at reducing OA symptoms similar to that of NSAIDs, and also possess a carry-over effect. Furthermore, 6-month randomised controlled trials (RCTs) using similar grade preparations have shown that CS 1200 mg/day plus glucosamine 1500 mg/day can provide significant pain relief over placebo [9] and comparable pain relief with celecoxib [10] in a subgroup of patients with moderate-to-severe knee pain.

CS is a natural product extracted from animal cartilage (e.g. bovine trachea). A recent Cochrane review concluded that CS, alone or in combination with glucosamine, has a beneficial effect on pain and joint space narrowing (JSN) in patients with knee OA [11]. Of note, different sources of CS with variable composition and purity have been used in these studies, which may explain some heterogeneity of results [12]. RCTs using pharmaceutical-grade preparations of CS have shown that at 800 mg/day the treatment significantly reduced JSN as assessed using X-ray imaging [13–15], and decreased cartilage volume loss as evaluated by magnetic resonance imaging (MRI) in a pilot study [16]. In OA joint tissues, CS has been shown to modify the chondrocyte death process, to improve the anabolic/catabolic balance of the extracellular cartilage matrix, to reduce some pro-inflammatory and catabolic factors, and to reduce the resorptive properties of subchondral bone osteoblasts [17–21]. These findings support the mode of action of CS at reducing OA structural change progression.

The aim of the current study was to ascertain whether CS at 1200 mg/day, the maximum and most commonly used therapeutic dosage of CS alone or in combination with other drugs/agents such as glucosamine, over a period of 24 months would reduce cartilage volume loss, as assessed by MRI. Celecoxib was chosen as the comparator for many reasons. First, it was shown in an RCT using MRI that celecoxib and placebo have a non-different effect on the progression of cartilage volume loss in knee OA patients [22]. Moreover, celecoxib has an established efficacy in knee OA treatment and widespread use [23]. It is preferred over other NSAIDs due to its lower incidence of gastrointestinal side effects.

Methods

Study design

This 24-month randomised, double-blind, double-dummy controlled study (ClinicalTrials.gov NCT01354145) of patients with symptomatic knee OA and clinical synovitis aimed to explore the effect of CS and celecoxib on knee OA cartilage volume loss. The study was performed in Quebec, Canada. Patients were recruited by physicians in four private clinics and one outpatient clinic (Service de rhumatologie, Centre hospitalier universitaire de Sherbrooke (CHUS), Sherbrooke, QC, Canada).

Patients

The study enrolled ambulatory men and women aged 40 years or older with primary symptomatic knee OA whose condition justified symptomatic treatment, as described previously [16]. They were diagnosed according to the clinical and radiological criteria of the American College of Rheumatology (ACR) [24], with clinical signs of synovitis (warmth, swelling, or effusion), a disease severity grade of 2–3 based on Kellgren–Lawrence radiographic scoring [25], a minimal medial joint space width of 2 mm on standing knee X-ray scan, and a visual analogue scale (VAS) pain index of at least 40 mm while walking. The X-ray inclusion criteria were selected not only to comply with ACR recommendations but also to avoid selection of patients with secondary OA and/or with too severe disease such as knee varus/valgus malalignment. Concomitant femoropatellar OA was not quantified by X-ray imaging. Participants were required to have no significant laboratory abnormalities. If both knees were affected by OA, the target knee with the most pronounced symptoms was selected if within the inclusion criteria. Full inclusion and exclusion criteria are presented in Additional file 1: Table S1.

Treatments

Patients were assigned sequentially in a 1:1 ratio according to a predefined randomisation scheme using a mathematical algorithm and a randomisation list (Ropack Pharmaceutical Packaging, Montreal, QC, Canada). The list contained assignment of sequential numbers to one of the two treatment groups, pharmaceutical-grade CS (Bioibérica S.A., Barcelona, Spain) 1200 mg (three 400 mg capsules in the morning) or celecoxib (Pfizer Canada, Saint-Laurent, QC, Canada) 200 mg (one 200 mg capsule + two placebo capsules in the morning) for 24 months. All products were over-encapsulated to have the same appearance, size, and colour. The patients, site personnel, and sponsor were blinded to treatment.

Patients were not permitted to take other NSAIDs during the study (or during the week before randomisation), but could take acetaminophen (up to 3 g/day) with consumption interrupted 48 hours preceding evaluations.

The prior and concomitant treatment, blinding, treatment compliance, and study schedule are described in Additional file 1: Methods.

Outcomes

The primary endpoint was percentage of cartilage volume loss over time in the lateral compartment (condyle and tibial plateau) of the target knee from baseline to 24 months. The decision for selecting this criterion was based on the findings of the pilot study [16] and those of other similar RCTs [26, 27]. The secondary endpoints included changes in percentage of cartilage volume loss in the medial compartment, synovitis severity (thickness of the synovial membrane), bone marrow lesion (BML) grade, and synovial fluid volume. The outcomes also included assessment on the VAS of knee pain, Western Ontario and McMaster Universities Osteoarthritis Index (WOMAC) scores, quality of life (QoL) Short Form-36 General Health (SF-36) scores, clinical evaluation (swelling, visual examination; effusion, bulge sign), analgesic consumption, and AEs, which were recorded during physical examinations at the baseline visit and follow-up visits at months 3, 6, 9, 12, 18, and 24. Safety outcomes included discontinuation of study treatment due to AEs, and changes in various laboratory measures and vital signs.

Knee MRI acquisitions

MRI was performed at baseline and at 12 and 24 months on 1.5 T scanners (Siemens, Erlangen, Germany; General Electric, Milwaukee, WI, USA) using a standard knee coil. The sequence acquisitions were as described previously for the cartilage [28] and synovial membrane [29].

The cartilage volume was measured by two experienced readers trained by musculoskeletal radiologists using the computer program Cartiscope™ (ArthroLab, Montreal, QC, Canada) as described previously [30, 31]. The readers were blinded to treatment and to MRI examination time points except for the baseline. The change in knee cartilage volume was obtained by subtracting the follow-up volume from the initial (baseline) volume. The reproducibility of the method has been demonstrated previously to be excellent: root mean square (RMS) coefficient of variation percentage (CV%) of 2.2 % for the global cartilage volume, 1.6 % for the medial compartment, and 2.6 % for the lateral compartment [30] and inter-reader and intra-reader intra-class correlation (ICC) of 0.94–0.99 [32]. In addition, the reproducibility of the reading is evaluated periodically using standard operating procedures (SOP; ArthroLab). The data show consistency of the method over time.

The extent of synovitis was assessed by measuring synovial thickness (mm) in four regions of interest (ROIs): the medial and lateral articular recess and the medial and lateral outer wall of the suprapatellar bursa [29]. The inter-reader and intra-reader correlation was excellent with ICC of 0.82–0.91 [29] and consistency of the method over time (SOP; ArthroLab). Of note, the measurement of the synovial membrane thickness according to this method relies on the presence of synovial fluid to localise the membrane in the different ROIs. An absence of synovial fluid, especially in the area of the medial suprapatellar bursa, thus accounts for missing values.

The synovial fluid was determined using a fully automated system as described previously [33]. Validation experiments revealed excellent coefficients of variation with a calibrated cylinder (1.4 %), sphere phantoms (0.8 %), manual quantification ($r = 0.98$, $p < 0.0001$), and comparison with direct aspiration ($r = 0.88$, $p = 0.0008$) [33].

BML were assessed in the same MRI sequences used for the cartilage [34]. The extent of the BML was evaluated in the global knee and each of the subregions using the following scale: 0, absence; 1, <25 %; 2, 25–50 %, 3, >50 % of the surface of the respective region regardless of the presence of additional smaller lesions. Reliability of the scoring system for BML changes was found to be excellent with ICC ranging from 0.88 to 0.93 [34] and consistency of the method over time (SOP; ArthroLab).

Statistical analysis

The study populations were carefully defined in the statistical analysis plan (SAP). The safety population included all randomised patients who received at least one dose of study treatment ($n = 194$ at baseline). The modified intention-to-treat (mITT) population comprised all randomised patients who received at least one dose of study medication and for whom at least one post-baseline efficacy MRI measurement was available. The according-to-protocol (ATP) population included patients who fully complied with the study's 24-month protocol and for whom all MRI evaluations were available. Data were entered into a computerised database using a blinded double-entry procedure, after which descriptive statistics for patient characteristics were tabulated. Before locking the database, the following actions were performed under conditions blinded for the type of intervention: the database was cleaned, all queries were resolved, a review meeting regarding blinded data was conducted, protocol deviations were identified, the SAP was developed, and signed approval was obtained. Following the final database lock, the statistical analysis was performed by an independent expert biostatistics firm (Inferential, Paris, France).

Descriptive variables at baseline are presented as number (percentage) or mean ± standard deviation (SD). Differences between the two treatment groups were assessed using a Kruskal–Wallis test or Student's t test for quantitative variables, and a chi-squared test or Fisher's exact test for categorical variables. Analgesic consumption was tallied and compared between the two groups. The primary efficacy outcome measure for structure modification was percentage cartilage volume loss in the lateral compartment of the target knee after 24 months of enrolment for the mITT population who had at least one post-baseline MRI measurement while using, as specified in the SAP, the imputation method of the last observation carried forward (mITT-LOCF). Because of the difference at baseline in body mass index (BMI) values between the two treatment groups (Table 1), an analysis of covariance (ANCOVA) including BMI as a covariate was performed on the mITT-LOCF population. In order to provide an additional measure of treatment efficacy, the ATP population (i.e. patients who completed the study according to the 24-month protocol) was also assessed using the ANCOVA method. Additionally, the data from the mITT and ATP populations were also analysed using a generalised linear mixed-model analysis. Secondary efficacy analyses of structural changes were done using the same methodology. Comparison of symptom changes using the WOMAC questionnaire, VAS pain, QoL SF-36, knee swelling and effusion, and safety were assessed on all available data as specified in the SAP.

No sample size estimation was carried out because this was an exploratory study. Statistical tests were two-sided and significance reached at $p < 0.05$. No statistical adjustments were made for multiple comparisons while analysing secondary outcomes. Statistical analyses were performed using SAS® software version 9.3 (SAS Institute, Cary, NC, USA).

Table 1 Randomised patient characteristics at baseline

	Chondroitin sulfate ($n = 97$)	Celecoxib ($n = 97$)
Female	53 (54.6)	61 (62.9)
Age (years)	61.4 ± 9.3	61.3 ± 8.5
Body mass index (kg/m^2)	30.1 ± 5.8	32.3 ± 5.8
At least one previous medical condition	86 (88.7)	86 (88.7)
At least one active medical condition	96 (99.0)	97 (100.0)
Cartilage volume (mm^3)		
Lateral compartment	4613 ± 1755	4405 ± 1157
Condyle	2621 ± 1073	2476 ± 716
Plateau	1993 ± 799	1930 ± 540
Medial compartment	4515 ± 1537	4255 ± 1217
Condyle	2807 ± 971	2646 ± 779
Plateau	1708 ± 623	1609 ± 489
Synovial membrane thickness (mm)	1.0 ± 0.2	1.0 ± 0.2
BML score (global knee)[a]	2.6 ± 3.0	2.7 ± 2.5
Synovial fluid volume (ml)	13.8 ± 14.6	10.8 ± 10.9
Joint swelling and effusion		
Swelling	76 (78.4)	78 (80.4)
Effusion	76 (78.4)	71 (73.2)
Both	59 (60.8)	55 (56.7)
Pain VAS (mm)[a]	62.42 ± 15.51	59.26 ± 18.10
WOMAC[a]		
Total score (0–240)	124.9 ± 38.1	126.7 ± 43.9
Pain score (0–50)	25.6 ± 8.1	25.5 ± 9.0
Stiffness score (0–20)	10.8 ± 3.7	11.7 ± 4.3
Physical function score (0–170)	88.5 ± 28.7	89.5 ± 32.5
Quality of life (SF-36)[a]		
Physical component summary	35.4 ± 7.8	35.7 ± 8.1
Mental component summary	51.7 ± 9.5	52.7 ± 11.0

Data shown as number of patients (%) or mean ± standard deviation
[a]Data were not available for two patients in the chondroitin sulfate group
BML bone marrow lesion, *SF-36* Short Form-36, *VAS* visual analogue scale, *WOMAC* Western Ontario and McMaster Universities Osteoarthritis Index

Results

Patients

The study was conducted from 21 June 2011 to 10 September 2014. A total of 194 patients were randomised to CS or celecoxib. The study populations used for analyses are as described in Fig. 1.

No differences were found in the baseline characteristics of the patient populations (Table 1) with the exception of BMI; although values for both groups were in the obesity category (≥30 kg/m^2), a higher value was found in the celecoxib group.

No significant difference between the treatment groups was found for previous or concomitant medications (Additional file 1: Table S2).

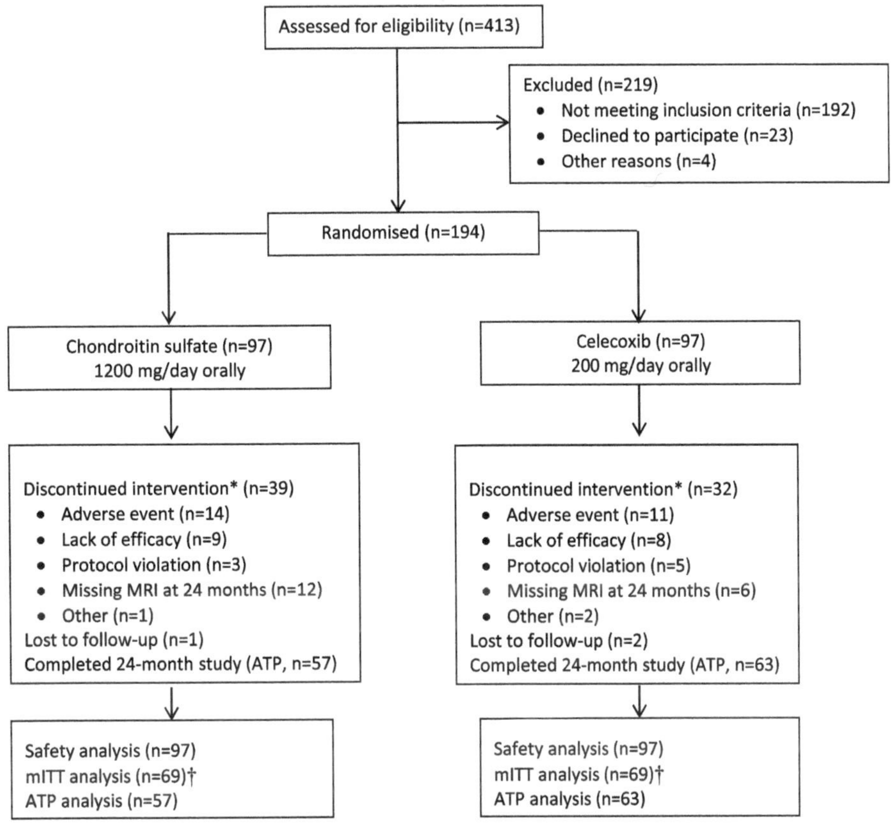

Fig. 1 Patient disposition. *Primary reasons for discontinuation. †mITT includes ATP patients plus those with MRI at 12 months but with MRI missing at final visit. *ATP* according-to-protocol, *mITT* modified intention-to-treat, *MRI* magnetic resonance imaging

Efficacy

Cartilage volume

In the adjusted mITT-LOCF analysis ($n = 138$), the percentage cartilage volume loss in the lateral compartment (primary endpoint) was not different in the CS ($n = 69$) and celecoxib ($n = 69$) groups at 24 months (Table 2). In the medial compartment and medial condyle, the cartilage volume loss was significantly less in the CS group at 24 months ($p = 0.018$ and $p = 0.008$, respectively) compared with celecoxib. The results from the generalised linear mixed-model analysis at 24 months showed $p = 0.038$ for the medial compartment and $p = 0.015$ for the medial condyle. However, the results of the adjusted analysis for the ATP population ($n = 120$; Table 2) showed a significant reduction in cartilage volume loss in CS-treated patients at 12 months for the medial compartment ($p = 0.049$) and at 24 months for the medial compartment and medial condyle ($p = 0.021$ and $p = 0.010$, respectively). The results from the generalised linear mixed-model analysis showed $p = 0.043$ and $p = 0.035$ for the medial compartment at 12 months and 24 months, respectively, and $p = 0.015$ for the medial condyle at 24 months.

Synovial membrane

The assessment of the mean synovial thickness in the global knee (four ROIs together) was not different between treatment groups at baseline (Table 1). The change in synovial membrane thickness between the two therapeutic groups was not different at any time point in both mITT ($n = 138$) and ATP ($n = 120$) population analyses (Table 2). However, in post-hoc analysis, we also examined the changes in synovial thickness in one of the four ROIs, the medial suprapatellar bursa ($n = 50$; Table 3). Because such measurement is reliant on the presence of synovial fluid to localise the membrane, the absence of synovial fluid accounts for missing values. Data showed, in patients for whom the assessment of thickness was possible at baseline and at 24 months, a numerical trend ($p = 0.076$) towards a decrease at 24 months in the CS group versus the celecoxib group. This is associated with a significant decrease ($p = 0.045$) in the cartilage volume loss in the medial compartment. Moreover, when analysed based on whether patients had experienced a decrease or increase in synovial membrane thickness from baseline to 24 months (Table 3),

Table 2 Changes in MRI parameters

mITT-LOCF population	24 months		
	Chondroitin sulfate (*n* = 69)	Celecoxib (*n* = 69)	*p* value[a]
Cartilage volume loss (%)			
Lateral compartment	−4.1 ± 3.1	−4.4 ± 3.0	0.814
Condyle	−3.0 ± 3.1	−4.1 ± 3.7	0.144
Plateau	−5.8 ± 4.7	−4.8 ± 3.5	0.182
Medial compartment	−6.3 ± 3.2	−8.1 ± 4.2	**0.018**
Condyle	−5.5 ± 3.9	−7.7 ± 4.7	**0.008**
Plateau	−7.6 ± 4.0	−8.6 ± 4.8	0.276
Synovial membrane thickness[b] (mm)	0.13 ± 0.25	0.14 ± 0.24	0.948
Synovial fluid volume (ml)	−2.6 ± 14.5	−2.0 ± 11.8	0.776
BML score[b]	1.1 ± 1.7	0.8 ± 1.7	0.322

ATP population	12 months			24 months		
	Chondroitin sulfate (*n* = 57)[c]	Celecoxib (*n* = 63)	*p* value[a]	Chondroitin sulfate (*n* = 57)[c]	Celecoxib (*n* = 63)	*p* value[a]
Cartilage volume loss (%)						
Lateral compartment	−3.4 ± 2.7	−3.3 ± 2.5	0.932	−4.6 ± 3.0	−4.4 ± 2.8	0.753
Condyle	−2.5 ± 3.2	−3.0 ± 3.0	0.234	−3.4 ± 3.0	−4.2 ± 3.6	0.316
Plateau	−4.6 ± 3.5	−3.8 ± 3.1	0.194	−6.3 ± 4.6	−4.8 ± 3.5	0.081
Medial compartment	−4.5 ± 2.6	−5.6 ± 3.0	**0.049**	−6.6 ± 3.3	−8.4 ± 4.2	**0.021**
Condyle	−3.8 ± 3.2	−5.0 ± 3.8	0.100	−5.7 ± 4.0	−8.1 ± 4.7	**0.010**
Plateau	−5.5 ± 3.0	−6.6 ± 3.8	0.155	−8.0 ± 4.2	−9.0 ± 4.8	0.334
Synovial membrane thickness[b] (mm)	0.03 ± 0.18	0.06 ± 0.18	0.579	0.15 ± 0.26	0.15 ± 0.24	0.731
Synovial fluid volume (ml)	−5.5 ± 12.6	−1.8 ± 9.2	0.326	−3.9 ± 15.4	−2.1 ± 12.2	0.945
BML score[b]	0.7 ± 1.4	0.3 ± 1.2	**0.051**	1.1 ± 1.7	0.8 ± 1.7	0.322

Data are mean ± standard deviation
[a]Analysis of covariance; model includes BMI as covariate; bold indicates statistical significance
[b]Global knee
[c]Among the 58 patients in the chondroitin sulfate group who completed the study, one patient did not complete the MRI at 24 months
ATP according-to-protocol, *BMI* body mass index, *BML* bone marrow lesion, *LOCF* last observation carried forward, *mITT* modified intention-to-treat, *MRI* magnetic resonance imaging

Table 3 Changes at 24 months in synovial membrane thickness and cartilage volume

				Decrease[a]			Increase[a]		
	Chondroitin sulfate (*n* = 26)[b]	Celecoxib (*n* = 24)[b]	*p* value[c]	Chondroitin sulfate (*n* = 12)	Celecoxib (*n* = 8)	*p* value[c]	Chondroitin sulfate (*n* = 12)	Celecoxib (*n* = 14)	*p* value[c]
Medial suprapatellar bursa									
Synovial membrane thickness loss (mm)	−0.66 ± 22.72	+17.96 ± 33.73	0.076	−0.23 ± 0.27	−0.14 ± 0.21	0.446	+0.13 ± 0.09	+0.25 ± 0.17	**0.030**
Medial compartment									
Cartilage volume loss (%)	−6.8 ± 3.5	−9.4 ± 4.7	**0.045**	−7.5 ± 3.7	−11.3 ± 3.5	**0.036**	−6.4 ± 3.4	−7.8 ± 4.8	0.404

Data are mean ± standard deviation
[a]Data from patients who presented a decrease or an increase in synovial membrane thickness at 24 months
[b]Synovial membrane thickness measurement is reliant on the presence of synovial fluid to localise the membrane; absence of synovial fluid accounts for missing values
[c]Student's *t* test or Wilcoxon Mann–Whitney test, bold indicates statistical significance

data showed that patients treated with CS had a significantly lesser increase ($p = 0.030$) in synovial membrane thickness compared with those in the celecoxib group. The patients in the CS group who experienced a decrease in synovial membrane thickness had significantly less cartilage volume loss ($p = 0.036$) than those in the celecoxib group.

Synovial fluid volume and BML score

Analyses showed no significant differences between the two treatment groups in baseline values (randomised patients, $n = 194$; Table 1) or in the changes (mITT, $n = 138$; ATP, $n = 120$; Table 2) in synovial fluid volume. For BML, the only significance was found in the changes at 12 months ($p = 0.051$) in the ATP population.

Joint effusion/swelling

The incidence of joint effusion and/or swelling decreased similarly in both groups during the study in the randomised patient population (all available data, baseline, $n = 194$; Additional file 1: Figure S1). A marked reduction in the incidence (%) of patients with joint swelling plus effusion was observed in both CS and celecoxib groups (42 % and 29 %, respectively) at 24 months.

Symptoms and function

Both therapeutic groups experienced a reduction in disease symptoms over time (all available data; baseline $n = 194$) (Fig. 2). The decrease in WOMAC scores (Fig. 2a–d) was slightly more pronounced in the celecoxib group compared with the CS group, mostly at earlier time points (months 3 and 6), but statistical significance was never reached except for the WOMAC total at month 3 (Fig. 2a) and stiffness at months 3 and 6 (Fig. 2c). At 24 months, the reduction in WOMAC pain (Fig. 2b) was 36 % for the CS group and 42 % for the celecoxib group. The level of pain on VAS decreased over time in both treatment groups (Fig. 2e). The reduction at 24 months was 38 % and 43 % for the CS and celecoxib groups, respectively (Fig. 2e).

With regards to the QoL SF-36 physical and mental component scores, an improvement in QoL was found for both groups without significant differences between them (data not shown).

The overall daily consumption of rescue analgesic (acetaminophen) was not different between the CS and celecoxib groups (584 versus 472 mg/day).

Safety

Study durations (mean ± SD) were 581 ± 254 and 579 ± 262 days in the CS and celecoxib groups, respectively ($n = 194$), and treatment durations were 543 ± 260 and 564 ± 263 days, respectively.

A total of 78 patients (80.4 %) in the CS group and 79 patients (81.4 %) in the celecoxib group reported at least one AE during the study. The most frequent AEs (Table 4) at the system organ class (SOC) level were musculoskeletal and connective tissue disorders, infections and infestations, and gastrointestinal disorders. The most common AEs by preferred term were nasopharyngitis, arthralgia, dyspepsia, headache, and back pain. Significant differences between the two groups were seen only for back pain and skin and subcutaneous tissue disorders (Table 4). The vascular disorders described in the table were hypertension (CS, $n = 4$; celecoxib, $n = 3$) and hot flush (CS, $n = 1$). Most emergent AEs were mild to moderate with no significant difference between treatment groups (Table 5). The overall frequency of patients with emergent AEs considered possibly or probably related to study treatment, including cardiovascular events (mainly hypertension; CS, $n = 4$, celecoxib, $n = 4$), was similar in the two groups. Findings regarding the AEs leading to study withdrawal were also similar in the two therapeutic groups. No death occurred during the study. Ten patients in the CS group versus six in the celecoxib group experienced at least one serious adverse event (SAE). One SAE (iron-deficiency anaemia) was considered by the investigator to be related to treatment in one patient in the CS group and two SAEs (pneumonia and pulmonary embolism) in one patient in the celecoxib group.

Discussion

In this 24-month RCT, although we found no statistically significant reduction in cartilage volume loss by CS treatment in the lateral compartment, which was the primary outcome of the study, CS at 1200 mg/day was found to have a beneficial effect versus celecoxib 200 mg/day on cartilage volume loss in the medial compartment in knee OA patients. Moreover, CS, to a greater extent than celecoxib, induced a lesser increase in synovial thickness in the medial suprapatellar bursa that was associated with a decrease in cartilage volume loss in the medial compartment. There was also no evidence of superiority of one treatment over the other at improving disease symptoms except joint stiffness in the early phase of the study, which was greater in celecoxib patients. These findings provide new information about the potential benefit of long-term treatment with CS in knee OA patients.

The reduction in cartilage volume loss found with CS in the current study is in line with several other RCTs [13–16] and meta-analyses and reviews [11, 35–38], in which MRI (cartilage volume) or X-ray imaging (JSN) were used to assess disease progression, a number of which used a placebo as a comparator [13–15], including a pilot study using MRI [16]. Of note, the results of a

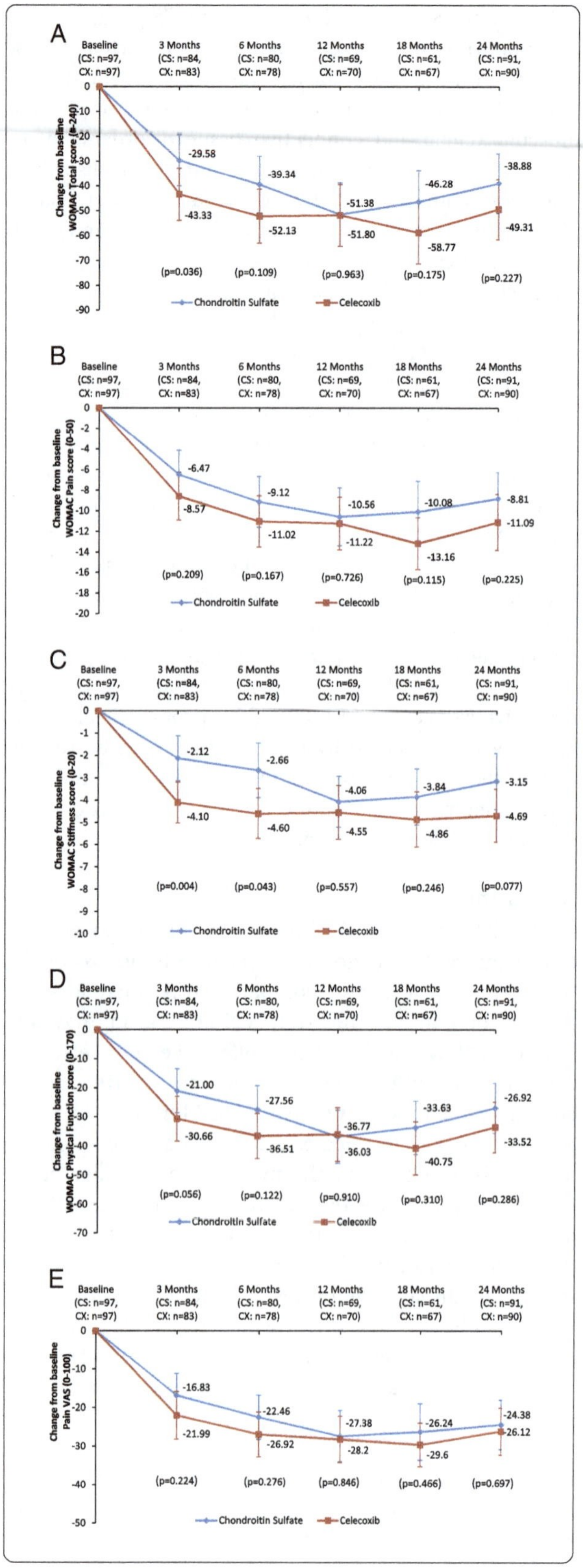

Fig. 2 Change in symptoms and function from baseline based on available data. WOMAC (**a**) total, (**b**) pain, (**c**) stiffness, and (**d**) function subscales, and (**e**) VAS, by visit. Data are mean of the relative change (%) from baseline. Statistical analyses comparing chondroitin sulfate and celecoxib were performed using Student's *t* test or the Kruskal–Wallis test. *CS* chondroitin sulfate, *CX* celecoxib, *WOMAC*, Western Ontario and McMaster Universities Osteoarthritis Index, *VAS* visual analogue scale

recent study in knee OA patients [39] reported a significant reduction in cartilage volume loss with CS plus glucosamine, but not with CS alone, compared with patients treated with placebo. The results of the latter [39], which used X-ray imaging and JSN to assess the disease-modifying osteoarthritis drug (DMOAD) effect, could possibly be explained by the fact that it was underpowered and of too short a duration for such imaging technology to allow an accurate assessment of possible changes related to treatment. Some other meta-analyses [40–42] have reported no beneficial effect of CS on JSN. Such findings can be at least partly explained by the heterogeneity between results of the studies included in the analyses, which may have been related, to some extent, to the use of non-pharmaceutical-grade CS as the therapeutic agent in some trials [12, 43, 44].

The change in cartilage volume in the lateral compartment was chosen as the primary endpoint based mainly on the results of the pilot study which reported significantly less cartilage volume loss in the lateral compartment with CS versus placebo [16], as well as two other knee OA RCTs using MRI [26, 27]. Here, the protective effect was found only in the medial compartment. This discrepancy could probably be explained by many factors including the difference in disease severity between the patients in each study. Patients in the current study had less severe disease than those in the pilot study [16], as evidenced by higher knee cartilage volume, particularly in the medial compartment. Because knee OA structural damage (cartilage volume loss) in such patients is predominantly seen in the medial compartment, disease progression in the lateral compartment may not have been sufficient for CS to demonstrate a significant therapeutic effect, as shown in a recent report [45]. Moreover, the duration of treatment in the pilot study of only 12 months and a lower dosage of CS (800 mg/day) may have precluded the finding of a positive effect in the medial compartment. Nevertheless, we believe that the present findings are of great importance from many aspects. First, they are very clinically relevant, as a recent consensus of experts recommends cartilage volume loss in the medial compartment as a clinical trial outcome [46]. The experts agree that it can predict knee replacement, is sensitive to change, and predicts outcome in a continuous manner. This is quite interesting in the

Table 4 Frequency of patients with at least one emergent adverse event (occurring in ≥5 % of patients): safety population

	Chondroitin sulfate ($n = 97$)		Celecoxib ($n = 97$)		p value[a]
	Events	n (%)	Events	n (%)	
Musculoskeletal and connective tissue disorders	72	37 (38.1)	59	38 (39.2)	>0.999
Arthralgia	19	14 (14.4)	14	11 (11.3)	0.669
Back pain	17	16 (16.5)	5	5 (5.2)	**0.019**
Pain in extremity	6	3 (3.1)	8	7 (7.2)	0.331
Infections and infestations	66	34 (35.1)	61	32 (33.0)	0.880
Nasopharyngitis	28	19 (19.6)	18	15 (15.5)	0.572
Gastrointestinal disorders	37	27 (27.8)	44	29 (29.9)	0.874
Dyspepsia	12	12 (12.4)	12	12 (12.4)	1.000
Gastroesophageal reflux disease	5	5 (5.2)	5	5 (5.2)	1.000
Nervous system disorders	21	16 (16.5)	22	21 (21.6)	0.465
Headache	15	12 (12.4)	10	10 (10.3)	0.821
Respiratory, thoracic, and mediastinal disorders	19	15 (15.5)	20	14 (14.4)	>0.999
Sinusitis	5	5 (5.2)	6	6 (6.2)	>0.999
Injury, poisoning, and procedural complications	18	14 (14.4)	18	13 (13.4)	>0.999
General disorders and administration site conditions	12	11 (11.3)	12	11 (11.3)	1.000
Skin and subcutaneous tissue disorders	3	3 (3.1)	11	11 (11.3)	**0.049**
Psychiatric disorders	4	4 (4.1)	9	9 (9.3)	0.250
Investigations	6	6 (6.2)	6	6 (6.2)	1.000
Surgical and medical procedures	8	5 (5.2)	8	6 (6.2)	>0.999
Vascular disorders[b]	7	6 (6.2)	5	4 (4.1)	0.747

Data shown are number of events or patients (%)
[a]Chi-squared test or Fisher's exact test for proportions (%), bold indicates statistical significance
[b]Vascular disorders include mainly hypertension, varicose veins, and ulcers

Table 5 Summary of emergent adverse events: safety population

	Chondroitin sulfate ($n = 97$)		Celecoxib ($n = 97$)		p value[a]
	Events	n (%)	Events	n (%)	
At least one AE	305	78 (80.4)	299	77 (79.4)	>0.999
Intensity					
Mild	203	61 (62.9)	215	61 (62.9)	1.000
Moderate	89	47 (48.5)	68	41 (42.3)	0.471
Severe	13	9 (9.3)	16	10 (10.3)	>0.999
SAE	16	10 (10.3)	9	6 (6.2)	0.435
Relationship to study treatment					
Not related	246	67 (69.1)	241	68 (70.1)	>0.999
Uncertain	20	14 (14.4)	23	13 (13.4)	>0.999
Related[b]	39	27 (27.8)	35	24 (24.7)	0.745
AE that led to study withdrawal	13	13 (13.4)	12	11 (11.3)	0.828
Ongoing[c]	95	50 (51.5)	100	50 (51.5)	1.000

[a]Chi-squared test for proportions (%)
[b]Relationship considered possible, probable, or very probable
[c]Not resolved/recovered at the end of the study
AE adverse event, *SAE* severe adverse event

context of the present study, because CS treatment was reported previously to have a beneficial effect on the need for total knee replacement in a 4-year follow-up study in knee OA [47]. A significant number of the patients ($n = 134$) who were randomised in the study are now being followed for a period of 4 years after study completion to evaluate the cumulative incidence of total knee replacement to ascertain whether the finding of our previous study [47] of the sparing effect of CS treatment on knee replacement could be confirmed. The results of the present study are also most helpful with regard to the selection of primary endpoints in future DMOAD RCTs. The selection of a very specific region of the knee in OA trials may not be the most optimal approach, as demonstrated in this study and in another recent RCT report [26]. This obviously needs to be examined more closely as results from additional RCTs become available.

The finding of a reduction in synovitis in the medial compartment by CS treatment in certain patients is interesting. It provides a hypothesis about the mechanism by which the effect of CS on cartilage volume loss is mediated. It also supports the findings of the pilot study regarding the effect of CS on synovitis [16].

The finding that CS had a beneficial effect comparable with that of celecoxib on pain, stiffness, physical function, and QoL is in line with a recent randomised trial in which CS in combination with glucosamine provided non-inferior pain relief to celecoxib [10] and supports findings from previous trials [13, 15, 48] and meta-analyses [11, 42, 49] that have also reported a significant beneficial effect of CS (with or without glucosamine) on pain. Of note is that not all clinical studies with CS have shown a significant effect on pain [14, 39], while others found a significant effect only in patients with moderate to severe pain [9]. Differences among the patient populations, product formulations that were studied, and follow-up times between studies may explain, to some extent, those discrepancies.

Regarding safety, this study confirmed the good tolerability of both treatments for up to 24 months, with no new safety issue, including cardiovascular events, arising for either treatment. These findings are similar to those observed in the MOVES study [10], which compared the symptomatic efficacy of CS plus glucosamine hydrochloride versus celecoxib in knee OA patients. It should, however, be taken into consideration that the patients included in this study and in the MOVES study [10] were those with low-risk cardiovascular and gastrointestinal diseases, which could have impacted the safety results.

As with all studies, the present study has some limitations. The relatively small sample size of this exploratory study and less severe disease severity in the patient population may have contributed to an underestimation of the effects of CS in the lateral compartment. Although patients with knee malalignment were excluded, such angulation was not assessed per se as an outcome variable and may be associated with the knee compartment in which cartilage volume loss could progress despite therapy. Additionally, although there is a well-known placebo effect in OA [50], we did not include a placebo group because it was felt that this would have been unethical, particularly in a 24-month study, and CS has already been shown to have a beneficial effect on JSN and/or pain in a number of placebo-controlled studies in knee OA [13–16, 48]. Similarly, celecoxib has proven pain efficacy over placebo in OA in several studies [51–53]. Moreover, celecoxib was found to have a neutral effect similar to placebo on cartilage volume loss in knee OA patients [16]. The interruption period for acetaminophen before evaluations was sufficient to have no effect on the studied pain outcomes.

Conclusion

This trial demonstrated, for the first time in a 24-month RCT using MRI, the superiority of CS over celecoxib at reducing the long-term progression of knee OA cartilage volume loss. Moreover, both drugs were found effective at reducing the symptoms of OA over the entire duration of the 24-month study, with no superiority of one over the other. These findings are interesting with regard to the potential usefulness of CS for long-term management of knee OA. A definitive study, however, will be required if one wishes to fully confirm the findings.

Abbreviations

ACR: American College of Rheumatology; AE: Adverse event; ANCOVA: Analysis of covariance; ATP: According-to-protocol; BMI: Body mass index; BML: Bone marrow lesion; DMOAD: Disease-modifying osteoarthritis drug; CS: Chondroitin sulfate; CV%: Coefficient of variation percentage; JSN: Joint space narrowing; LOCF: Last observation carried forward; mITT: Modified intention-to-treat; MRI: Magnetic resonance imaging; NSAID: Non-steroidal anti-inflammatory drug; OA: Osteoarthritis; qMRI: Quantitative magnetic resonance imaging; QoL: Quality of life; RCT: Randomised controlled trial; RMS: Root mean square; ROI: Region of interest; SAE: Serious adverse event; SD: Standard deviation; SYSADOA: Symptomatic slow-acting drug for osteoarthritis; VAS: Visual analogue scale; WOMAC: Western Ontario and McMaster Universities Osteoarthritis Index

Acknowledgements

Jenny Lloyd and Sophie Rushton-Smith (MedLink Healthcare Communications Ltd) provided medical writing support. The authors thank André Pelletier and Josée Thériault for the MRI reading, and Marie-Josée Berthiaume, MD, and Thomas Moser, MD, expert musculoskeletal radiologists at the University of Montreal, for the training and supervision in the MRI reading. Virginia Wallis assisted with manuscript preparation.

Funding

This trial was funded by Bioibérica SA, Barcelona, Spain. The sponsor provided all of the study medication free of charge and met the expenses that arose during the course of the study. The sponsor also participated in the study design and data analysis (safety only).

Authors' contributions

J-PP conceived the study, was responsible for the data collection and analysis, interpreted the data, undertook the literature search, was involved in the drafting or critical revision of the manuscript, and approved the final submitted version. J-PR conceived the study, was responsible for the data collection and analysis, interpreted the data, undertook the literature search, was involved in the drafting or critical revision of the manuscript, and approved the final submitted version. ADB was responsible for the data collection and analysis, was involved in the drafting or critical revision of the manuscript, and approved the final submitted version. LB was responsible for the data collection and analysis, was involved in the drafting or critical revision of the manuscript, and approved the final submitted version. FM was responsible for the data collection and analysis, was involved in the drafting or critical revision of the manuscript, and approved the final submitted version. AJdB-F was responsible for the data collection and analysis, was involved in the drafting or critical revision of the manuscript, and approved the final submitted version. PD was responsible for the data collection and analysis, was involved in the drafting or critical revision of the manuscript, and approved the final submitted version. MD was responsible for the data collection and analysis, was involved in the drafting or critical revision of the manuscript, and approved the final submitted version. PP was responsible for the data collection and analysis, was involved in the drafting or critical revision of the manuscript, and approved the final submitted version. FA was responsible for the data collection and analysis, interpreted the data, undertook the literature search, was involved in the drafting or critical revision of the manuscript, and approved the final submitted version. JM-P conceived the study, was responsible for the data collection and analysis, interpreted the data, undertook the literature search, was involved in the drafting or critical revision of the manuscript, and approved the final submitted version.

Authors' information

Not applicable.

Competing interests

J-PP is a shareholder in ArthroLab and consultant for Bioibérica. J-PR is a consultant for ArthroLab. MD is a consultant for ArthroLab. PD, PP, and FA are employees of ArthroLab. JM-P is a shareholder in ArthroLab and consultant for Bioibérica. No non-financial conflicts of interest exist for any of the authors.

Author details

[1]Osteoarthritis Research Unit, University of Montreal Hospital Research Centre (CRCHUM), 900 Saint-Denis, Suite R11.412, Montreal, Quebec H2X 0A9, Canada. [2]Institut de rhumatologie de Montréal, Montreal, Quebec, Canada. [3]Centre de rhumatologie St-Louis, Sainte-Foy, Quebec, Canada. [4]Groupe de recherche en Rhumatologie et Maladies Osseuses Inc., Sainte-Foy, Quebec, Canada. [5]Centre de recherche musculo-squelettique, Trois-Rivières, Quebec, Canada. [6]Service de rhumatologie, Centre hospitalier universitaire de Sherbrooke (CHUS), Sherbrooke, Quebec, Canada. [7]ArthroLab Inc., Montreal, Quebec, Canada. [8]StatSciences Inc., Notre-Dame de l'Île-Perrot, Quebec, Canada.

References

1. Murray CJ, Vos T, Lozano R, Naghavi M, Flaxman AD, Michaud C, Ezzati M, Shibuya K, Salomon JA, Abdalla S, et al. Disability-adjusted life years (DALYs) for 291 diseases and injuries in 21 regions, 1990-2010: a systematic analysis for the Global Burden of Disease Study 2010. Lancet. 2012;380(9859):2197–223.
2. Woolf AD, Pfleger B. Burden of major musculoskeletal conditions. Bull World Health Organ. 2003;81(9):646–56.
3. Bruyere O, Cooper C, Pelletier JP, Branco J, Luisa Brandi M, Guillemin F, Hochberg MC, Kanis JA, Kvien TK, Martel-Pelletier J, et al. An algorithm recommendation for the management of knee osteoarthritis in Europe and internationally: a report from a task force of the European Society for Clinical and Economic Aspects of Osteoporosis and Osteoarthritis (ESCEO). Semin Arthritis Rheum. 2014;44(3):253–63.
4. Bhatia D, Bejarano T, Novo M. Current interventions in the management of knee osteoarthritis. J Pharm Bioallied Sci. 2013;5(1):30–8.
and internationally: a report from a task force of the European Society for Clinical and Economic Aspects of Osteoporosis and Osteoarthritis (ESCEO). Semin Arthritis Rheum. 2014;44(3):253–63.
4. Bhatia D, Bejarano T, Novo M. Current interventions in the management of knee osteoarthritis. J Pharm Bioallied Sci. 2013;5(1):30–8.
5. Jordan KM, Arden NK, Doherty M, Bannwarth B, Bijlsma JW, Dieppe P, Gunther K, Hauselmann H, Herrero-Beaumont G, Kaklamanis P, et al. EULAR Recommendations 2003: an evidence based approach to the management of knee osteoarthritis: report of a Task Force of the Standing Committee for International Clinical Studies Including Therapeutic Trials (ESCISIT). Ann Rheum Dis. 2003;62(12):1145–55.
6. Hochberg MC, Altman RD, April KT, Benkhalti M, Guyatt G, McGowan J, Towheed T, Welch V, Wells G, Tugwell P. American College of Rheumatology 2012 recommendations for the use of nonpharmacologic and pharmacologic therapies in osteoarthritis of the hand, hip, and knee. Arthritis Care Res (Hoboken). 2012;64(4):465–74.
7. McAlindon TE, Bannuru RR, Sullivan MC, Arden NK, Berenbaum F, Bierma-Zeinstra SM, Hawker GA, Henrotin Y, Hunter DJ, Kawaguchi H, et al. OARSI guidelines for the non-surgical management of knee osteoarthritis. Osteoarthritis Cartilage. 2014;22(3):363–88.
8. Roberts E, Delgado Nunes V, Buckner S, Latchem S, Constanti M, Miller P, Doherty M, Zhang W, Birrell F, Porcheret M, et al. Paracetamol: not as safe as we thought? A systematic literature review of observational studies. Ann Rheum Dis. 2016;75(3):552–9.
9. Clegg DO, Reda DJ, Harris CL, Klein MA, O'Dell JR, Hooper MM, Bradley JD, Bingham CO, Weisman MH, Jackson CG, et al. Glucosamine, chondroitin sulfate, and the two in combination for painful knee osteoarthritis. N Engl J Med. 2006;354(8):795–808.
10. Hochberg MC, Martel-Pelletier J, Monfort J, Moller I, Castillo JR, Arden N, Berenbaum F, Blanco FJ, Conaghan PG, Domenech G, et al. Combined chondroitin sulfate and glucosamine for painful knee osteoarthritis: a multicentre, randomised, double-blind, non-inferiority trial versus celecoxib. Ann Rheum Dis. 2016;75(1):37–44.
11. Singh JA, Noorbaloochi S, MacDonald R, Maxwell LJ. Chondroitin for osteoarthritis. Cochrane Database Syst Rev. 2015;1, CD005614.
12. Martel-Pelletier J, Farran A, Montell E, Verges J, Pelletier JP. Discrepancies in composition and biological effects of different formulations of chondroitin sulfate. Molecules. 2015;20(3):4277–89.
13. Kahan A, Uebelhart D, De Vathaire F, Delmas PD, Reginster JY. Long-term effects of chondroitins 4 and 6 sulfate on knee osteoarthritis: The study on osteoarthritis progression prevention, a two-year, randomized, double-blind, placebo-controlled trial. Arthritis Rheum. 2009;60(2):524–33.
14. Michel BA, Stucki G, Frey D, De Vathaire F, Vignon E, Bruehlmann P, Uebelhart D. Chondroitins 4 and 6 sulfate in osteoarthritis of the knee: a randomized, controlled trial. Arthritis Rheum. 2005;52(3):779–86.
15. Uebelhart D, Malaise M, Marcolongo R, DeVathaire F, Piperno M, Mailleux E, Fioravanti A, Matoso L, Vignon E. Intermittent treatment of knee osteoarthritis with oral chondroitin sulfate: a one-year, randomized, double-blind, multicenter study versus placebo. Osteoarthritis Cartilage. 2004;12(4):269–76.
16. Wildi LM, Raynauld JP, Martel-Pelletier J, Beaulieu A, Bessette L, Morin F, Abram F, Dorais M, Pelletier JP. Chondroitin sulphate reduces both cartilage volume loss and bone marrow lesions in knee osteoarthritis patients starting as early as 6 months after initiation of therapy: a randomised, double-blind, placebo-controlled pilot study using MRI. Ann Rheum Dis. 2011;70(6):982–9.
17. Chan PS, Caron JP, Orth MW. Effect of glucosamine and chondroitin sulfate on regulation of gene expression of proteolytic enzymes and their inhibitors in interleukin-1-challenged bovine articular cartilage explants. Am J Vet Res. 2005;66(11):1870–6.
18. Tat SK, Pelletier JP, Vergés J, Montell E, Lajeunesse D, Fahmi H, Lavigne M, Martel-Pelletier J. Chondroitin and glucosamine sulfate in combination decrease the pro-resorptive properties of human osteoarthritis subchondral bone osteoblasts. Arthritis Res Ther. 2007;9:R117.
19. Monfort J, Pelletier J-P, Garcia-Giralt N, Martel-Pelletier J. Biochemical basis of the effect of chondroitin sulfate on osteoarthritis articular tissues. Ann Rheum Dis. 2008;67:735–40.
20. du Souich P, Garcia AG, Verges J, Montell E. Immunomodulatory and anti-inflammatory effects of chondroitin sulphate. J Cell Mol Med. 2009;13(8A):1451–63.

21. Martel-Pelletier J, Kwan Tat S, Pelletier JP. Effects of chondroitin sulfate in the pathophysiology of the osteoarthritic joint: a narrative review. Osteoarthritis Cartilage. 2010;18 Suppl 1:S7–11.
22. Raynauld JP, Martel-Pelletier J, Beaulieu A, Bessette L, Morin F, Choquette D, Haraoui B, Abram F, Pelletier JP. An open-label pilot study evaluating by magnetic resonance imaging the potential for a disease-modifying effect of celecoxib compared to a modelized historical control cohort in the treatment of knee osteoarthritis. Semin Arthritis Rheum. 2010;40(3):185–92.
23. Bensen WG, Fiechtner JJ, McMillen JI, Zhao WW, Yu SS, Woods EM, Hubbard RC, Isakson PC, Verburg KM, Geis GS. Treatment of osteoarthritis with celecoxib, a cyclooxygenase-2 inhibitor: a randomized controlled trial. Mayo Clin Proc. 1999;74(11):1095–105.
24. Altman RD, Asch E, Bloch DA, Bole G, Borenstein D, Brandt KD, Christy W, Cooke TD, Greenwald R, Hochberg M, et al. Development of criteria for the classification and reporting of osteoarthritis. Classification of osteoarthritis of the knee. Arthritis Rheum. 1986;29:1039–49.
25. Kellgren JH, Lawrence JS. Radiological assessment of osteoarthosis. Ann Rheum Dis. 1957;16:494–502.
26. Lohmander LS, Hellot S, Dreher D, Krantz EF, Kruger DS, Guermazi A, Eckstein F. Intraarticular sprifermin (recombinant human fibroblast growth factor 18) in knee osteoarthritis: a randomized, double-blind, placebo-controlled trial. Arthritis Rheumatol. 2014;66(7):1820–31.
27. Raynauld JP, Martel-Pelletier J, Bias P, Laufer S, Haraoui B, Choquette D, Beaulieu AD, Abram F, Dorais M, Vignon E, et al. Protective effects of licofelone, a 5-lipoxygenase and cyclo-oxygenase inhibitor, versus naproxen on cartilage loss in knee osteoarthritis: a first multicentre clinical trial using quantitative MRI. Ann Rheum Dis. 2009;68(6):938–47.
28. Wildi LM, Martel-Pelletier J, Abram F, Moser T, Raynauld JP, Pelletier JP. Assessment of cartilage changes over time in knee osteoarthritis disease-modifying osteoarthritis drug trials using semiquantitative and quantitative methods: pros and cons. Arthritis Care Res (Hoboken). 2013;65(5):686–94.
29. Pelletier JP, Raynauld JP, Abram F, Haraoui B, Choquette D, Martel-Pelletier J. A new non-invasive method to assess synovitis severity in relation to symptoms and cartilage volume loss in knee osteoarthritis patients using MRI. Osteoarthritis Cartilage. 2008;16 Suppl 3:S8–13.
30. Raynauld JP, Martel-Pelletier J, Berthiaume MJ, Labonté F, Beaudoin G, de Guise JA, Bloch DA, Choquette D, Haraoui B, Altman RD, et al. Quantitative magnetic resonance imaging evaluation of knee osteoarthritis progression over two years and correlation with clinical symptoms and radiologic changes. Arthritis Rheum. 2004;50:476–87.
31. Kauffmann C, Gravel P, Godbout B, Gravel A, Beaudoin G, Raynauld JP, Martel-Pelletier J, Pelletier JP, de Guise JA. Computer-aided method for quantification of cartilage thickness and volume changes using MRI: validation study using a synthetic model. IEEE Trans Biomed Eng. 2003; 50(8):978–88.
32. Raynauld JP, Kauffmann C, Beaudoin G, Berthiaume MJ, de Guise JA, Bloch DA, Camacho F, Godbout B, Altman RD, Hochberg M, et al. Reliability of a quantification imaging system using magnetic resonance images to measure cartilage thickness and volume in human normal and osteoarthritic knees. Osteoarthritis Cartilage. 2003;11(5):351–60.
33. Li W, Abram F, Pelletier JP, Raynauld JP, Dorais M, d'Anjou MA, Martel-Pelletier J. Fully automated system for the quantification of human osteoarthritic knee joint effusion volume using magnetic resonance imaging. Arthritis Res Ther. 2010;12(5):R173.
34. Raynauld JP, Martel-Pelletier J, Berthiaume MJ, Beaudoin G, Choquette D, Haraoui B, Tannenbaum H, Meyer JM, Beary JF, Cline GA, et al. Long term evaluation of disease progression through the quantitative magnetic resonance imaging of symptomatic knee osteoarthritis patients: correlation with clinical symptoms and radiographic changes. Arthritis Res Ther. 2006;8(1):R21.
35. Gallagher B, Tjoumakaris FP, Harwood MI, Good RP, Ciccotti MG, Freedman KB. Chondroprotection and the prevention of osteoarthritis progression of the knee: a systematic review of treatment agents. Am J Sports Med. 2015;43(3):734–44.
36. Hochberg M, Chevalier X, Henrotin Y, Hunter DJ, Uebelhart D. Symptom and structure modification in osteoarthritis with pharmaceutical-grade chondroitin sulfate: what's the evidence? Curr Med Res Opin. 2013;29(3):259–67.
37. Hochberg MC. Structure-modifying effects of chondroitin sulfate in knee osteoarthritis: an updated meta-analysis of randomized placebo-controlled trials of 2-year duration. Osteoarthritis Cartilage. 2010;18 Suppl 1:S28–31.
38. Lee YH, Woo JH, Choi SJ, Ji JD, Song GG. Effect of glucosamine or chondroitin sulfate on the osteoarthritis progression: a meta-analysis. Rheumatol Int. 2010;30(3):357–63.
39. Fransen M, Agaliotis M, Nairn L, Votrubec M, Bridgett L, Su S, Jan S, March L, Edmonds J, Norton R, et al. Glucosamine and chondroitin for knee osteoarthritis: a double-blind randomised placebo-controlled clinical trial evaluating single and combination regimens. Ann Rheum Dis. 2015;74(5):851–8.
40. Wandel S, Juni P, Tendal B, Nuesch E, Villiger PM, Welton NJ, Reichenbach S, Trelle S. Effects of glucosamine, chondroitin, or placebo in patients with osteoarthritis of hip or knee: network meta-analysis. BMJ. 2010;341:c4675.
41. Reichenbach S, Sterchi R, Scherer M, Trelle S, Burgi E, Burgi U, Dieppe PA, Juni P. Meta-analysis: chondroitin for osteoarthritis of the knee or hip. Ann Intern Med. 2007;146(8):580–90.
42. Richy F, Bruyere O, Ethgen O, Cucherat M, Henrotin Y, Reginster JY. Structural and symptomatic efficacy of glucosamine and chondroitin in knee osteoarthritis: a comprehensive meta-analysis. Arch Intern Med. 2003;163(13):1514–22.
43. Henrotin YE. Interpretation of metaanalyses: pitfalls should be more widely recognized. J Rheumatol. 2012;39(6):1107–9.
44. Rainsford KD. Importance of pharmaceutical composition and evidence from clinical trials and pharmacological studies in determining effectiveness of chondroitin sulphate and other glycosaminoglycans: a critique. J Pharm Pharmacol. 2009;61(10):1263–70.
45. Roubille C, Martel-Pelletier J, Abram F, Dorais M, Delorme P, Raynauld JP, Pelletier JP. Impact of disease treatments on the progression of knee osteoarthritis structural changes related to meniscal extrusion: data from the OAI progression cohort. Semin Arthritis Rheum. 2015;45(3):257–67.
46. Pelletier JP, Cooper C, Peterfy C, Reginster JY, Brandi ML, Bruyere O, Chapurlat R, Cicuttini F, Conaghan PG, Doherty M, et al. What is the predictive value of MRI for the occurrence of knee replacement surgery in knee osteoarthritis? Ann Rheum Dis. 2013;72(10):1594–604.
47. Raynauld JP, Martel-Pelletier J, Dorais M, Haraoui B, Choquette D, Abram F, Beaulieu A, Bessette L, Morin F, Wildi LM, et al. Total knee replacement as a knee osteoarthritis outcome: predictors derived from a 4 year long-term observation following a randomized clinical trial using chondroitin sulfate. Cartilage. 2013;4(3):219–26.
48. Moller I, Perez M, Monfort J, Benito P, Cuevas J, Perna C, Domenech G, Herrero M, Montell E, Verges J. Effectiveness of chondroitin sulphate in patients with concomitant knee osteoarthritis and psoriasis: a randomized, double-blind, placebo-controlled study. Osteoarthritis Cartilage. 2010;18 Suppl 1:S32–40.
49. Schneider H, Maheu E, Cucherat M. Symptom-modifying effect of chondroitin sulfate in knee osteoarthritis: a meta-analysis of randomized placebo-controlled trials performed with structum®. Open Rheumatol J. 2012;6:183–9.
50. de Campos GC. Placebo effect in osteoarthritis: Why not use it to our advantage? World J Orthop. 2015;6(5):416–20.
51. Conaghan PG, Dickson J, Bolten W, Cevc G, Rother M. A multicentre, randomized, placebo- and active-controlled trial comparing the efficacy and safety of topical ketoprofen in Transfersome gel (IDEA-033) with ketoprofen-free vehicle (TDT 064) and oral celecoxib for knee pain associated with osteoarthritis. Rheumatology (Oxford). 2013;52(7):1303–12.
52. Bingham 3rd CO, Sebba AI, Rubin BR, Ruoff GE, Kremer J, Bird S, Smugar SS, Fitzgerald BJ, O'Brien K, Tershakovec AM. Efficacy and safety of etoricoxib 30 mg and celecoxib 200 mg in the treatment of osteoarthritis in two identically designed, randomized, placebo-controlled, non-inferiority studies. Rheumatology (Oxford). 2007;46(3):496–507.
53. Tannenbaum H, Berenbaum F, Reginster JY, Zacher J, Robinson J, Poor G, Bliddal H, Uebelhart D, Adami S, Navarro F, et al. Lumiracoxib is effective in the treatment of osteoarthritis of the knee: a 13 week, randomised, double blind study versus placebo and celecoxib. Ann Rheum Dis. 2004;63(11):1419–26.

11

Efficacy and safety of adult human bone marrow-derived, cultured, pooled, allogeneic mesenchymal stromal cells (Stempeucel®): preclinical and clinical trial in osteoarthritis ofthe knee joint

Pawan Kumar Gupta[1*], Anoop Chullikana[1], Mathiyazhagan Rengasamy[1], Naresh Shetty[2], Vivek Pandey[3], Vikas Agarwal[4], Shrikant Yeshwant Wagh[5], Prasanth Kulapurathu Vellotare[1], Devi Damodaran[1], Pachaiyappan Viswanathan[1], Charan Thej[1,6], Sudha Balasubramanian[1] and Anish Sen Majumdar[1*]

Abstract

Background: Osteoarthritis (OA) is a common and debilitating chronic degenerative disease of the joints. Currently, cell-based therapy is being explored to address the repair of damaged articular cartilage in the knee joint.

Methods: The in vitro differentiation potential of adult human bone marrow-derived, cultured, pooled, allogeneic mesenchymal stromal cells (Stempeucel®) was determined by differentiating the cells toward the chondrogenic lineage and quantifying sulfated glycosaminoglycan (sGAG). The mono-iodoacetate (MIA)-induced preclinical model of OA has been used to demonstrate pain reduction and cartilage formation. In the clinical study, 60 OA patients were randomized to receive different doses of cells (25, 50, 75, or 150 million cells) or placebo. Stempeucel® was administered by intra-articular (IA) injection into the knee joint, followed by 2 ml hyaluronic acid (20 mg). Subjective evaluations—visual analog scale (VAS) for pain, intermittent and constant osteoarthritis pain (ICOAP), and Western Ontario and McMaster Universities Osteoarthritis (WOMAC-OA) index—were performed at baseline and at 1, 3, 6, and 12 months of follow-up. Magnetic resonance imaging of the knee was performed at baseline, and at 6 and 12 months follow-up for cartilage evaluation.

Results: Stempeucel® differentiated into the chondrogenic lineage in vitro with downregulation of Sox9 and upregulation of Col2A genes. Furthermore, Stempeucel® differentiated into chondrocytes and synthesized a significant amount of sGAG (30 ± 1.8 μg/μg GAG/DNA). In the preclinical model of OA, Stempeucel® reduced pain significantly and also repaired damaged articular cartilage in rats. In the clinical study, IA administration of Stempeucel® was safe, and a trend towards improvement was seen in the 25-million-cell dose group in all subjective parameters (VAS, ICOAP, andWOMAC-OA scores), although this was not statistically significant when compared to placebo. Adverse events were predominant in the higher dose groups (50, 75, and 150 million cells). Knee pain and swelling were the most common adverse events. The whole-organ magnetic resonance imaging score of the knee did not reveal any difference from baseline and the placebo group.

(Continued on next page)

* Correspondence: pawan.gupta@stempeutics.com; anish.majumdar@stempeutics.com
[1]Stempeutics Research Pvt Ltd, Akshay Tech Park, No. 72 & 73, 2nd Floor, EPIP Zone, Phase I-Area, Whitefield, Bangalore 560066, India
Full list of author information is available at the end of the article

(Continued from previous page)

Conclusion: Intra-articular administration of Stempeucel® is safe. A twenty-five-million-cell dose may be the most effective among the doses tested for pain reduction. Clinical studies with a larger patient population are required to demonstrate a robust therapeutic efficacy of Stempeucel® in OA.

Keywords: Mesenchymal stromal cells, Osteoarthritis, Cell therapy

Background

Osteoarthritis (OA) is a common and debilitating chronic degenerative disease of large joints, especially the hip and knee, characterized by a loss of articular cartilage, subchondral sclerosis, and marginal osteophyte formation. Worldwide, approximately 9.6% of men and 18% of women aged ≥60 years have symptomatic osteoarthritis [1]. Current treatment in early-stage OA includes weight reduction, quadriceps strengthening exercises, non-steroidal anti-inflammatory drugs, intra-articular (IA) glucocorticoid injections, viscosupplements, and bracing [2–4]. Total joint arthroplasty is the mainstay treatment for end-stage OA of the knee joint, which is often associated with serious and life-threatening complications including increase risk of infection [5].

Currently, cell therapy- and tissue engineering-based approaches are being used to address the issue of repair of damaged articular cartilage. This includes autologous cultured chondrocytes and mesenchymal stromal cells (MSCs) obtained from various tissues that are used for transplantation into the cartilage lesion. Autologous chondrocyte implantation has inherent disadvantages such as a two-stage surgical procedure (harvesting healthy cartilage and transplanting culture-expanded chondrocytes from that sample) that may cause further cartilage damage and degeneration [6, 7], and chondrocyte dedifferentiation during culture that might result in fibrocartilage rather than hyaline cartilage formation [6, 8]. Thus, autologous or allogeneic MSCs are rapidly emerging as an investigational product for cartilage repair [9–11]. The anti-inflammatory and immunomodulatory properties of MSCs suggest that these cells can reduce inflammation and pain reduction in the knee. Concurrently, MSCs may initiate the repair process of the damaged cartilage by differentiating into chondrocytes, as well as by inducing proliferation and maturation of the remaining healthy chondrocytes or by inducing differentiation of chondroprogenitors [12]. A whole host of growth factors, biological modulators, and extracellular matrix proteins produced by MSCs may play a pivotal role in enhancing neocartilage formation [12].

Several preclinical studies and clinical trials have been conducted using MSCs which have reported the safety and therapeutic effect of its administration in patients with OA, although the majority of these studies have been conducted as single-dose, single-arm pilot studies [13–15]. Hence, there is a need for randomized, double-blind, controlled clinical trials. We have carried out in vitro studies to show the differentiation efficiency of adult human bone marrow-derived, cultured, pooled, allogeneic mesenchymal stromal cells (Stempeucel®) into the chondrogenic lineage and the expression of chondrocyte-specific markers. In order to determine if Stempeucel® is efficacious in a preclinical model, we have administered these cells intra-articularly into the knee joints of rats with mono-iodoacetate (MIA)-induced OA. After completion of these studies, a phase 2 dose-finding clinical study was initiated to evaluate the safety (primary endpoint), potential efficacy, and appropriate dose (secondary endpoints) of IA administration of Stempeucel® in patients with OA of the knee joint.

Methods

Production and characterization of Stempeucel® and placebo

Stempeucel® is a bone marrow-derived, ex vivo expanded, pooled, allogeneic human MSC population that has been characterized previously [16, 17]. The pooled cells were manufactured in an approved Good Manufacturing Practice (GMP) facility from bone marrow-derived MSCs (BMMSCs) of three different healthy volunteers to produce a working cell bank (WCB). The pooled MSCs from the WCB were further expanded to manufacture the investigational medicinal product, Stempeucel®. The cells expressed all markers characteristic of MSC, were negative for hematopoietic surface antigens, and also efficiently differentiated into osteocytes, chondrocytes, and adipocytes in vitro [16]. Two hundred million expanded BMMSCs were cryopreserved and stored in 15 ml PLASMA-LYTE A (Baxter, Deerfield, Illinois) containing 5% human serum albumin and 10% dimethyl sulfoxide (DMSO) in cryobags (MacoPharma, Mouvaux, France). Placebo contained 15 ml PLASMA-LYTE A in similar cryobags. The investigational medicinal product (IMP) specification is given in Table 1.

In vitro studies show differentiation of Stempeucel® to the chondrogenic lineage and quantification of sulfated glycosaminoglycan

The chondrogenic differentiation potential of six Stempeucel® batches was evaluated in monolayer cultures using chondrogenesis induction medium (catalog no. A10071-01; Gibco).

Table 1 Investigational medicinal product (IMP) specification

S. no	Description	Specifications	
1	Morphology	Cells are fibroblastic and spindle-shaped in active growing conditions Cells are intact and round in shape after trypsin action	
2.	Cell count	180 to 220 million cells per bag	
3.	Viability	≥85%	
4.	Cell phenotype	CD 73 >80% CD105 > 80% CD 90 > 80% CD 166 > 80%	CD 34 <5% CD 45 < 5% CD 133 < 5% CD 14 < 5% CD19 < 5% HLA-DR < 5%
5.	Karyotyping	Normal, 46 XY	
6.	Mycoplasma PCR ELISA	Not detected	
7.	Sterility test	Must comply	
8.	Differentiation assay to adiopocyte, osteocyte, and chondrocyte	Confirmation of differentiation	

Cells were plated at a density of 1000 cells/cm^2 in six-well plates and cultured in DMEM-KO with 10% fetal bovine serum (FBS) and 2 ng/mL basic fibroblast growth factor (bFGF) until 80% confluency. The cells were induced to differentiation in chondrogenic induction medium (Gibco) for 21 days; the medium was replenished every 3 days and uninduced cells were harvested at 80% confluency and served as the corresponding control for background estimation. After 21 days of differentiation, the cells were trypsinized and pelleted by centrifugation at 1000 rpm and the chondrogenic differentiation was quantified by measuring the amount of sulfated glycosaminoglycan (sGAG) using a Blyscan kit (catalog no. B1000; Bicolor). The final sGAG content was represented after normalizing with total DNA content estimated using a Quant-iT Pico green kit (P7589; ThermoFisher, USA).

Quantitative RT-PCR for chondrogenic-specific gene markers

Total cellular RNA was isolated using an RNeasy mini kit (Qiagen) from the undifferentiated and the differentiated BMMSCs for chondroyte lineage (described above). The RNA samples were treated with RNAse free DNase I (Ambion), and reverse-transcribed into cDNA using a high-capacity cDNA reverse transcription kit (Applied Biosystems) according to the manufacturer's instructions. Real-time PCR was carried out using the SYBR green kit (catalog no. 4309155; Applied Biosystems) using step one plus (Applied Biosystems). Beta actin served as the internal control. The sequences for the gene-specific primers are as follows: Sox9, forward TTTCCAAGACACAAACATGA, reverse AAAGTCCAGTTTCTCGTTGA; Col2A, forward TTTCCCA GGTCAAGATGGTC, reverse TCACCTGGTTTTCCACCTTC. Ct values were normalized to the housekeeping gene β-actin.

Preclinical model of osteoarthritis

Ten-week-old male Wistar rats ($n = 80$) weighing between 175 and 285 g were used for the preclinical study. The experimental protocol was approved by the Institutional Animal Ethics Committee (IAEC), and the experiment was carried out at a CRO animal facility.

Bilateral osteoarthritis was induced in rats ($n = 74$) by injection of MIA (Sigma-Aldrich, USA) into the knee joints according to published methods [18–20]. Briefly, the animals were anesthetized with 3% isoflurane; 1 mg MIA dissolved in 50 μl saline was delivered into the articular cavity. The rats ($n = 6$) receiving only the saline solution served as sham control animals (group I) throughout the experiment. The pain sensitivity of the knee joints was measured before MIA injection and once every week after MIA injection as described by Di Cesare et al. [21]. The Pressure Application Measurement device (PAM; Ugo Basile, Italy) was used to measure the mechanical pain threshold of the knee joints. The gram-force (gf) that elicited the limb withdrawal was recorded. Three weeks after MIA injection, animals displaying PAM values that ranged between 272 and 601 gf were considered to have developed OA and were selected for the study ($n = 60$). Prior to performing the experiment described in this paper, we had conducted a validation study in which the range of PAM values was evaluated against gross pathology and histological evidence of OA in rats (data not shown). The range of PAM values was selected accordingly prior to randomizing the animals in the current study. Rats were divided into four different groups and each group consisted of 15 rats (Table 2). Sham control animals (group I) showed an average PAM value of 870 ± 138 gf.

Stempeucel® administration in MIA-induced rats

At day 0, animals in both groups 1 (sham control) and group 2 (vehicle control) received 60 μl vehicle

Table 2 Animal grouping and sacrifice schedule

Group		Animals sacrificed (no of rats)*		
		4 weeks	8 weeks	12 weeks
Group 1	Sham control	2	2	2
Group 2	Vehicle control	3	6	6
Group 3	Hyaluronic acid (HA)	3	6	6
Group 4	Stempeucel® low dose + HA (6×10^5 cells/joint)	3	6	6
Group 5	Stempeucel® high dose + HA (1.3×10^6 cells/joint)	3	6	6

*Number of animals sacrificed at each time point after Stempeucel® administration

(Plasmalyte A; Baxter) through the IA route delivered by a 27-gauge needle. For group 3 animals, 30 μl hyaluronic acid (HA; Hyalgan®; Fidia Pharmaceuticals, Italy) was injected followed by 30 μl vehicle. For group 4 and 5 rats, freshly-thawed Stempeucel® was used after washing in Plasmalyte A to remove DMSO and resuspending in Plasmalyte A. Stempeucel® was administered at two different doses: 6×10^5 cells/joint (low dose; human equivalent dose (HED) of 25 million cells) and 1.3×10^6 cells/joint (high dose; HED of 50 million cells). Both doses were formulated in 30 μl Plasmalyte A and injected into group 4 (low-dose group) and group 5 (high-dose group) animals, respectively. Cell administration was immediately followed by 30 μl HA injection. In order to reduce the xenogeneic rejection of cells, cyclosporine A (CsA; Novartis, Switzerland) was injected subcutaneously into all the experimental animals at a dose of 10 mg/kg daily for an initial 1 week starting at day −3 of cell injection, after which daily CsA administration was continued orally at the same dose until the end of the study. The pain response was measured at weekly intervals up to week 10. The final measurements were taken at week 12.

Gross and histological evaluation of cartilage repair in preclinical model

The treatment regimen and the number of animals sacrificed after BMMSC administration at various time points are shown in Table 2. Rats from all the groups were sacrificed at 4, 8, and 12 weeks after vehicle/HA/Stempeucel® administration. The knee joints were dissected and the cartilage surface was visualized macroscopically on the exposed joints, and the distal femur from the right joints was dissected and processed for histological analysis.

All joint specimens were fixed in 10% formalin buffer and then decalcified in 10% EDTA (RFCL, India) for 2 weeks; the decalcification solution was changed twice in a week. The joints were embedded in paraffin; serial sagittal sections (5-μm thick) were prepared and stained with hematoxylin and eosin (H&E) and Safranin-O fast green staining for proteoglycan visualization and estimation [22]. The severity of articular damage was evaluated using the Osteoarthritis Research Society International (OARSI) grading system [23, 24] on the H&E-stained sections. The binding intensity of Safranin-O to the sGAG was quantified using imageJ software [25]. The region of interest (ROI) around the cartilage area ($n = 3$ per section) was selected, and the intensity of red (R), green (G), and blue (B) were measured and the proportion of red staining was calculated using the equation $r = R/(R^2 + G^2 + B^2)^{1/2}$ where, R is the intensity of red and 'r' refers to the intensity of the red fraction with respect to other primary colors [26]. The sections were graded and quantified by an independent observer blinded to the treatment groups.

Clinical study design and enrollment criteria

This was a randomized, double-blind, multicentric, placebo-controlled, phase II study assessing the safety and efficacy of IA Stempeucel® in patients with OA of knee. The study was conducted in accordance with the Good Clinical Practice (GCP) guidelines as issued by the International Conference on Harmonization (ICH/135/95, July 2002), Schedule Y of the Drugs and Cosmetics Rules, 1945, Ethical guidelines for biomedical research on human participants prepared by the Indian Council of Medical Research in 2006 and the Declaration of Helsinki (64th WMA General Assembly, Fortaleza, Brazil, October 2013). Approval was obtained from the Central Drugs Standard Control Organization (Indian FDA) and the institutional ethics committees of the five participating hospitals. The study was registered in the National Institute of Health registry of clinical trials (https://clinicaltrials.gov/ct2/show/NCT01453738). An independent data safety monitoring board was formed comprising of drug safety physicians and an expert in the therapeutic area to monitor the safety data at predefined intervals during the progress of the study. The study was conducted from November 2011 to November 2013. Written informed consent was obtained from all participants before screening. Of the 82 patients screened, 62 patients were randomized to the study from five centers. Two patients dropped out from the study after randomization but before IMP administration; thus 60 patients received the IMP. Four dose levels were studied in this trial: 25, 50, 75, and 150 million cells (25 M, 50 M, 75 M, and 150 M, respectively). At each dose level, 15 patients were randomized into two groups (Stempeucel® and placebo) in a 2:1 ratio using a computer generated randomization. Thus, 10 subjects received Stempeucel® and 5 subjects received placebo at each dose level (Fig. 1). As this was the first study of IA administration of Stempeucel® in OA patients, no formal sample size calculation was performed. Eligibility criteria of the patients in the trial are given in Table 3.

Preparation of IMP at the clinical trial sites

Block randomization (block size 5) was performed centrally by a biostatistician using PROC PLAN in SAS. The IMP (Stempeucel® or placebo) was shipped in a cryoshipper (temperature −185 to −196 °C) to clinical trial sites whenever each patient was eligible for the study. Preparation of IMP for injection was performed under a validated biosafety cabinet by a trained person independent of the investigator's team. A cryobag containing IMP was thawed at 37 °C in a water bath. The cell suspension was diluted to 100 ml using PLASMA-LYTE A using two 50-ml centrifuge tubes. The cell pellet was resuspended in 2 ml PLASMA-LYTE A (for the 25- and 50-million-cell dose groups) and in 4 ml PLASMA-LYTE A (for the 75- and 150-million-cell dose groups) based on the viable cell count and was loaded to a blinded syringe. For the placebo preparation, a similar amount of PLASMA-LYTE A was loaded to a blinded syringe. The IMP (Stempeucel® or placebo) was presented to the investigators in a blinded syringe (using semitransparent tape) in a temperature-controlled transport box at 2–8 °C. It was not possible to distinguish between Stempeucel® and placebo upon visual inspection of the blinded syringes.

Injection protocol for the clinical study

Pre-medication (hydrocortisone 100 mg IV and pheniramine maleate 45.5 mg IV) was administered 15–30 min before administration of the IMP to prevent the possibility of a potential anaphylactic reaction to the allogeneic cells. The IA injections were performed by qualified and experienced investigators (either orthopedician or rheumatologist) using a 2.0-inch (5.1-cm) 20-gauge needle as a lateral midpatellar injection (an injection into the patellofemoral joint). IMP injection was followed by injection of 2 ml hyaluronic acid (20 mg; Hyalgan, Fidia Farmaceutici S.p.A., Italy). Patients were hospitalized for the procedure, and were monitored for 24 h after the injection. Patients were discharged after inspection of the target joint, a general physical examination, and vital signs evaluation.

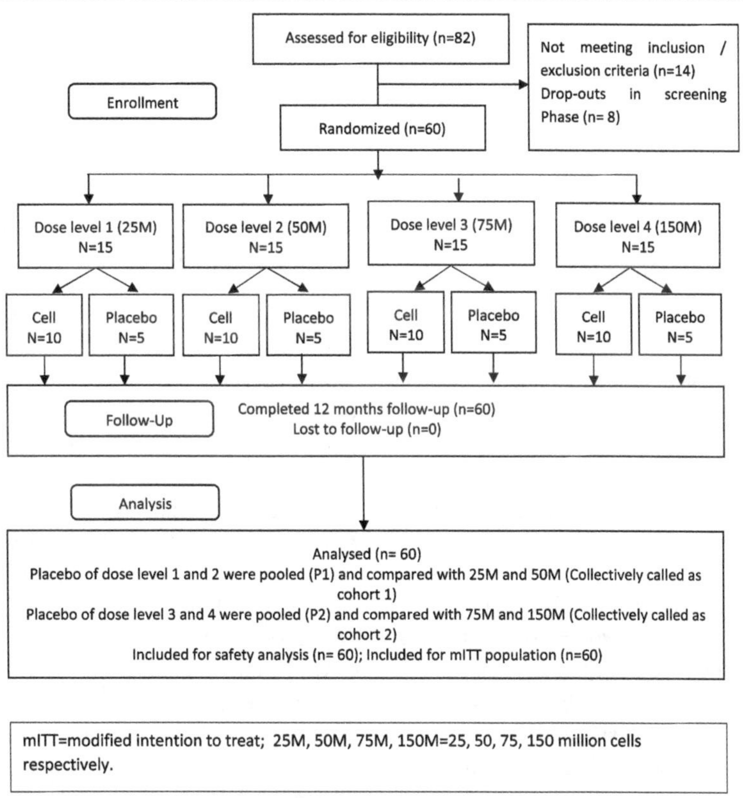

Fig. 1 CONSORT flow chart showing the number of patients randomized, followed-up, and analyzed. *M* million cells, *Cell* Stempeucel®, *mITT* modified intention to treat

Table 3 Subject eligibility criteria

Inclusion criteria
1. Males or females in the age range 40–70 years (both inclusive)
2. Radiographic evidence of grade 2 to 3 osteoarthritis (OA) based on the Kellgren and Lawrence radiographic entry criteria*
3. History of primary idiopathic OA of the knee characterized by pain which required intake of analgesics
4. Self-reported difficulty in at least one of the following activities attributed to knee pain: lifting and carrying groceries, walking 400 meters, getting in and out of a chair, or going up and down stairs
5. Patients who had been on stable medication, including non-steroidal anti-inflammatory drugs (NSAIDs)/opioid or opiate analgesics, for the past 3 months
6. Female patients of childbearing age who agreed to use accepted methods of contraception during the course of the study
7. Ability to provide written informed consent
Exclusion criteria
1. Prior or ongoing medical conditions (e.g., concomitant illness, psychiatric condition, alcoholism, drug abuse), medical history, physical findings, electrocardiogram (ECG) findings, or laboratory abnormality that, in the investigator's opinion, could adversely affect the safety of the subject, makes it unlikely that the course of treatment or follow-up would be completed or could impair the assessment of study results
2. History of surgery or major trauma to the study joint
3. Arthroscopy on the study joint in the previous 12 months
4. Signs of active study joint inflammation including redness, warmth, and/or, if qualifying with OA of the knee, a large, bulging effusion of the study knee joint with the loss of normal contour of the joint at the screening visit or at the baseline examination
5. Patients who received intra-articular steroids or hyaluronan within the last 3 months
6. Infections in or around the knee
7. Patients awaiting a replacement knee or hip joint
8. Patients with other conditions that caused pain
9. Patients with deformity of the knee joint
10. Significantly incapacitated or disabled and would be categorized as ACR Functional Class IV (largely or wholly incapacitated) or unable to walk without assistive devices
11. Patients with other known rheumatic or inflammatory disease such as rheumatoid arthritis
12. Other pathologic lesions on X-rays of knee
13. Positive hepatitis B surface antigen, hepatitis C antibody test, anti-HIV antibody test, or Rapid Plasma Reagin (RPR)
14. History of bleeding disorders
15. Known hypersensitivity to hyaluronan or animal sera
16. For women of child-bearing potential: positive pregnancy test or lactating (females who were planning pregnancy within the next year were excluded)

*If both knees of a patient were eligible to be included in the study, the knee to be included was as per investigator judgment

Follow-up for the clinical trial patients

Patients were followed up at 1 week, and 1, 3, and 6 months after injection of IMP. The clinical data were unblinded after 6 months and patients were further followed-up for both safety and efficacy until 12 months after the injection. Safety assessments included monitoring of all adverse events (AEs), assessment of electrocardiogram (ECG) parameters, hematological (complete blood count including erythrocyte sedimentation rate) and biochemical (liver function tests, kidney function tests, and lipid profile) values, physical examination, and vital signs measurements. Adverse events were captured by interviewing the subjects and laboratory data evaluations during the visits. The efficacy endpoints included improvement in pain from OA graded on a visual analog scale (VAS) from 0 to 10 (0 = no pain; 10 = worst pain); also, the Western Ontario and McMaster Universities Osteoarthritis (WOMAC-OA) index (total score, pain, stiffness, and physical function scores) and intermittent and constant osteoarthritis pain (ICOAP) was used (constant and intermittent pain score) to evaluate pain and function of the joint. X-ray of the knee was carried out at baseline, and at 3 and 6 months follow-up. Magnetic resonance imaging (MRI) of the knee was carried out at baseline, and at 6 and 12 months follow-up. MRI of the knee was performed using a 1.5-T whole body scanner and a circumferential eight-channel knee coil. Proton density T2-weighted sequences were captured: sagittal intermediate, axial intermediate, and coronal intermediate for assessing osteophytes and cartilage (for scoring cartilage signal and morphology, marginal osteophytes, subarticular bone marrow abnormality, subarticular cysts, and subarticular bone attrition); sagittal PD FS for assessing menisci and cruciate ligaments (for scoring of ACL, PCL, medial, and lateral menisci); and sagittal 3D FIESTA-C for assessing cartilage surface and superficial erosions (for scoring cartilage signal and morphology). Images were scored to assess the whole-organ magnetic resonance imaging score (WORMS) by two experienced radiologists using combined reads. In case of non-concurrence, advice was taken from a third independent radiologist whose report was considered final. WORMS scoring used in this study was modified for calculation of total WORMS score. The parameters included were articular surface features which include cartilage signal and morphology, subarticular bone marrow abnormality, subarticular cysts, subarticular bone attrition, and marginal osteophytes. They were scored for all 14 compartments of the knee joint. The compartment totals were added to obtain the overall knee joint score [27].

Statistical analysis

Preclinical data

GraphPad Prism software was used to calculate the statistical significance of all preclinical experimental data. The data are expressed as the mean ± SEM. Quantitative RT-PCR data analysis was performed using Student's *t* test. Pain threshold differences between various treatment groups and the Safranin-O quantification were examined for statistical significance using two-way analysis of variance followed by a Bonferroni post-hoc test. The OARSI grade analysis was performed using one-way analysis followed by Kruskal–Wallis test. $P < 0.05$ denoted the presence of a significant difference between groups.

Clinical trial data

The SAS package (SAS® Institute Inc., USA, version 9.2) was used for statistical evaluation. For analysis purpose, subjects were grouped as follows: four treatment groups (25 M, 50 M, 75 M, and 150 M cell dose), and two placebo groups. Patients who received placebo in 25 M and 50 M dose levels were grouped into one placebo group (both received the IMP in 2 ml PLASMA-LYTE A; P1) and those who received placebo corresponding to the 75 M and 150 M dose groups (both received the IMP in 4 ml PLASMA-LYTE A) were grouped into another group (P2). Thus, there were four treatment groups and two placebo groups forming a total of six groups. The treatment groups 25 M and 50 M were compared with P1 (the three groups collectively called cohort 1) and treatment groups 75 M and 150 M were compared with P2 (the three groups collectively called cohort 2). AEs were coded by the Medical Dictionary for Regulatory Activities (MedDRA) primary system organ class (SOC) and preferred term (PT). AEs were summarized descriptively by total number of AE(s) and compared between the six study groups. Continuous variables are presented as mean ± SD. The data distribution was visually examined for normality before applying the statistical tool for analysis. Comparisons among groups were conducted using Kruskal–Wallis test, with alpha set at 0.05 for significance.

Results

Differentiation efficiency of Stempeucel® into chondrogenic lineage in vitro

We evaluated the chondrogenic differentiation potential of Stempeucel® batches in monolayer cultures. The extent of differentiation was also assessed by mRNA expression of Sox9 and Col2A. We observed a significant downregulation of Sox9, which is an early inducer of chondrogenesis in the differentiated cells compared to the control ($P < 0.02$, $n = 6$), and upregulation of Col2A, the gene that encodes for type 2 collagen, a major cartilage matrix protein and a mature chondrocyte marker (Fig. 2a and b). Chondrogenic differentiation of BMMSCs was quantified by measuring the amalgamation of sGAG which is known to play a central role in cartilage homeostasis [28]. All six batches of Stempeucel® differentiated to chondrocytes and synthesized significant amount of sGAG (30 ± 1.8 μg/μg GAG/DNA) compared to that produced by the undifferentiated cells (12.07 ± 5.6 μg/μg GAG/DNA; $P < 0.001$, $n = 6$) (Fig. 2c). These data suggest that the pooled BMMSC samples efficiently differentiated into the chondrogenic lineage, confirming the presence of mature chondrocytes after differentiation.

Intra-articular administration of Stempeucel® ameliorates OA-induced joint pain in a preclinical model

The MIA-induced OA model was the first validated pain model of OA used to evaluate the analgesic and anti-inflammatory properties of therapeutic agents [20]. In our study, the mechanical pain threshold was measured weekly by PAM test. Pain threshold values from various time points are shown in Fig. 3a. Analysis of PAM scores indicates that animals treated with both low and high doses of Stempeucel® showed improvement in pain threshold from week 2 onwards as compared to vehicle or HA-treated animals and continued to improve until 8 weeks after cell injection. While the pain improvement appeared to reach saturation by 8 weeks with the low dose of cells, it continued to improve until 12 weeks in the animals that received a high dose of Stempeucel® (Fig. 3a). Animals treated with HA alone showed some improvement in pain threshold at the initial time period (week 3); however, this improvement was not found to be consistent. When comparing the PAM scores between the HA- and Stempeucel®-treated groups, animals treated with the high dose of cells exhibited a significant pain-reduction effect at week 4 ($P < 0.001$), week 8 ($P < 0.001$) and week 12 ($P < 0.05$), whereas the low-dose group showed a significant effect at week 4 ($P < 0.05$) and week 8 ($P < 0.001$), but not at week 12. These results clearly demonstrate that intra-articularly injected Stempeucel® is able to reduce the pain significantly in the MIA-induced OA rat model.

Cartilage repair induced by Stempeucel® administration in a preclinical model

Macroscopic evaluation of articular cartilage was performed in rats at 4, 8, and 12 weeks after cell injection. Varying degrees of cartilage damage were observed in animals injected with MIA and subsequently administered with vehicle. These degenerative changes include cartilage fibrillation, erosion, and osteophyte formation (data not shown). The degree of cartilage damage was progressively reduced with both low and high doses of Stempeucel® + HA treatment, while only marginal change was noticed in a few HA-treated animals.

Based on H&E staining of the cartilage tissue, we scored the femoral condyle section of rats using the OARSI grading system. As expected, sham control animals showed a normal histological appearance of the cartilage throughout the study (Fig. 3b, panels a, f, and k for weeks 4, 8, and 12, respectively). In the vehicle-treated animals, the OA joints showed fibrillation, and appreciable loss of chondrocytes was observed at both weeks 4 and 8 (Fig. 3b, panels b and g). By week 12, the cartilage damage was found to be severe and the hyaline tissue was replaced with fibrocartilage (Fig. 3b, panel l). The HA-treated animals showed marginal improvement in cartilage architecture (Fig. 3b, panels c, h, and m). In contrast, animals receiving both low and high doses of Stempeucel® showed almost intact cartilage with a larger number of chondrocytes (Fig. 3b, panels d, i, and n for a low dose of cells and panels e, j, and o for a high dose of cells). The calculated OARSI grades of the different treatment groups were compared at week 12. Although,

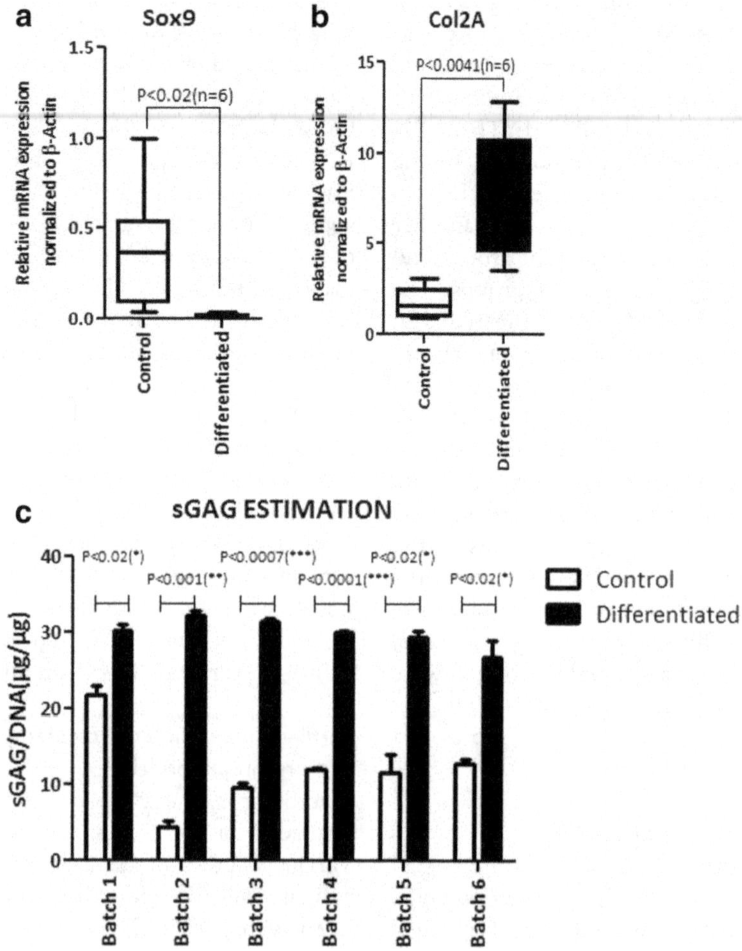

Fig. 2 Quantification of gene expression and sGAG. Quantitative mRNA expression of **a** SOX9 and **b** Col2A in the control (*white bar*) and chondrogenically differentiated Stempeucel® (*black bar*) by real-time PCR analysis ($n = 6$). **c** Sulfated glycosaminoglycan (*sGAG*) content in the control (*white bar*) and chondrogenically differentiated Stempeucel® (*black bar*) by DMMB dye-binding assay. The sGAG values were normalized to the DNA content in the control and chondrogenically differentiated Stempeucel® ($n = 6$). Results are represented as mean with SEM

both low- and high-cell doses showed histological improvement, a statistically significant reduction in OARSI grade was observed only in the high-dose Stempeucel®-treated animals ($P < 0.05$) in comparison to animals in the vehicle group. The Safranin-O stained area of the cartilage was greater in both the cell-treated groups (Fig. 4a, panels d, i, and n for the low dose and panels e, j, and o for the high dose). It is important to note that the intensity of Safranin-O staining increased progressively with both doses of Stempeucel®. In fact, at week 12, Safranin-O staining intensity was found to be comparable between the high- and low-cell dose animals and sham controls (Fig. 4a). In comparison to the HA- and vehicle-treated groups, sGAG intensity was found to be significantly higher in Stempeucel®-treated and in sham control animals at week 12 (Fig. 4b). These findings suggest that intra-articularly injected Stempeucel® + HA repaired MIA-induced articular cartilage damage in rats with OA of the knee joint.

Clinical study

Demographics and baseline characteristics of patients

The demographics and other baseline characteristics of the enrolled patients are presented in Table 4. All six groups were mostly comparable in terms of baseline characteristics. Sixty patients were included in the modified intention to treat analysis (mITT) group. There was no premature unblinding of any patient. The patients' age, sex, weight, height, and body mass index (BMI) were balanced across groups. High scores for VAS, WOMAC, and ICOAP suggest that these patients had severe pain and were balanced across all groups.

Procedural safety

All patients tolerated the procedure well in cohort 1 (25 M, 50 M, and P1) and cohort 2 (75 M, 150 M, and P2). Ten patients (1 in 50 M, 6 in 75 M, and 3 in 150 M dose groups) experienced pain and swelling at the injection site.

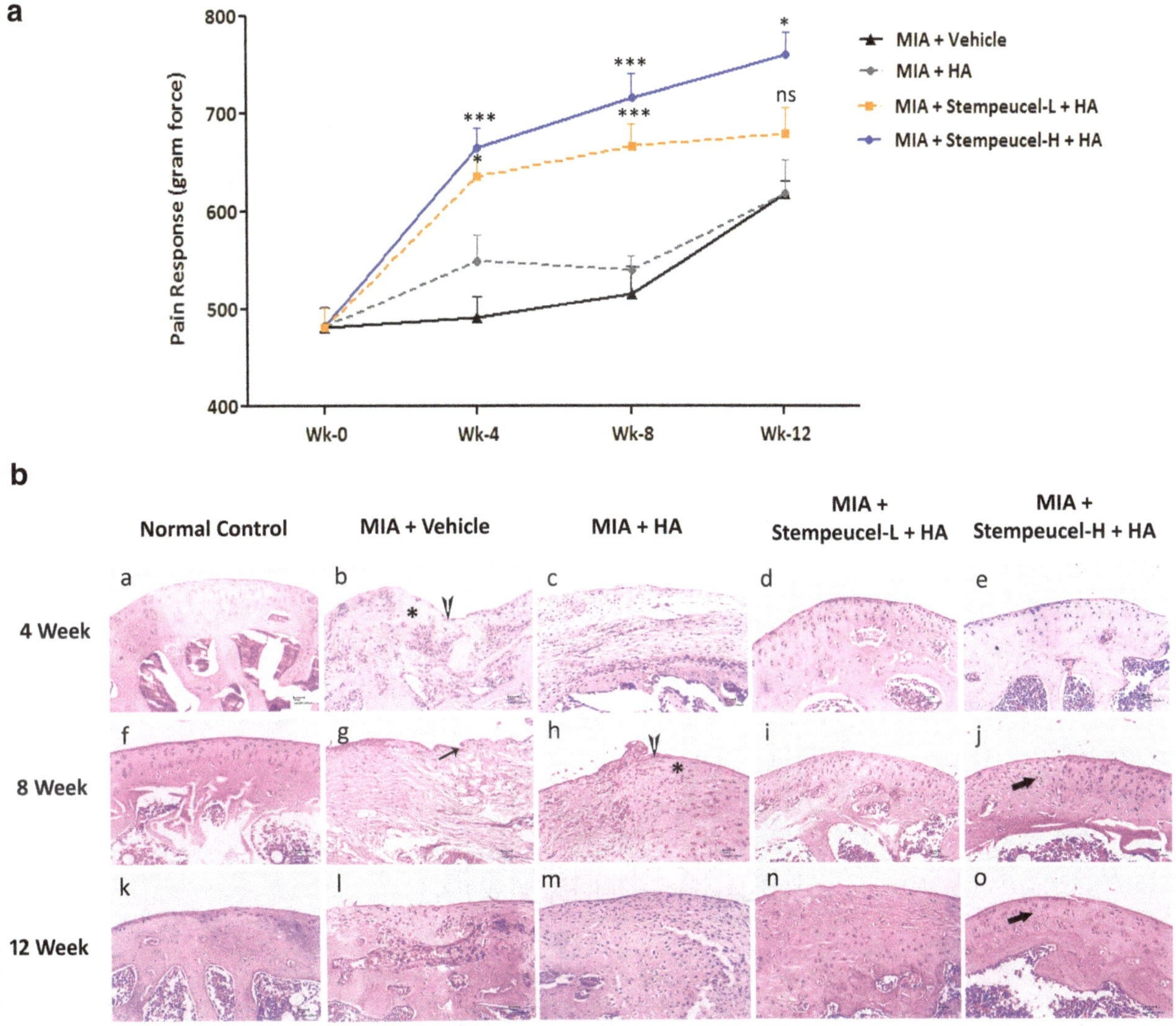

Fig. 3 Effect of intra-articular injection of Stempeucel® on pain reduction and cartilage repair in an osteoarthritic rat model. **a** The effect of Stempeucel® on pain reduction at week 0 (before cell injection), and at weeks 4, 8, and 12 after cell injection. Data are presented as mean ± SEM. $*P < 0.05$, $***P < 0.001$ versus hyaluronic acid (*HA*)-treated group. **b** Photomicrographs of representative joint sections of femoral condyle stained with H&E at 4 (a–e), 8 (f–j), and 12 weeks (k–o) after Stempeucel® treatment. Osteoarthritic changes, such as loss of chondrocytes (*), loss of cartilage (*vertical arrow*), and fibrillation (*thin arrow*) are evident in vehicle-treated and HA-treated joints. Proliferation of chondrocytes (*thick arrow*), regeneration, and repair of cartilage tissue was evident in Stempeucel®-treated groups. *Scale bars* = 100 μm, magnification 10×. *H* high dose of Stempeucel®, *L* Low dose of Stempeucel®, *MIA* mono-iodoacetate, *ns* not significant

The events were mild to moderate in severity, assessed as related to the IMP, and recovered upon conservative therapy. Among the 10 patients, one subject (150 M dose group) had IMP-related synovial effusion requiring hospitalization for one additional day of observation, thus meeting the criteria of a serious adverse event (SAE). Other SAEs in the study were determined to be unrelated to the IMP and were as follows: hysterectomy for menorrhagia in one subject in the 25 M group, suture-related complication and varicose vein in one subject in the P1 group, and hemorrhoidal hemorrhage and umbilical hernia, respectively, in one subject each in the P2 group.

Overall evaluation of adverse events

A total of 97 AEs were reported in 40 subjects (Table 5). The distribution of AEs in the different dose groups was as follows: 24 (25 M), 13 (50 M), 21 (P1), 17 (75 M), 11 (150 M), and 11 (P2). No patient died or was withdrawn from the study due to an AE. Most of the AEs were mild to moderate in severity. One severe AE was reported in each of 25 M (dyslipidemia), 50 M (anemia), 150 M (muscle hemorrhage), and P2 (umbilical hernia) groups. Physical examination and vital signs data were unremarkable after the injection. In cohort 1, most of the AEs observed in the study were related to the SOC

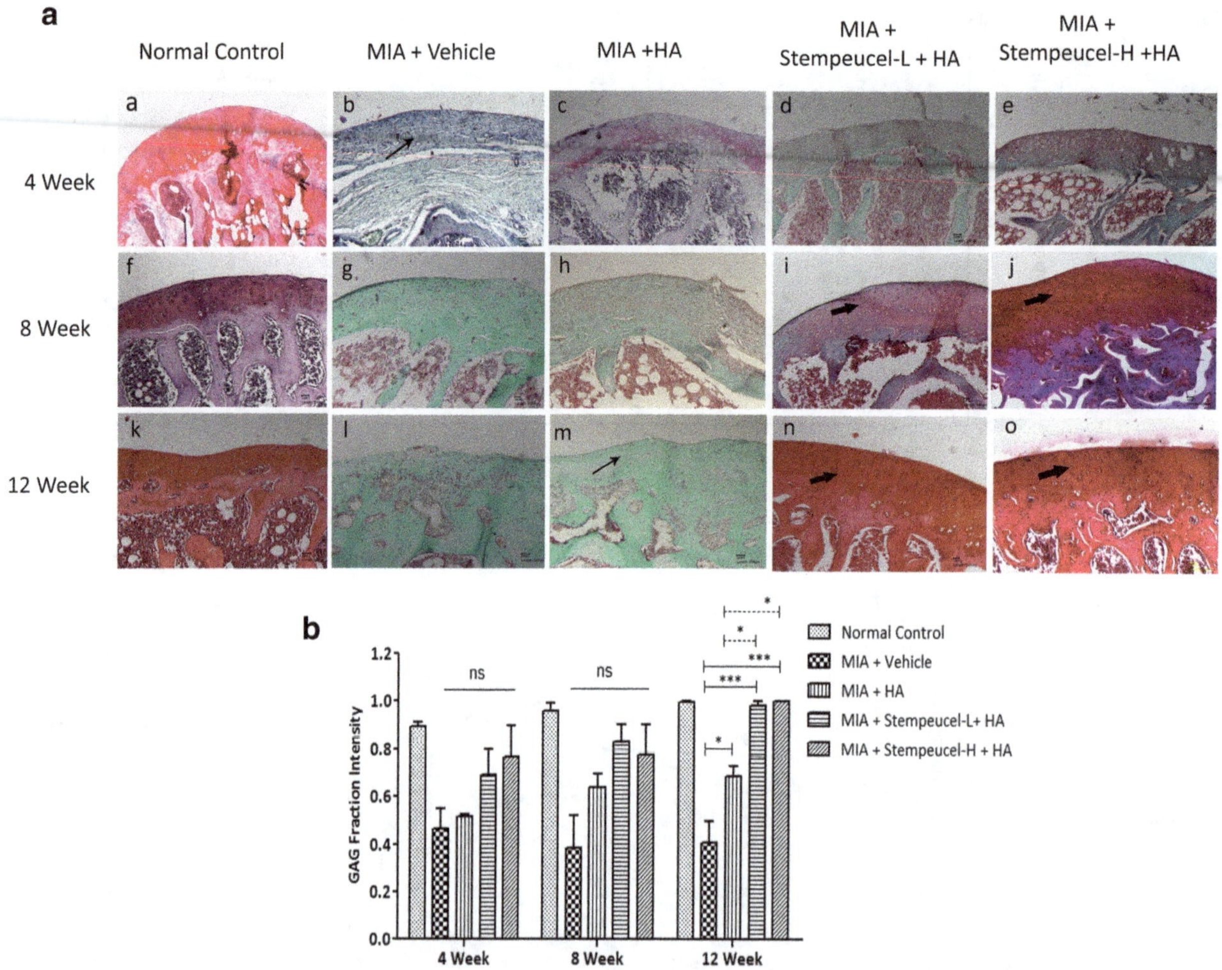

Fig. 4 Histological evaluation of Safranin-O stained joint sections. **a** Photomicrographs of representative joint specimens of femoral condyle stained with Safranin-O at 4 (a–e), 8 (f–j), and 12 weeks (k–o) after Stempeucel® treatment. Loss of articular surface, roughening of cartilage and reduced staining of Safranin-O (*thin arrow*) were observed in vehicle- and HA-treated joints. Strongly stained Safranin-O-positive cartilage (*thick arrow*) with increased numbers of chondrocytes was seen in the Stempeucel®-treated groups. *Scale bars* = 100 μm, magnification 10×. **b** Sulfated glycosaminoglycan (*GAG*) fraction intensity was measured from histological images of Safranin-O-stained sections at weeks 4, 8, and 12. The intensity of Safranin-O staining is represented graphically, and the data are represented as mean ± SEM. At 12 weeks, the Stempeucel®-treated groups (both low (*L*) and high (*H*) dose) showed a significant improvement in the sGAG content compared to the disease control (mono-iodoacetate; *MIA*) and hyaluronic acid (*HA*)-treated groups. *$P < 0.05$, *** $P < 0.001$. *ns* not significant

(musculoskeletal and connective tissue disorders); the most common AE was arthralgia. In cohort 2, most of the AE(s) observed in the study were related to the SOC (general disorders and administration site conditions). The most common AEs in the 75 M group were injection site pain and arthralgia. Three events of arthralgia were experienced by two subjects (one subject had two episodes of arthralgia due to OA) and four events of injection site joint pain were experienced by four subjects in the 75 M dose group. One event of hypersensitivity to IMP (joint swelling) was experienced by a subject in the 75 M dose group. Three events of hypersensitivity to IMP (joint swelling) were experienced by three subjects in the 150 M group. All events of joint pain and swelling recovered completely upon symptomatic treatment. Hematology, serum chemistry, serology, urine analyses, and ECG evaluation did not reveal any significant abnormalities.

Efficacy results

VAS scores decreased over the study period for all the treatment groups except for patients in the 150 M group. The maximum reduction in the VAS score was seen in the 25 M group at 12 months compared to the other groups of patients (40.3 ± 17.3, 30.3 ± 31.0, and 21.3 ± 28.3 cm in 25 M, 50 M, and P1, respectively; $P = 0.3833$). VAS decreased by 67.4% in the 25 M group compared to 41.4% and 36.0% in the 50 M group and P1, respectively ($P = 0.0587$) (Fig. 5).

Table 4 Summary of Demographic Characteristics at Baseline

	Cohort 1				Cohort 2			
Parameter	25 M (*n* = 10)	50 M (*n* = 10)	P1 (*n* = 10)	*P* value	75 M (*n* = 10)	150 M (*n* = 10)	P2 (*n* = 10)	*P* value
Age (years)	58.10 ± 8.23	57.30 ± 9.45	54.90 ± 8.27	0.73	55.00 ± 6.72	54.00 ± 6.73	56.70 ± 5.19	0.6
Female (*n*)	7	8	10	NA	8	5	7	NA
Male (*n*)	3	2	0	NA	2	5	3	NA
Height (cm)	156.85 ± 9.64	157.30 ± 12.23	152.25 ± 9.72	0.39	158.40 ± 8.86	158.88 ± 9.30	159.70 ± 10.67	0.9
Weight (kg)	73.10 ± 15.86	69.00 ± 14.62	66.10 ± 7.67	0.45	71.30 ± 9.09	66.00 ± 9.13	66.90 ± 8.57	0.39
BMI (kg/m^2)	29.73 ± 6.09	27.74 ± 4.16	28.84 ± 4.91	0.76	28.38 ± 2.38	26.33 ± 4.48	26.40 ± 3.99	0.3
WOMAC total	1315.8 ± 444.8	1498.4 ± 407.4	1239.6 ± 472.2	0.28	1470.6 ± 471.0	1388.1 ± 508.8	1382.0 ± 324.7	0.9
ICOAP total	45.7 ± 19.2	59.3 ± 21.7	49.3 ± 18.7	0.38	58.4 ± 20.7	46.4 ± 22.0	54.8 ± 17.8	0.54
VAS	60.9 ± 19.7	73.7 ± 15.2	61.0 ± 23.8	0.24	57.4 ± 29.0	46.6 ± 23.6	65.3 ± 12.2	0.11
WORMS total score	67.0 ± 19.8	78.8 ± 40.9	76.5 ± 23.5	0.65	71.3 ± 21.4	62.0 ± 17.9	70.8 ± 14.7	0.48
Kellgren and Lawrence Grade 2 (*n*)	4	1	3	NA	1	3	2	NA
Kellgren and Lawrence Grade 3 (*n*)	6	9	7	NA	9	7	8	NA

Values are shown as mean ± SD unless indicated otherwise
25 M, 50 M, 75 M, 150 M = 25, 50, 75, and 150 million cells, respectively
P1, P2 = placebo 1 and placebo 2, respectively
BMI body mass index, ICOAP intermittent and constant osteoarthritis pain, NA statistical comparisons for these groups have not been conducted due to too few samples, VAS visual analog scale, WOMAC Western Ontario and McMaster Universities

Table 5 Summary of adverse events

	Cohort 1			Cohort 2		
System organ class	25 M (*n* = 10)	50 M (*n* = 10)	P1 (*n* = 10)	75 M (*n* = 10)	150 M (*n* = 10)	P2 (*n* = 10)
Any adverse event	24 (7)	13 (7)	21 (7)	17 (7)	11 (6)	11 (6)
Blood and lymphatic system disorders	0	1 (1)	1 (1)	0	0	0
Endocrine disorders	0	0	0	1 (1)	0	0
Eye disorders	0	1 (1)	0	0	0	0
Gastrointestinal disorders	1 (1)	0	2 (2)	1 (1)	0	3 (3)
General disorders and administration site conditions	2 (1)	4 (2)	0	9 (6)	4 (3)	0
Infections and infestations	3 (3)	1 (1)	4 (3)	0	1 (1)	1 (1)
Injury, poisoning, and procedural complications	0	0	1 (1)	2 (1)	3 (3)	0
Investigations	2 (2)	1 (1)	1 (1)	0	1 (1)	2 (2)
Metabolism and nutrition disorders	4 (3)	0	3 (3)	0	0	1 (1)
Musculoskeletal and connective tissue disorders	6 (3)	3 (3)	5 (4)	4 (2)	2 (2)	3 (2)
Nervous system disorders	1 (1)	0	1 (1)	0	0	0
Renal and urinary disorders	0	1 (1)	0	0	0	0
Reproductive system and breast disorders	1 (1)	0	0	0	0	0
Respiratory, thoracic, and mediastinal disorders	0	0	0	0	0	1 (1)
Skin and subcutaneous tissue disorders	1 (1)	0	1 (1)	0	0	0
Surgical and medical procedures	2 (1)	0	0	0	0	0
Vascular disorders	1 (1)	1 (1)	2 (1)	0	0	0

Values are shown as number of events (number of patients)
25 M, 50 M, 75 M, 150 M = 25, 50, 75, and 150 million cells, respectively
P1, P2 = placebo 1 and placebo 2, respectively

The WOMAC composite index score decreased over the study period for all the treatment groups. The maximum reduction in the WOMAC composite score was seen in the 25 M group at 12 months compared to the other groups (717.8 ± 503.8, 359.9 ± 786.4, and 233.8 ± 641.9 in the 25 M, 50 M, and P1 groups, respectively; $P = 0.2651$). The WOMAC composite index decreased by an mean of 64.8% in the 25 M patients compared to 14.4% and 49.3% in the 50 M and P1, respectively ($P = 0.1793$). A similar trend was observed in all the WOMAC subscores (WOMAC pain reduced by 145.1 ± 105.2, 74.1 ± 167.2, and 57.4 ± 151.3 ($P = 0.3484$); WOMAC stiffness reduced by 69.6 ± 44.7, 4.5 ± 87.2, and 25.8 ± 53.4 ($P = 0.0324$); and WOMAC physical function reduced by 503.1 ± 375.1, 290.3 ± 559.2, and 150.6 ± 457.8 ($P = 0.2939$) in the 25 M, 50 M, and P1 groups, respectively) (Fig. 6).

ICOAP total scores decreased over the study period for all the treatment groups, except the 150 M group. The maximum reduction in the ICOAP total score was seen in the 25 M group at 12 months (21.4 ± 21.2, 12.3 ± 27.4, and 7.5 ± 27.1 in the 25 M, 50 M, and P1 groups, respectively; $P = 0.5271$) (Fig. 7). ICOAP total decreased by 34.6% in the 25 M group compared to 29.0% and 22.2% in the 50 M and P1 groups, respectively ($P = 0.3844$). A similar trend was seen in ICOAP subscores (constant pain reduced by 26.5 ± 25.3, 20.5 ± 30.2, and 12 ± 31.8 ($P = 0.6140$); intermittent pain reduced by 17.1 ± 28.4, 5.4 ± 33.1, and 3.8 ± 26.3 ($P = 0.6215$) in the 25 M, 50 M, and P1 groups, respectively).

Thus, overall the patients in the 25 M group consistently showed pain reduction in all subjective parameters measured in the study. Due to the small sample size, none of the efficacy parameters were statistically significant as the study was not powered for establishing efficacy. There were no clinically meaningful changes in the X-ray parameters at follow-up visits compared to baseline (data not presented). In the MRI evaluation, overall, there was no perceptible change in WORMS score including cartilage signal and morphology from baseline to follow-up visits in any of the groups of patients (Table 6).

Discussion

The propensity of MSCs to differentiate into chondrocytes in vitro [29] and their ability to repair articular cartilage has been shown in various preclinical models of OA [30–32]. In several studies, MSCs were prepared and injected with sodium hyaluronan to increase the engraftment and chondrogenic activity [30, 33]. In the present study, the efficacy of Stempeucel® was evaluated in a well-validated animal model of OA that was induced by MIA injection into the knee joints. Both low and high doses of Stempeucel® + HA treatment showed significant improvement in the pain threshold from week 2 onwards when compared to animals treated only with HA; treatment with only HA provided a short-term benefit on pain reduction, which corroborates with an earlier publication [34]. We did not observe a significant difference between the two Stempeucel® treatment groups of animals (low and high dose) on pain reduction. However, it is important to note that the pain reduction in the high-dose animals continued to improve until the end of the study (12 weeks). Although the exact mechanism of action of MSCs on pain reduction is not known, anti-inflammatory activity has been attributed to this effect. To date, some studies have demonstrated the role of MSCs on OA-induced pain behavior [35–37]. Van Buul et al. reported improvement of weight-bearing joints of the affected limb after intra-articular application of both rat and human BMMSCs in MIA-induced OA rats [37]. However, unlike the results presented in this study, the authors did not observe cartilage regeneration. Furthermore, in several animal studies, it has been shown that the increased levels of pro-inflammatory cytokines might have contributed to pain increase. Intra-

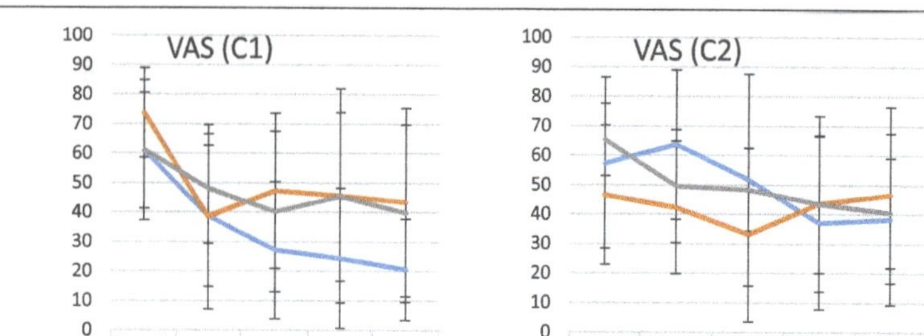

	Baseline	1M	3M	6M	12M
25M	60.9	38.7	27.1	24.4	20.6
50M	73.7	38.4	47.3	45.6	43.4
P1	61	48	40.2	45.3	39.7

	Baseline	1M	3M	6M	12M
75M	57.4	63.6	51.7	37.1	38.3
150M	46.6	42.3	33.1	43.6	46.6
P2	65.3	49.5	48.3	43.4	40.5

Fig. 5 Visual analog scale values. Data are presented as mean ± SD. 1 M, 3 M, 6 M, and 12 M = 1, 3, 6, and 12 months, respectively; *C1* cohort 1, *C2* cohort 2, *M* million cells, *P* placebo, *VAS* visual analog scale

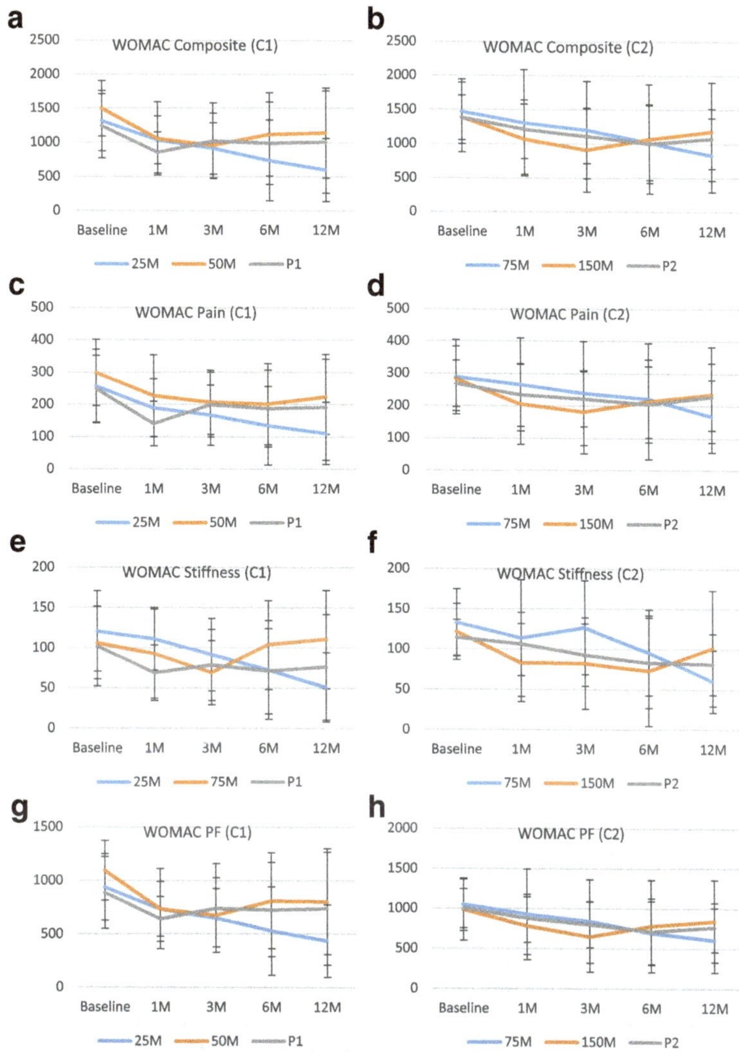

Fig. 6 WOMAC results. WOMAC **a**, **b** composite, **c**, **d** pain, **e**, **f** stiffness, and **g**, **h** physical function (*PF*) results are shown for cohorts 1 (**a**, **c**, **e** and **g**) and 2 (**b**, **d**, **f**, and **h**). Data are presented as mean ± SD. 1 M, 3 M, 6 M, and 12 M = 1, 3, 6, and 12 months, respectively; *C1* cohort 1, *C2* cohort 2, *M* million cells, *P* placebo, *WOMAC* Western Ontario and McMaster Universities

articularly administered MSCs probably play an important role in attenuating the inflammation-induced pain by secreting a wide range of anti-inflammatory cytokines and analgesic peptides [38], and Stempeucel® might have also contributed to pain reduction through a similar mechanism.

We also demonstrated that the pooled BMMSC population are efficient in differentiating into chondrocytes in vitro, and secrete a significant amount of sGAG (Fig. 2c). When these cells were administered intra-articularly into OA-affected joints, we observed a progressive increase in proteoglycan staining. The improvement in cartilage repair was observed both macroscopically and microscopically. The sGAG intensity data revealed that the total proteoglycan content was significantly higher in both the cell + HA treated groups compared to animals treated only with HA. One of the short comings of the preclinical results is that we did not determine the therapeutic effect of BMMSCs without HA. However, based on the published data it appears that administration of MSCs in combination with HA provided better therapeutic benefit than either HA or MSC treatment alone in an experimental animal model of OA [30]. The concomitant reduction in MIA-induced pain followed by an increase in cartilage regeneration observed in this study suggests that human bioactive factors synthesized by BMMSCs may be responsible for both the reduction in inflammation and promotion of endogenous cartilage regeneration via a paracrine mechanism [12].

This clinical study met its predefined endpoint of safety of intra-articular administration of Stempeucel® in osteoarthritis of the knee joint. Adverse events were

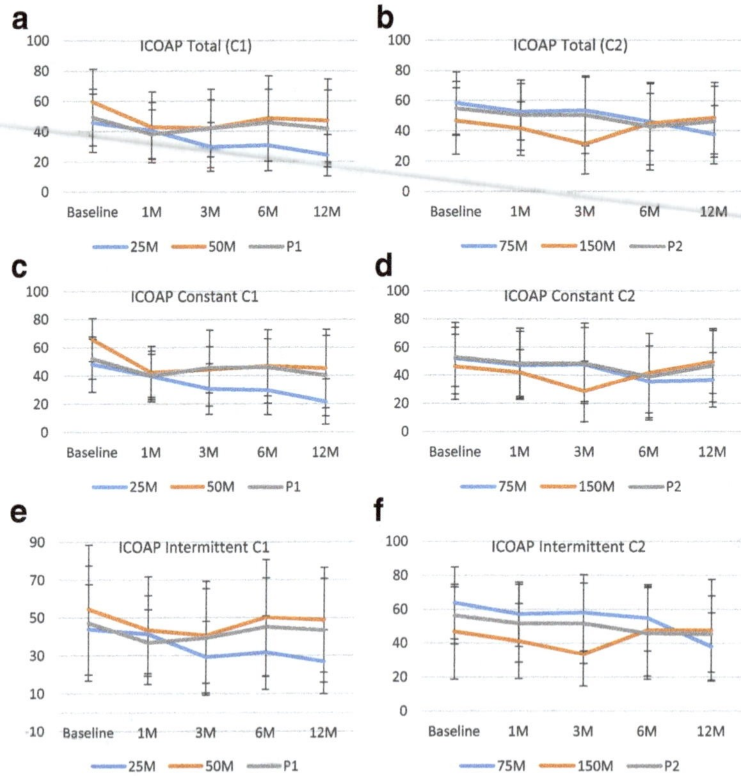

Fig. 7 ICOAP results. ICOAP **a, b** total, **c, d** constant pain, and **e, f** intermittent pain results are shown for cohorts 1 (**a**, **c**, and **e**) and 2 (**b**, **d**, and **f**). Data are presented as mean ± SD. 1 M, 3 M, 6 M, and 12 M = 1, 3, 6, and 12 months, respectively; *C1* cohort 1, *C2* cohort 2, *ICOAP* intermittent and constant osteoarthritis pain, *M* million cells, *P* placebo

predominantly local pain and swelling, particularly seen in patients randomized to the higher dose groups (75 M and 150 M) and they resolved completely upon symptomatic treatment. There was no evidence of ectopic tissue or tumor formation locally at 1-year follow-up. Hematological, biochemical, and serological parameters were comparable in both the cell and placebo arm in all groups of patients. Limited joint space, higher dose, and volume of injection (6 ml) may be the reason for increased joint swelling and pain seen in cohort 2 (75 M and 150 M). Furthermore, it can be assumed that a proportion of the cells injected into the joint space have not survived and this phenomenon was more pronounced with higher cell doses. Probably, such non-viable cells produce an inflammatory reaction causing pain and swelling, as reported earlier [39]. The frequency of these complications was similar to a report from another study using culture-expanded bone marrow-derived MSCs [40]. In another study using allogeneic non-HLA matched BMMSCs in two different doses (50 and 150 million cells) which were pre-mixed with hyaluronic acid (5 ml) and administered in partial medial meniscectomy patients [10], the adverse events were similar to those seen in our study, with the most frequently reported AE by system organ class being musculoskeletal and connective tissue disorders [10]; however, the adverse events did not differ between the two doses tested. Recently, Vega et al. have conducted a study using IA injection of allogeneic BMMSCs (40 million cells suspended in 8 ml of Ringer-Lactate) in OA of the knee joint [11]. Post-

Table 6 WORMS scoring of MRI of the knee at each visit

WORMS	25 M	50 M	P1	*P* value	75 M	150 M	P2	*P* value
Baseline	67.0 (19.8)	78.8 (40.9)	76.5 (23.5)	–	71.3 (21.4)	62.0 (17.9)	70.8 (14.7)	–
6 months	67.5 (20.5)	77.9 (41.2)	74.9 (22.4)	0.5521	71.4 (20.9)	62.0 (17.7)	69.9 (14.3)	0.7360
12 months	66.1 (19.2)	78.0 (41.1)	74.9 (22.5)	0.5310	67.0 (20.9)	60.6 (15.7)	72.3 (15.2)	0.0609

Values are shown as mean (SD)
The range of WORMS score used in this study was 0–314
25 M, 50 M, 75 M, 150 M = 25, 50, 75, 150 million cells, respectively
P1, P2 = Placebo 1 and 2, respectively
MRI magnetic resonance imaging, WORMS whole-organ magnetic resonance imaging score

implantation pain was observed in 53% to 60% of patients in both the experimental and control groups. The pain responded to analgesics and improved within 1 to 6 days. Hence, pain and local swelling may be the most common post-injection complication in patients after IA injection of MSCs which responds within a few days of symptomatic treatment.

One of the most important factors influencing the clinical outcome of a study is to determine the optimal treatment dose. In this study, patients in the low-dose group (25 million cells) showed improved outcomes in the pain measurement scores, whereas those in the higher dose groups did not. The VAS and WOMAC composite index scores decreased by 64% and 64.4% in the 25-million-cell arm as compared to 36% and 49.3% in the active controls with HA, respectively, at 12 months follow-up. In a proof of concept study, three doses of autologous adipose tissue-derived MSCs (AD-MSCs) were used: 10 million, 50 million, and 100 million cells. The WOMAC score improved at 6 months follow-up in the high-dose group [14]. In another study using allogeneic BMMSCs at a dose of 40 million cells, improvement in pain, disability, quality of life, and cartilage quality by MRI was noted in the cell-treated group [11]. Several reasons are hypothesized for this effect in the low-dose group of patients as observed in this study. Firstly, a dose of 25 M cells may be optimum with the volume of hyaluronic acid (2 ml) used in the study as a supporting matrix. Secondly, the 25-million-cell dose maybe optimal for the limited IA space in the knee joint. Thirdly, doses higher than 25 million might cause cell aggregation due to a high cell concentration or insufficient space in the knee joint and subsequently cause cell death. Fourthly, the 25-million-cell dose may be lying in the upper range of the efficacy dose since numerous studies reports that doses in the range of 10 to 25 million BMSCs may be efficacious in OA of the knee joint [15, 41–45]. Finally, higher doses of MSCs may activate the MSCs to function as an M1-type cell with a pro-inflammatory response [46], whereas the 25 M dose may be the optimal concentration of cells which gives rise to an M2-type MSC with an anti-inflammatory/immunosuppressive response. Hence, which cell dose will lead to the best outcome cannot be determined until a series of dose-finding studies are carried out.

Various studies are ongoing to determine the optimal tissue source of MSCs for therapeutic repair of the cartilage tissue. The combination of MSCs with scaffolds, growth factors, platelet-rich plasma (PRP), and genetic modification have also been studied. It is not clear which source of stem cells, or a combination product, will be the best for the disease condition. Studies have shown that adipose tissue-derived stem cells are both safe and efficacious [13, 14, 47–49], whereas other studies have shown that bone marrow-derived cells are equally efficacious [10, 11, 50–52]. A current focus for knee cartilage repair is to use scaffolds that provide a three-dimensional environment for guiding and supporting the cells for cartilage repair. An advantage for using a scaffold is containment of the implanted cells on the lesion, and these biomaterials may act as barriers for fibroblast invasion of the graft [53, 54]. Koh et al. have used PRP as a scaffold as it acts as an MSC accelerator for clinical chondrogenesis, is non-immunogeneic and bioabsorbable, and can be easily prepared preoperatively [13]. In another study, fibrin glue has been used as a scaffold in MSC implantation to induce improved cell survival, proliferation, gene expression, differentiation, and matrix synthesis leading to repair of the cartilage lesion [55]. Cartistem® (MEDIPOST Co. Ltd., South Korea) is a combination product of human umbilical cord blood-derived mesenchymal stem cells and hyaluronic acid [56]. This acts as a biodegradable matrix in MSC implantation as it facilitates the migration and adherence of cells to the damaged cartilage, leading to better healing of the damaged lesion. Hence, more studies are required to pinpoint the best source of stem cells and the scaffold to be used to demonstrate both safety and efficacy.

The method of delivery of cells—either by direct intra-articular injection or by open arthroscopy injection—into the joint cavity is also important and may be one of the factors for deriving efficacy. In one of the initial studies, Wakitani et al. transplanted cells of bone marrow embedded in collagen gel into the articular cartilage defect at the time of high tibial osteotomy [43]. Cartistem®, a combination product approved by the Korean FDA, has been applied to the damaged area through arthroscopy after conducting a microfracture [57]. These open surgical methods have their disadvantages such as pain, longer hospital stay, and higher cost. Minimally invasive techniques such as intra-articular injection have been adopted by different groups [14, 15, 41, 45, 50]. IA injection is patient-friendly in terms of being less invasive, with reduced hospital stay, and are likely to reach a larger patient population as it can be performed in peripheral hospitals. Ultrasound guidance of knee injections could be a better option to more precisely deliver the cells intra-articularly. Berkoff et al. have reported that ultrasound guidance of knee injections resulted in better IA accuracy of needle placement than anatomical guidance (95.8% versus 77.8%; $P < 0.001$) [58]. This enhanced injection accuracy achieved with ultrasound needle guidance directly improves patient-related clinical outcomes. However, in developing countries, ultrasound-guided intra-articular injection may be a challenge due to limited access to the instrument.

The present study, though it has shown good subjective improvement in pain and functional scores, did not demonstrate improvement in cartilage signal and morphology by MRI. We have used the WORMS scoring system, which is a semiquantitative MRI system for evaluating structural change in knee OA. WORMS scoring has been extensively studied for the prevalence and severity of cartilage loss, bone marrow lesions, and meniscal damage [59, 60], and has seldom been studied for cartilage regeneration. Koh et al. studied the effect of adipose-derived MSCs with PRP in OA of the knee joint and found that WORMS score significantly improved from 60.0 points to 48.3 points and cartilage subscore improved from 28.3 points to 21.7 points at 24 months follow-up ($P < 0.001$) as compared to baseline [13]. However, in our study, the cartilage subscore did not demonstrate any significant worsening or improvement of the cartilage in any of the subgroups. The reason for the WORMS score differences between these two studies could be due to several reasons: the type of MSCs used are different, better complementarity between adipose-derived MSC and PRP, or the length of follow-up time (24 months vs. 12 months) after cell administration. The limited number of patients used in this study for MRI analysis might have contributed as well. Regardless of these differences, Stempeucel® administration in the preclinical model clearly suggested the ability of these cells in combination with HA to trigger adequate proteoglycan synthesis for cartilage repair. Future clinical trials of Stempeucel® in OA patients should consider using guided delivery of cells in and around the lesion site or by arthroscopy, followed by MRI measurements using delayed gadolinium-enhanced MRI of cartilage (dGEMRIC) or T2 mapping to perform compositional (sGAG) analysis of the cartilage before and after cell administration. One of the limitations of this study was unblinding of the trial after 6 months follow-up, particularly given that the subjective measurements of clinical data (VAS, WOMAC, and ICOAP) were the secondary endpoints.

Conclusions

This clinical study satisfied the primary endpoints of safety of Stempeucel® administration in OA patients at all four doses tested. In addition, a trend towards pain reduction at the lowest cell dose of 25 M was observed by VAS, WOMAC, and ICOAP pain scoring criteria, but this was not statistically significant when compared to placebo. Analysis of the remaining secondary endpoints did not reveal therapeutic efficacy which could be attributed to the low number of patients enrolled in the study. The fact that a pooled population of allogeneic BMMSCs could elicit pain reduction and cartilage regeneration in a preclinical model of OA coupled with the safety profile observed in human patients with a positive trend in pain reduction (in one of the cell doses tested) warrants further study in a large number of patients to investigate the therapeutic role of Stempeucel® in cartilage regeneration in OA patients.

Abbreviations

AE: Adverse event; BMI: Body mass index; BMMSC: Bone marrow-derived mesenchymal stromal cell; dGEMRIC: Delayed gadolinium-enhanced magnetic resonance imaging of cartilage; DMSO: Dimethyl sulfoxide; GCP: Good Clinical Practice; GMP: Good Manufacturing Practice; HA: Hyaluronic acid; HED: Human equivalent dose; IA: Intraarticular; ICH: International Conference on Harmonization; ICOAP: Intermittent and constant osteoarthritis pain; IMP: Investigational medicinal product; MedDRA: Medical Dictionary for Regulatory Activities; MIA: Mono-iodoacetate; mITT: Modified intention to treat; MRI: Magnetic resonance imaging; MSC: Mesenchymal stromal cell; OA: Osteoarthritis; PAM: Pressure Application Measurement; PT: Preferred term; SAE: Serious adverse event; sGAG: sulfated glycosaminoglycan; SOC: System organ class; VAS: Visual analog scale; WCB: Working cell bank; WOMAC-OA: Western Ontario and McMaster Universities Osteoarthritis; WORMS: Whole-organ magnetic resonance imaging score

Acknowledgments

This study was funded by Stempeutics Research Pvt. Ltd.

Funding

This study has been funded by Stempeutics Research Pvt. Ltd., Bangalore.

Authors' contributions

PKG participated in the design of the study, analyzed the data, and drafted, edited, and revised the manuscript. AC participated in the design of the study, analyzed the data, and drafted, edited, and revised the manuscript. MR designed and conducted preclinical studies of Stempeucel®, analyzed and interpreted data, and drafted and edited the manuscript. NS participated in the design of the study, recruited and followed-up the patients, collected the data, and edited the manuscript. VP participated in the design of the study, recruited and followed-up the patients, collected the data, and edited the manuscript. SYW participated in the design of the study, recruited and followed-up the patients, collected the data, and edited the manuscript. VA participated in the design of the study, recruited and followed-up the patients, collected the data, and edited the manuscript. PKV participated in the design of the study, coordinated and collected the clinical trial data, and reviewed and edited the manuscript. DD participated in the isolation, expansion, and cryopreservation of Stempeucel®, processed the cells before administration to patients in the clinical trial, and reviewed and edited the manuscript. PV conducted the quality check of Stempeucel® before release for clinical trials, and reviewed and edited the manuscript. CT conducted the in vitro assays of Stempeucel®, and reviewed and edited the manuscript. SB conducted the in vitro assay, and preclinical studies of Stempeucel®, and reviewed and edited the manuscript. ASM participated in the design of the study, analyzed the data, and drafted, edited, and revised the manuscript. All authors reviewed and approved the final manuscript.

Authors' information

Not applicable.

Competing interests

PKG, AC, MR, PKV, CT, SB, DD, PV, and ASM are employees of Stempeutics Research Pvt. Ltd. The remaining authors declare that they no competing interests.

Author details
[1]Stempeutics Research Pvt Ltd, Akshay Tech Park, No. 72 & 73, 2nd Floor, EPIP Zone, Phase I-Area, Whitefield, Bangalore 560066, India. [2]M.S Ramaiah Medical College & Hospitals, MSR Nagar, MSRIT Post, Bangalore 560054, India. [3]Kasturba Medical College and Hospital, Madhav Nagar, Manipal 576104, India. [4]Sanjay Gandhi Post Graduate Institute of Medical Sciences, Raebareli Road, Lucknow 226014, India. [5]Jehangir Clinical Development Center, Jehangir Hospital, 33, Sasoon Road, Pune 411001, India. [6]Manipal University, Manipal, India.

References

1. Murray C, Lopez A. The global burden of disease: a comprehensive assessment of mortality and disability from disease, injuries and risk factors in 1990 and projected to 2020. Boston: Harvard University Press; 1996.
2. Osteoarthritis: care and management. https://www.nice.org.uk/guidance/cg177. Accessed 8 May 2016.
3. Hochberg MC, Altman RD, April KT, Benkhalti M, Guyatt G, McGowan J, et al. American College of Rheumatology 2012 recommendations for the use of nonpharmacologic and pharmacologic therapies in osteoarthritis of the hand, hip, and knee. Arthritis Care Res. 2012;64(4):465–74.
4. Jordan KM, Arden NK, Doherty M, Bannwarth B, Bijlsma JWJ, Dieppe P, et al. EULAR Recommendations 2003: an evidence based approach to the management of knee osteoarthritis: report of a Task Force of the Standing Committee for International Clinical Studies Including Therapeutic Trials (ESCISIT). Ann Rheum Dis. 2003;62(12):1145–55.
5. Schrama JC, Espehaug B, Hallan G, Engesæter LB, Furnes O, Havelin LI, et al. Risk of revision for infection in primary total hip and knee arthroplasty in patients with rheumatoid arthritis compared with osteoarthritis: a prospective, population-based study on 108,786 hip and knee joint arthroplasties from the Norwegian Arthroplasty Register. Arthritis Care Res. 2010;62(4):473–9.
6. Knutsen G, Drogset JO, Engebretsen L, Grøntvedt T, Isaksen V, Ludvigsen TC, et al. A randomized trial comparing autologous chondrocyte implantation with microfracture. J Bone Jt Surg. 2007;89(10):2105–12.
7. Brittberg M, Lindahl A, Nilsson A, Ohlsson C, Isaksson O, Peterson L. Treatment of deep cartilage defects in the knee with autologous chondrocyte transplantation. N Engl J Med. 1994;331(14):889–95.
8. Von der Mark K, Gauss V, von der Mark H, Müller P. Relationship between cell shape and type of collagen synthesised as chondrocytes lose their cartilage phenotype in culture. Nature. 1977;267(5611):531–2.
9. Veronesi F, Giavaresi G, Tschon M, Borsari V, Nicoli Aldini N, Fini M. Clinical use of bone marrow, bone marrow concentrate, and expanded bone marrow mesenchymal stem cells in cartilage disease. Stem Cells Dev. 2013; 22(2):181–92.
10. Vangsness CT, Farr J, Boyd J, Dellaero DT, Mills CR, LeRoux-Williams M. Adult human mesenchymal stem cells delivered via intra-articular injection to the knee following partial medial meniscectomy: a randomized, double-blind, controlled study. J Bone Joint Surg Am. 2014;96(2):90–8.
11. Vega A, Martín-Ferrero MA, Del Canto F, Alberca M, García V, Munar A, et al. Treatment of knee osteoarthritis with allogeneic bone marrow mesenchymal stem cells: a randomized controlled trial. Transplantation. 2015;99(8):1681–90.
12. Gupta PK, Das AK, Chullikana A, Majumdar AS. Mesenchymal stem cells for cartilage repair in osteoarthritis. Stem Cell Res Ther. 2012;3:25.
13. Koh Y-G, Jo S-B, Kwon O-R, Suh D-S, Lee S-W, Park S-H, et al. Mesenchymal stem cell injections improve symptoms of knee osteoarthritis. Arthroscopy. 2013;29(4):748–55.
14. Jo CH, Lee YG, Shin WH, Kim H, Chai JW, Jeong EC, et al. Intra-articular injection of mesenchymal stem cells for the treatment of osteoarthritis of the knee: a proof-of-concept clinical trial. Stem Cells Dayt Ohio. 2014;32(5):1254–66.
15. Emadedin M, Aghdami N, Taghiyar L, Fazeli R, Moghadasali R, Jahangir S, et al. Intra-articular injection of autologous mesenchymal stem cells in six patients with knee osteoarthritis. Arch Iran Med. 2012;15(7):422–8.
16. Mamidi MK, Nathan KG, Singh G, Thrichelvam ST, Mohd Yusof NAN, Fakharuzi NA, et al. Comparative cellular and molecular analyses of pooled bone marrow multipotent mesenchymal stromal cells during continuous passaging and after successive cryopreservation. J Cell Biochem. 2012;113(10):3153–64.
17. Gupta PK, Chullikana A, Parakh R, Desai S, Das A, Gottipamula S, et al. A double blind randomized placebo controlled phase I/II study assessing the safety and efficacy of allogeneic bone marrow derived mesenchymal stem cell in critical limb ischemia. J Transl Med. 2013;11:143.
18. Guingamp C, Gegout-Pottie P, Philippe L, Terlain B, Netter P, Gillet P. Mono-iodoacetate-induced experimental osteoarthritis. A dose-response study of loss of mobility, morphology, and biochemistry. Arthritis Rheum. 1997;40(9):1670–9.
19. Pomonis JD, Boulet JM, Gottshall SL, Phillips S, Sellers R, Bunton T, et al. Development and pharmacological characterization of a rat model of osteoarthritis pain. Pain. 2005;114(3):339–46.
20. Vermeirsch H, Biermans R, Salmon PL, Meert TF. Evaluation of pain behavior and bone destruction in two arthritic models in guinea pig and rat. Pharmacol Biochem Behav. 2007;87(3):349–59.
21. Di Cesare ML, Micheli L, Zanardelli M, Ghelardini C. Low dose native type II collagen prevents pain in a rat osteoarthritis model. BMC Musculoskelet Disord. 2013;14:228.
22. Schmitz N, Laverty S, Kraus VB, Aigner T. Basic methods in histopathology of joint tissues. Osteoarthritis Cartilage. 2010;18 Suppl 3:113–6.
23. Pritzker KPH, Gay S, Jimenez SA, Ostergaard K, Pelletier J-P, Revell PA, et al. Osteoarthritis cartilage histopathology: grading and staging. Osteoarthritis Cartilage. 2006;14(1):13–29.
24. Gerwin N, Bendele AM, Glasson S, Carlson CS. The OARSI histopathology initiative—recommendations for histological assessments of osteoarthritis in the rat. Osteoarthritis Cartilage. 2010;18(3):24–34.
25. Moyer JT, Priest R, Bouman T, Abraham AC, Donahue TLH. Indentation properties and glycosaminoglycan content of human menisci in the deep zone. Acta Biomater. 2013;9(5):6624–9.
26. Villegas DF, Hansen TA, Liu DF, Donahue TLH. A quantitative study of the microstructure and biochemistry of the medial meniscal horn attachments. Ann Biomed Eng. 2008;36(1):123–31.
27. Peterfy CG, Guermazi A, Zaim S, Tirman PFJ, Miaux Y, White D, et al. Whole-Organ Magnetic Resonance Imaging Score (WORMS) of the knee in osteoarthritis. Osteoarthritis Cartilage. 2004;12(3):177–90.
28. Stubendorff JJ, Lammentausta E, Struglics A, Lindberg L, Heinegård D, Dahlberg LE. Is cartilage sGAG content related to early changes in cartilage disease? Implications for interpretation of dGEMRIC. Osteoarthritis Cartilage. 2012;20(5):396–404.
29. Wu L, Leijten JCH, Georgi N, Post JN, van Blitterswijk CA, Karperien M. Trophic effects of mesenchymal stem cells increase chondrocyte proliferation and matrix formation. Tissue Eng Part A. 2011;17(9-10): 1425–36.
30. Sato M, Uchida K, Nakajima H, Miyazaki T, Guerrero AR, Watanabe S, et al. Direct transplantation of mesenchymal stem cells into the knee joints of Hartley strain guinea pigs with spontaneous osteoarthritis. Arthritis Res Ther. 2012;14:R31.
31. Mokbel AN, El Tookhy OS, Shamaa AA, Rashed LA, Sabry D, El Sayed AM. Homing and reparative effect of intra-articular injection of autologus mesenchymal stem cells in osteoarthritic animal model. BMC Musculoskelet Disord. 2011;12:259.
32. Nam HY, Karunanithi P, Loo WCP, Naveen SV, Chen HC, Hussin P, et al. The effects of staged intra-articular injection of cultured autologous mesenchymal stromal cells on the repair of damaged cartilage: a pilot study in caprine model. Arthritis Res Ther. 2013;15:R129.
33. Murphy JM, Fink DJ, Hunziker EB, Barry FP. Stem cell therapy in a caprine model of osteoarthritis. Arthritis Rheum. 2003;48(12):3464–74.
34. Suhaeb AM, Naveen S, Mansor A, Kamarul T. Hyaluronic acid with or without bone marrow derived-mesenchymal stem cells improves osteoarthritic knee changes in rat model: a preliminary report. Indian J Exp Biol. 2012;50(6):383–90.
35. Black LL, Gaynor J, Adams C, Dhupa S, Sams AE, Taylor R, et al. Effect of intraarticular injection of autologous adipose-derived mesenchymal stem and regenerative cells on clinical signs of chronic osteoarthritis of the elbow joint in dogs. Vet Ther. 2008;9(3):192–200.
36. Frisbie DD, Kisiday JD, Kawcak CE, Werpy NM, McIlwraith CW. Evaluation of adipose-derived stromal vascular fraction or bone marrow-derived mesenchymal stem cells for treatment of osteoarthritis. J Orthop Res. 2009; 27(12):1675–80.
37. Van Buul GM, Siebelt M, Leijs MJC, Bos PK, Waarsing JH, Kops N, et al. Mesenchymal stem cells reduce pain but not degenerative changes in a mono-iodoacetate rat model of osteoarthritis. J Orthop Res. 2014;32(9):1167–74.
38. Guo W, Wang H, Zou S, Gu M, Watanabe M, Wei F, et al. Bone marrow stromal cells produce long-term pain relief in rat models of persistent pain. Stem Cells Dayt Ohio. 2011;29(8):1294–303.

39. Rock KL, Kono H. The inflammatory response to cell death. Annu Rev Pathol. 2008;3:99–126.
40. Centeno CJ, Schultz JR, Cheever M, Freeman M, Faulkner S, Robinson B, et al. Safety and complications reporting update on the re-implantation of culture-expanded mesenchymal stem cells using autologous platelet lysate technique. Curr Stem Cell Res Ther. 2011;6(4):368–78.
41. Davatchi F, Abdollahi BS, Mohyeddin M, Shahram F, Nikbin B. Mesenchymal stem cell therapy for knee osteoarthritis. Preliminary report of four patients. Int J Rheum Dis. 2011;14(2):211–5.
42. Nejadnik H, Hui JH, Feng Choong EP, Tai B-C, Lee EH. Autologous bone marrow-derived mesenchymal stem cells versus autologous chondrocyte implantation: an observational cohort study. Am J Sports Med. 2010;38(6): 1110–6.
43. Wakitani S, Imoto K, Yamamoto T, Saito M, Murata N, Yoneda M. Human autologous culture expanded bone marrow mesenchymal cell transplantation for repair of cartilage defects in osteoarthritic knees. Osteoarthritis Cartilage. 2002;10(3):199–206.
44. Wong KL, Lee KBL, Tai BC, Law P, Lee EH, Hui JHP. Injectable cultured bone marrow-derived mesenchymal stem cells in varus knees with cartilage defects undergoing high tibial osteotomy: a prospective, randomized controlled clinical trial with 2 years' follow-up. Arthroscopy. 2013;29(12):2020–8.
45. Centeno CJ, Busse D, Kisiday J, Keohan C, Freeman MM. Increased knee cartilage volume in degenerative joint disease using percutaneously implanted, autologous mesenchymal stem cells, platelet lysate and dexamethasone. Ann Transplant. 2008;9:246–51.
46. Saether EE, Chamberlain CS, Leiferman EM, Kondratko-Mittnacht JR, Li WJ, Brickson SL, et al. Enhanced medial collateral ligament healing using mesenchymal stem cells: dosage effects on cellular response and cytokine profile. Stem Cell Rev. 2014;10(1):86–96.
47. Koh Y-G, Choi Y-J, Kwon S-K, Kim Y-S, Yeo J-E. Clinical results and second-look arthroscopic findings after treatment with adipose-derived stem cells for knee osteoarthritis. Knee Surg Sports Traumatol Arthrosc. 2015;23(5):1308–16.
48. Koh Y-G, Choi Y-J. Infrapatellar fat pad-derived mesenchymal stem cell therapy for knee osteoarthritis. Knee. 2012;19(6):902–7.
49. Ruiz M, Cosenza S, Maumus M, Jorgensen C, Noël D. Therapeutic application of mesenchymal stem cells in osteoarthritis. Expert Opin Biol Ther. 2015;1–10.
50. Orozco L, Munar A, Soler R, Alberca M, Soler F, Huguet M, et al. Treatment of knee osteoarthritis with autologous mesenchymal stem cells: a pilot study. Transplant J. 2013;95(12):1535–41.
51. Centeno CJ, Busse D, Kisiday J, Keohan C, Freeman M, Karli D. Regeneration of meniscus cartilage in a knee treated with percutaneously implanted autologous mesenchymal stem cells. Med Hypotheses. 2008;71(6):900–8.
52. Huang JI, Kazmi N, Durbhakula MM, Hering TM, Yoo JU, Johnstone B. Chondrogenic potential of progenitor cells derived from human bone marrow and adipose tissue: a patient-matched comparison. J Orthop Res. 2005;23(6):1383–9.
53. Frenkel SR, Toolan B, Menche D, Pitman MI, Pachence JM. Chondrocyte transplantation using a collagen bilayer matrix for cartilage repair. J Bone Joint Surg (Br). 1997;79(5):831–6.
54. Iwasa J, Engebretsen L, Shima Y, Ochi M. Clinical application of scaffolds for cartilage tissue engineering. Knee Surg Sports Traumatol Arthrosc. 2009; 17(6):561–77.
55. Kim YS, Choi YJ, Suh DS, Heo DB, Kim YI, Ryu J-S, et al. Mesenchymal stem cell implantation in osteoarthritic knees: is fibrin glue effective as a scaffold? Am J Sports Med. 2015;43(1):176–85.
56. CARTISTEM®, mesenchymal stem cells for treatment of osteoarthritis—LifeMap Discovery. http://discovery.lifemapsc.com/regenerative-medicine/cell-therapy-applications/cartilage-cartistem-mesenchymal-stem-cells-for-treatment-of-osteoarthritis. Accessed 13 Nov 2015.
57. Rush University Medical Center announces human clinical trial for Cartistem. http://www.stemcellsfreak.com/2013/01/Cartistem-clinical-trial.html. Accessed 14 Nov 2015.
58. Berkoff DJ, Miller LE, Block JE. Clinical utility of ultrasound guidance for intra-articular knee injections: a review. Clin Interv Aging. 2012;7:89–95.
59. Lynch JA, Roemer FW, Nevitt MC, Felson DT, Niu J, Eaton CB, et al. Comparison of BLOKS and WORMS scoring systems part I. Cross sectional comparison of methods to assess cartilage morphology, meniscal damage and bone marrow lesions on knee MRI: data from the osteoarthritis initiative. Osteoarthritis Cartilage. 2010;18(11):1393–401.
60. Felson DT, Lynch J, Guermazi A, Roemer FW, Niu J, McAlindon T, et al. Comparison of BLOKS and WORMS scoring systems part II. Longitudinal assessment of knee MRIs for osteoarthritis and suggested approach based on their performance: data from the Osteoarthritis Initiative. Osteoarthritis Cartilage. 2010;18(11):1402–7.

12

The immediate effect of a soft knee brace on pain, activity limitations, self-reported knee instability, and self-reported knee confidence in patients with knee osteoarthritis

Tomasz Cudejko[1,2], Martin van der Esch[2*], Marike van der Leeden[1,2], Josien C. van den Noort[1,3], Leo D. Roorda[2], Willem Lems[4,5], Jos Twisk[6,7], Martijn Steultjens[8], James Woodburn[8], Jaap Harlaar[1,9] and Joost Dekker[1,10]

Abstract

Background: We aimed to (i) evaluate the immediate effect of a soft knee brace on pain, activity limitations, self-reported knee instability, and self-reported knee confidence, and (ii) to assess the difference in effect between a non-tight and a tight soft brace in patients with knee osteoarthritis (OA).

Methods: Forty-four patients with knee OA and self-reported knee instability participated in the single-session, laboratory, experimental study. A within-subject design was used, comparing a soft brace with no brace, and comparing a non-tight with a tight soft brace. The outcome measures were pain, self-reported knee instability and knee confidence during level and perturbed walking on the treadmill and activity limitations (10-m walk test and the get up and go (GUG) test). Linear mixed-effect model analysis for continuous outcomes and logistic generalized estimating equations for categorical outcomes were used to evaluate the effect of wearing a soft brace.

Results: Wearing a soft brace significantly reduced pain during level walking ($B - 0.60$, $P = 0.001$) and perturbed walking ($B - 0.80$, $P < 0.001$), reduced the time to complete the 10-m walk ($B - 0.23$, $P < 0.001$) and the GUG tests ($B - 0.23$, $P = 0.004$), reduced self-reported knee instability during level walking (OR 0.41, $P = 0.002$) and perturbed walking (OR 0.36, $P < 0.001$), and reduced lack of confidence in the knees during level walking (OR 0.45, $P < 0.001$) and perturbed walking (OR 0.56, $P < 0.001$), compared with not wearing a soft brace. There was no difference in effects between a non-tight and tight brace, except for the 10-m walk test. Wearing a tight brace significantly reduced the time to complete the 10-m walk test in comparison with wearing a non-tight brace ($B - 0.11$, $P = 0.03$).

Conclusion: The results of this study indicate that a soft brace is an efficacious intervention targeting pain, activity limitations, self-reported knee instability, and knee confidence in the immediate term in patients with knee OA. Further studies are needed evaluating the mode of action based on exerted pressure, and on the generalization to functioning in daily life.

Keywords: Knee, Osteoarthritis, Brace, Orthotics

* Correspondence: m.vd.esch@reade.nl
[2]Amsterdam Rehabilitation Research Centre Reade, Dr. J. van Breemenstraat 2, 1056 AB Amsterdam, P.O. Box 58271, 1040 HG Amsterdam, The Netherlands
Full list of author information is available at the end of the article

Background

Soft braces are elastic, non-adhesive orthoses recommended in the non-surgical management of patients with knee osteoarthritis (OA) [1]. Because of ease of use, lack of complications, and low cost, soft braces are commonly used with the aim of reducing pain and activity limitations [1]. Soft brace efficacy and effectiveness has been assessed in laboratory [2, 3] and ambulatory settings [4, 5]. A laboratory setting allows the assessment of the immediate efficacy of an intervention under controlled conditions, while an ambulatory setting allows the assessment of the effectiveness in real life, where uncontrollable factors may be present. The evidence for immediate efficacy of a soft brace in patients with knee OA is limited. A recent systematic review with meta-analyses on soft bracing in knee OA showed an immediate, moderate improvement in pain when wearing a soft brace [6]. As the results were based on only two studies of low to moderate quality, however, further studies are needed.

It is not well-understood how a soft brace might reduce activity limitations and pain in patients with knee OA. A decrease in pain might be due to sensory stimulation of the skin, leading to a reduction in transmission of pain signals [7]. It is also assumed that a soft brace stimulates cutaneous mechanoreceptors, resulting in improved joint proprioception accuracy, which may have an impact on knee joint stability [2]. Improved knee joint stability might reduce activity limitations [8, 9]. To our knowledge, there is only one study that showed that a soft brace improves self-reported knee instability [3], while the effect of a soft brace on instability-related lack of confidence in the knee [10] is unknown. Externally applied perturbations challenge knee stabilization strategies in patients with knee OA [11, 13]. Perturbed conditions therefore provide a powerful test of soft braces. However, whether a soft brace has an effect on knee stability and knee confidence in perturbed conditions has not been assessed yet. Given the high prevalence of self-reported knee instability and lack of confidence in the knee in patients with knee OA [9, 14], there is a need to study the effect of a soft brace on knee stability and knee confidence during both level and perturbed walk.

Hassan et al. [15] reported that a non-tight soft brace was more effective than a tight brace in reducing pain and improving postural sway in patients with knee OA. The authors suggested that a non-tight brace provides more recurrent stimuli to cutaneous mechanoreceptors, whereas a tight brace provides constant pressure, to which skin mechanoreceptors adapt [15]. There is a clear need to replicate this study in order to determine whether the level of tightness has an effect on activity limitations, knee stability and knee confidence.

The currently available evidence for the use of soft braces in patients with knee OA is limited and of low quality. Thus, the aims of the study were to (i) evaluate the immediate effect of a soft brace on pain, activity limitations, and self-reported knee instability and knee confidence, and to (ii) assess the difference in effect between a non-tight and a tight soft brace in patients with knee OA. We hypothesized that (i) a soft brace reduces pain, activity limitations, and self-reported knee instability, and improves knee confidence, and that (ii) a non-tight soft brace has a greater effect than a tight soft brace.

Methods

Trial design

In this single-session, laboratory, experimental study, a within-subject design was used, comparing a soft brace with no soft brace, and comparing a non-tight with a tight soft brace. The order of the non-tight and tight brace was randomized, using a computer generated random sequence made prior to the study. All participants were blinded to the type of brace (non-tight or tight).

Participants

Participants were recruited from the Amsterdam Osteoarthritis (AMS-OA) cohort through telephone-based screening between August 2015 and April 2016. The AMS-OA cohort consists of participants with established knee and/or hip OA according to the American College of Rheumatology (ACR) criteria [16], who had been referred to an outpatient rehabilitation center (Reade, Center for Rehabilitation and Rheumatology, Amsterdam, the Netherlands). Participants were assessed by rheumatologists, radiologists, and rehabilitation physicians. According to the ACR criteria, knee OA is diagnosed if knee pain is present and three of the following six parameters are present: age > 50 years, morning stiffness < 30 minutes, crepitus, bony tenderness, bony enlargement and no palpable warmth. The inclusion criteria for the present study were (i) diagnosis of bilateral or unilateral knee OA according to the ACR criteria [16], (ii) age between 50 and 80 years, and (iii) presence of self-reported knee instability in the past 3 months. Self-reported knee instability was defined as at least one episode of buckling, shifting, or giving way of the knee in the last three months, reported by participants [17].

The exclusion criteria for the AMS-OA cohort were total knee replacement and/or inflammatory arthritis (including rheumatoid arthritis, crystal arthropathy, septic arthritis, and spondylarthropathy). Additional exclusion criteria for the present study were (i) radiographic patello-femoral (PF) joint OA (PFOA), and (ii) presence of comorbidity resulting in severe activity limitations. The soft brace in the current study did not involve patellar opening, thus, to avoid applying pressure on the PF compartment, we excluded patients with PFOA.

Interventions

A commercially available soft brace (GENUTEX A2, Human I; Bleiswijk, The Netherlands) was used. The following sizes of the soft brace were available: S: 30–35 cm, M: 35–40 cm, L: 40–45 cm, XL: 45–50 cm, and XXL: 50–55 cm. These sizes were used to differentiate between a non-tight and tight soft brace. A tight brace was defined as one fitted based on shank and thigh circumferences measured according to instructions provided by the distributor. A non-tight brace was defined as one a size larger than a tight brace. Fitting and positioning of the brace were performed by a trained investigator (TC) according to instructions provided by the distributor. Both knees were braced regardless of the knee OA status. Participants were allowed to become accustomed to the brace before treadmill walking. Participants were blinded to the type of brace by informing them that the study was a comparison of two different braces, without mentioning differences in tightness. Braces were identical in appearance.

Primary outcome measure

Pain

Knee pain during walking on the treadmill was assessed using the Dutch-translated 11-point numerical rating scale (NRS) (0–10), with higher scores representing more pain [18]. The following question was asked during both level and perturbed walking: "On a scale from 0 to 10, how would you score the level of your left/right knee pain while walking on the treadmill?" The Dutch translated NRS has been frequently used in the Netherlands [17, 19, 20].

Secondary outcome measures

Activity limitations

Activity limitations were assessed with two standardized physical performance tests: the 10-m walk test [21] and the get up and go (GUG) test [22]. The 10-m walk test assesses the time to walk a distance of 10 m along a level and unobstructed corridor [21]. Participants were instructed to walk as fast as possible and timed with a stopwatch. The GUG test measures the time a person takes to get up from a chair and walk 15 m as fast as possible along a level and unobstructed corridor [23]. The intraclass correlation coefficient (ICC) for the GUG test is 0.98 for intra-tester reliability and 0.98 for inter-tester reliability [22].

Self-reported knee instability

Self-reported knee instability was assessed with the Dutch version of the questionnaire developed by Irrgang et al. [24]. Self-reported knee instability was assessed with a question on the number of episodes during walking on the treadmill of perceived buckling, shifting, or giving way, separately for the right and left knee. The following question was asked during both level and perturbed walking: "How many times have you had a sensation of left/right knee buckling, shifting, or giving way while walking on the treadmill?" Self-reported knee instability was dichotomized into no episode of knee instability versus one or more episodes of knee instability. The translated Dutch version of the questionnaire has been previously used by our research group [20, 25].

Self-reported knee confidence

Knee confidence was assessed using a 5-point Likert scale (not at all, mildly, moderately, severely, and extremely) in response to the question asked during both level and perturbed walking: "How much were you troubled with lack of confidence in your left/right knee while walking on the treadmill?" This is a single item from the Dutch-validated Knee injury and Osteoarthritis Outcome Score (KOOS) [26–28]. Self-reported knee confidence was dichotomized into lack (mildly, moderately, severely, or extremely troubled) versus full (not troubled at all) knee confidence.

Other measures

Participants' demographic and clinical characteristics were recorded prior to testing and included: age, gender, duration of symptoms, body-mass index (BMI), knee OA radiographic severity, and muscle strength. BMI was calculated as body mass in kilograms divided by height in square meters. The Kellgren and Lawrence score (KL score) from the more severely affected knee was used to assess the radiographic severity of the disease [29]. Conventional radiographs of tibiofemoral joints were made by a weight-bearing posterior-anterior view according to Buckland-Wright et al. [30]. Two independent observers graded radiographs: a bone and joint radiologist and an epidemiologist trained by two musculoskeletal radiologists. Muscle strength (in Newton meters per kilogram of body weight (Nm/kg)) was assessed for flexion and extension of the knee using an isokinetic dynamometer (Humac Norm, CSMi, Boston, USA) according to a previously described protocol [11]. The mean strength of the quadriceps and hamstring muscles of the left and right knee was reported. The Dutch translation of the Western Ontario and McMaster Universities Osteoarthritis Index (WOMAC) was used to assess self-reported knee pain, stiffness, and activity limitations of the most affected knee [12, 13].

Sample size

The study was powered on self-reported pain. An expected effect size of 0.5 was calculated from the change in pain and its confidence interval reported in the study of Hassan et al. [15]. With effect size = 0.5, alpha = 0.05, power (1-β) = 0.80, and a two-sided test, the minimum number of subjects required was n = 33. Allowing for an attrition rate of 10% during the course of the study [31], this study needed to include at least 36 patients.

Procedure

The study procedure is presented in Table 1. Participants of the study attended a single testing session. Outcome measures, with the exception of the 10-m walk and GUG tests, were assessed on the treadmill, which is integrated into the GRAIL system. The GRAIL system is made up of a treadmill with a dual belt, placed in a virtual reality environment (GRAIL system, MOTEKForce Link, The Netherlands). Walking on the treadmill was initially performed with no brace. Patients had a familiarization session on the treadmill lasting at least one minute, during which walking speed was determined. They were instructed to walk at a comfortable, self-selected pace while shod and wearing a safety harness. Following the familiarization session, participants were subjected to two tasks (without wearing a brace): (i) level walking for 2 minutes and (ii) walking with mechanical perturbations on the treadmill. Mechanical perturbations on the treadmill comprised five lateral-medial translations (2 cm displacements) of the treadmill belts during the stance phase of a gait cycle. For safety reasons, participants were informed about mechanical perturbations in advance. The mechanical perturbations of the treadmill occurred at random moments. Immediately following each of the two tasks, participants reported their average levels of knee pain, number of knee instability episodes, and perceived knee confidence. Subsequently, participants were randomized to receive a non-tight or tight brace and the two tasks were repeated while wearing a brace. Prior to testing on the treadmill, the 10-m walk and GUG tests were performed without the brace. Following testing on the treadmill, the 10-m walk and GUG tests were repeated with the brace (non-tight or tight).

After a 30-minute rest, the procedure crossed over to the second part of the assessments but with another type of soft brace (tight or non-tight). By counterbalancing the order of the type of brace we controlled the potential confounding effect of fatigue and learning effects on the comparison between a non-tight versus tight brace.

Statistical analysis

Descriptive statistics were used to characterize the study population. Numbers (percentages) were used for categorical variables, and means (SD) for continuous variables. Prior to the statistical analysis, outcome measures were checked for normality using the Shapiro–Wilk and Kolmogorov–Smirnov tests. Pain and self-reported knee instability and knee confidence were obtained for each knee separately (knee-level variable), and data from both knees were used in the statistical analysis. Data on the 10-m walk and GUG tests were analyzed as person-level variables. Four comparisons were analyzed: (i) brace versus no brace, (ii) tight brace versus no brace (i.e., baseline before tight), (iii) non-tight brace versus no brace (i.e., baseline before non-tight), and (iv) non-tight brace versus tight brace. Linear mixed-effect model analysis for repeated measurements within participants was used for continuous outcome measures (pain, 10-m walk test, GUG test). Logistic generalized estimating equations (GEE) analysis with an exchangeable working correlation matrix was used for dichotomous outcome measures (self-reported knee instability and knee confidence). No covariates were included in the models, because addition of a covariate to a repeated measures analysis does not alter the main effects of a within-subject factor (e.g., age, gender, etc. are the same at each data point) [32]. Statistical significance was accepted at $P < 0.05$. All analyses were performed using SPSS software, version 22.0 (SPSS, Chicago, IL, USA).

Results

There were 214 persons from the AMS-OA cohort initially contacted for eligibility; 144 persons declined to participate and 26 did not meet the inclusion criteria for the following reasons: absence of self-reported knee instability in the last 3 months (n = 13), comorbidity severely affecting daily functioning (n = 8), or age not

Table 1 Study procedure

Baseline assessment without an SB	Intervention assessment with an SB[a]	Rest[b]	Baseline assessment without an SB	Intervention assessment with an SB[a]
1. 10-m walk test	1. Level walk		1. 10-m walk test	1. Level walk
2. GUG test	A. Pain		2. GUG test	A. Pain
3. Level walk	B. SKI and SCI		3. Level walk	B. SKI and SCI
A. Pain	2. Perturbed walk		A. Pain	2. Perturbed walk
B. SKI and SCI	A. Pain		B. SKI and SCI	A. Pain
4. Perturbed walk	B. SKI and SCI		4. Perturbed walk	B. SKI and SCI
A. Pain	3. 10-m walk test		A. Pain	3. 10-m walk test
B. SKI and SCI	4. GUG test		B. SKI and SCI	4. GUG test

SB soft brace, *SKI* self-reported knee instability, *GUG* get up and go test, *SCI* self-reported knee confidence
[a]Tight or non-tight soft brace
[b]Rest of 30 minutes

between 50 and 80 years (n = 5). In total, 44 patients with knee OA and self-reported knee instability participated in the study. Demographics and clinical characteristics of the participants are shown in Table 2. The participants had a mean ± SD age of 65.7 ± 9.3 years, a mean ± SD BMI of 29.8 ± 5.5 kg/m^2, and 29 (65.9%) were women.

Descriptive data on pain and activity limitations by the conditions are presented in Table 3. The results of the statistical evaluation of the outcomes are presented in Table 4. Wearing a soft brace significantly reduced pain during level walking (*B* – 0.60, *P* = 0.001) and perturbed walking (*B* – 0.80, *P* < 0.001), reduced the time to complete the 10-m walk test (B – 0.23, *P* < 0.001) and GUG test (*B* – 0.23, *P* = 0.004), reduced self-reported knee instability during level walking (OR 0.41, *P* = 0.002) and perturbed walking (OR 0.36, *P* < 0.001), and reduced lack of confidence in the knees during level walking (OR 0.45, *P* < 0.001) and perturbed walking (OR 0.56, *P* < 0.001), compared with not wearing a soft brace (Table 4, column 2).

Whether the brace was non-tight or tight, the effects were similar (Table 4, columns 3 and 4). There was no difference in effects between a non-tight and tight brace, except for the 10-m walk test. Wearing a tight brace significantly reduced the time to complete the 10-m walk test in comparison with wearing a non-tight brace (*B* – 0.11, *P* = 0.03) (Table 4, column 5).

To determine whether the beneficial effects were in most participants or predominantly due to large effects in a few, the effect of wearing a soft brace on the outcome measures has been calculated per individual and presented on the histograms. The distribution of the individual effects per outcomes was fairly normal indicating that the overall beneficial effects are not attributable to large effects in a few participants [33].

Table 2 Descriptive statistics of the study participants (n = 44)

Variable	Value
Age (years)	65.7 (9.3)
Female, number (%)	29 (65.9)
Body mass index (kg/m^2)	29.8 (5.5)
Duration of symptoms (years)	13.0 (10.3)
Pain last week (NRS, range 0–10)	4.7 (1.9)
WOMAC, pain (range 0–20)	8.8 (4.0)
WOMAC, stiffness (range 0–8)	4.6 (1.7)
WOMAC, physical function (range 0–68)	32.5 (12.7)
WOMAC, total score (range 0–96)	45.9 (17.5)
Muscle strength, (Nm/kg)	0.88 (0.33)
Walking speed on the treadmill, (m/s)	0.74 (0.24)
KL grade, number (%)	
0 (none)	3 (7.0)
1 (doubtful)	16 (37.2)
2 (mild)	9 (20.9)
3 (moderate)	10 (23.3)
4 (severe)	5 (11.6)
Self-reported knee instability < 3 months, number (%)	
Rarely (1–2 times)	13 (29.5)
Regularly (3–4 times)	18 (40.9)
Very often (>4 times)	13 (29.5)

Categorical variables are presented as numbers (percentage); continuous variables are presented as means ± SD
NRS numeric rating scale, *WOMAC* Western Ontario and McMaster Universities Osteoarthritis Index *KL* Kellgren–Lawrence score

Discussion

In this study, we found that a soft brace reduced activity limitations and pain, and improved self-reported knee stability and knee confidence in patients with knee OA. We did not find significant differences between a non-tight and a tight brace, with the exception of performing the 10-m walk test. The results support the use of a soft brace as an efficacious treatment option in the immediate management of patients with knee OA.

This is the first high-quality study reporting on the immediate effect of wearing a soft brace, on pain, activity limitations, and self-reported knee instability, and knee confidence in patients with knee OA. The results of the recent systematic review on soft bracing in knee OA [6] showed that the quality of previous studies [2, 3, 15] ranged from low [3, 15] to fair [2] according to the Downs and Black scale [34]. If our study is scored according to the same criteria [34], the study is scored as a good-quality study (i.e., study quality percentage 68%). Compared to previous studies, our study received a higher score in the Downs and Black scale in statistical analysis, representativeness of the study population, and reporting on the facilities where patients were assessed.

The size of the effect on pain in our study is comparable to those observed in previous studies [2, 3, 15]. Bryk et al. [2] observed a 0.6 mm reduction in the visual analog scale (VAS) for pain during the Stair Climb Power Test (SCPT), while Schween et al. [3] and Hassan et al. [15] reported a similar decrease in the VAS for pain during level walking. We observed a 0.6-point (95% CI −0.97–0.23) and 0.8-point (95% CI −1.11–0.43) decrease in pain on the NRS for level and perturbed walking, respectively. This effect is close to the 1-point threshold for the minimal clinically important difference for NRS pain [35].

To our knowledge, only Bryk et al. [2] used performance-based physical tests to evaluate the immediate effect of a soft brace on activity limitations in patients with knee OA. Our study confirms their findings [2]. We found that wearing a soft brace significantly

Table 3 Pain and activity limitations by the conditions, mean (SD)

Outcomes	No brace	Brace	No brace	Tight brace	No brace	Non-tight brace	Tight brace	Non-tight brace
Pain, level walk[a]	3.28 (2.8)	2.67 (2.7)	3.44 (3.0)	2.83 (2.7)	3.14 (2.7)	2.53 (2.7)	2.79 (2.7)	2.55 (2.7)
Pain, perturbed walk[a]	3.41 (2.9)	2.60 (2.8)	3.51 (2.9)	2.76 (2.9)	3.33 (2.9)	2.47 (2.6)	2.72 (2.9)	2.50 (2.6)
10-m walk test[b]	7.04 (1.8)	6.81 (2.0)	6.89 (1.7)	6.67 (1.9)	7.11 (2.0)	6.89 (2.1)	6.75 (1.9)	6.86 (2.1)
GUG test[b]	10.89 (3.2)	10.66 (3.6)	10.65 (2.8)	10.57 (3.5)	11.13 (3.5)	10.75 (3.7)	10.58 (3.5)	10.70 (3.7)

GUG get up and go test
[a]Numeric rating scale (range 0–10)
[b]Seconds

reduced time to complete both the 10-m walk and GUG tests by 0.23 s (95% CI −0.31–0.13 and −0.38–0.07, respectively). In the absence of information on the minimal clinically important change in these measures, the clinical relevance of these effects cannot be evaluated. Furthermore, these effects should be viewed in the light of this being a laboratory-based study and the short duration of brace use. Further research on generalization to functioning in daily life and the clinical relevance of these effects in daily life is indicated.

Previously, only one study had observed that a soft brace improved self-reported knee instability [3], while the effect on knee confidence had not been studied before. The present study confirms that a soft brace improves self-reported knee stability, and is the first study to show that a soft brace improved confidence in the knees, in patients with knee OA. These results are noteworthy, given that self-reported knee instability has been reported in the majority (>60%) of patients with knee OA [9, 14], and that it may affect their quality of life [9, 25]. Knee confidence may influence decisions about participation in physical activity. Lack of confidence may force patients with knee OA to alter their daily activities, to avoid knee buckling and pain [36]. A soft brace may therefore indirectly influence daily activities via the improvement of knee instability and knee confidence.

This is the first study using external perturbations on the treadmill to evaluate the effect of a soft brace on pain, and on self-reported knee instability and knee confidence. External perturbations provide a more stimulating and challenging environment for knee stability [37], and simulate situations in which patients might experience increased knee instability and lack of confidence. Knee OA could affect the ability of the neuromuscular system to execute appropriate commands in response to external challenges, resulting in joint instability [37]. It is therefore important to show that, even when participants were subjected to external perturbations, the effect of wearing a soft brace on pain and self-reported knee instability and knee confidence continued.

The second aim of this study was to assess the difference in effect between a non-tight and a tight brace. We hypothesized that a non-tight brace would elicit stronger effects than a tight brace. This hypothesis was based on

Table 4 Statistical evaluation of the outcome measures by the comparisons

	Brace vs. no brace	*P* value	Tight brace vs. no brace	*P* value	Non-tight brace vs. no brace	*P* value	Non-tight vs. tight brace	*P* value
Outcomes, *B* (95% CI)[a]								
Pain, level walk	−0.60 (−0.97–0.23)	0.001*	−0.60 (−1.01–0.06)	0.028*	−0.60 (−1.01–0.07)	0.026*	−0.24 (−0.77 0.29)	0.37
Pain, perturbed walk	−0.80 (−1.11–0.43)	<0.001**	−0.75 (−1.31–0.02)	0.012*	−0.86 (−1.36–0.36)	0.001*	−0.21 (−0.44 0.30)	0.41
10 m walk test	−0.23 (−0.31–0.13)	<0.001**	−0.22 (−0.33–0.10)	<0.001**	−0.23 (−0.31–0.14)	<0.001**	0.11 (0.01 0.20)	0.03*
GUG test	−0.23 (−0.38–0.07)	0.004*	−0.08 (−0.25 0.08)	0.335	−0.38 (−0.57–0.17)	<0.001**	0.12 (−0.03 0.27)	0.13
Outcomes, OR (95% CI)[b]								
Knee instability, level walk	0.41 (0.23 0.66)	0.002*	0.37 (0.19 0.68)	0.002*	0.46 (0.22 0.93)	0.018*	1.06 (0.65 1.73)	0.79
Knee instability, perturbed walk	0.36 (0.22 0.59)	<0.001**	0.34 (0.18 0.62)	0.001*	0.39 (0.22 0.67)	0.001*	1.15 (0.66 2.0)	0.59
Knee confidence, level walk	0.45 (0.31 0.65)	<0.001**	0.48 (0.31 0.74)	0.001*	0.42 (0.27 0.65)	<0.001**	1.07 (0.75 1.51)	0.69
Knee confidence, perturbed walk	0.56 (0.38 0.82)	<0.001**	0.62 (0.35 0.77)	0.004*	0.63 (0.40 0.96)	0.033*	0.97 (0.60 1.56)	0.91

[a]Beta (B) coefficients (95% CI): negative value indicates reduced mean value of the outcome measure when wearing a brace
[b]Odds ratios (OR) (95% CI): value <1 indicates reduced chance of self-reported knee instability and lack of confidence in the knees when wearing a brace
*Significant at a *P* value <0.05; **significant at a *P* value <0.001

a study reporting that a non-tight brace reduced pain and improved postural sway more than a tight brace [15]. Hassan et al. [15] speculated that a non-tight brace provided more recurrent stimuli, by allowing movement between the brace and the skin, and thus elicited continuous response from cutaneous receptors. By contrast, a tight brace might provide constant pressure, to which skin mechanoreceptors adapt. Our hypothesis was not confirmed. Differences in the type of the brace may be an explanation. Hassan et al. [15] used a tubigrip elastic bandage, whereas we used a soft brace specifically designed for the knee joint. More importantly, we are unaware whether the level of pressure exerted on the skin by our soft brace was comparable to that used by Hassan et al. [15]. There is therefore a need to develop a reliable and valid measure of tightness.

Because a soft brace is an efficacious intervention, there is a need to understand the mechanisms underlying the effect. Soft braces might reduce self-reported knee instability by altering proprioceptive feedback [15] and enhancing muscle activity [38]. Mild compression provided by a soft brace [2, 39] might result in an improved sense of joint stability and greater confidence in the knee joint [10]. It has been suggested that soft braces reduce joint contact forces, due to less muscle co-contraction [3, 40]. Another mechanism could be an increase in skin temperature [39, 40]. Heat therapies are widely used in clinical practice to obtain analgesia, decrease muscle spasm, and encourage regional blood flow [41]. Thus, a soft brace, by providing warmth to the skin, may lead to less muscle contracture and therefore to reduced knee joint compressive forces. Finally, a placebo effect is a mechanism that should be considered [4, 42]. To better understand how soft braces work in knee OA, studies exploring the potential mechanisms underlying the observed effects are warranted.

Some limitations should be acknowledged. First, it was not possible to blind participants to the brace; however, it should be noted that blinding to the intervention in this type of studies is generally not possible. Second, our study provided information on effect in the laboratory. Thus, we do not know whether the observed effects can be generalized to the daily life of patients with knee OA. In light of limited evidence in this area, this should be a priority for future research in order to determine whether wearing a soft brace has long-term effects in daily life in patients with knee OA. Finally, assessment of the outcomes was performed first without a brace and then with a brace. This order may have led to bias because of possible learning effects.

Conclusions

In conclusion, the results of this study indicate that a soft brace is an efficacious intervention, targeting pain, activity limitations, and self-reported knee instability and knee confidence in the immediate-term in patients with knee OA. Although the results can potentially impact clinical practice, we acknowledge that studies on the generalization to functioning in daily life are required to support a soft brace as an established treatment option.

Abbreviations

ACR: American College of Rheumatology; AMS-OA: Amsterdam Osteoarthritis cohort; BMI: Body mass index; CI: Confidence interval; GEE: Generalized estimating equations analysis; GUG: Get up and go test; ICC: Intraclass correlation coefficient; K&L: Kellgren & Lawrence; KL: Kellgren–Lawrence score; KOOS: Knee Osteoarthritis Outcome Score; NRS: Numeric rating scale; OA: Osteoarthritis; PFOA: Patello-femoral joint osteoarthritis; ROA: Radiographic knee osteoarthritis; SCI: Self-reported knee confidence; SCPT: Stair Climb Power Test; SD: Standard deviation; SKI: Self-reported knee instability; VAS: Visual analog scale; WOMAC: Western Ontario and McMaster Universities Osteoarthritis Index

Acknowledgments

We gratefully thank Djody van Swaal, from Centrum Orthopedie Rotterdam, for providing the soft braces. We gratefully acknowledge Marjolein Booij, MSc, Linda van Gardner, MSc, and Anke Hofste, MSc, for their help during data collection. We thank Johannes Gijsbers, PhD for his help in the development of the application for treadmill perturbations.

Funding

This work was supported by the European Union, Seventh Framework Programme, under grant agreement number 607510. The European Union did not contribute to the design, interpretation of data, drafting, and final approval of the manuscript.

Authors' contributions

Study conception and design: TC, MvdE, and JD. Acquisition of data: TC, MvdE, and JD. Analysis and interpretation of data; TC, MvdE, MvdL, JvdN, LR, WL, JT, MS, JW, JH, and JD. Drafting the article or revising it critically for important intellectual content: TC, MvdE, MvdL, JvdN, LR, WL, JT, MS, JW, JH, and JD. Final approval of the version of the article to be published: TC, MvdE, MvdL, JvdN, LR, WL, JT, MS, JW, JH, and JD.

Competing interests

The authors declare that they have no competing interests.

Author details

[1]Department of Rehabilitation Medicine, VU University Medical Center, Amsterdam, The Netherlands. [2]Amsterdam Rehabilitation Research Centre Reade, Dr. J. van Breemenstraat 2, 1056 AB Amsterdam, P.O. Box 58271, 1040 HG Amsterdam, The Netherlands. [3]Department of Radiology and Nuclear Medicine, Musculoskeletal Imaging Quantification Center (MIQC), Academic Medical Center, Amsterdam, The Netherlands. [4]Amsterdam Rheumatology & Immunology Center, Amsterdam Medical Center, Reade, VU University Medical Center, Amsterdam, The Netherlands. [5]Jan van Breemen Research Institute, Reade, Amsterdam, The Netherlands. [6]Department of Health Sciences, VU University Amsterdam, Amsterdam, The Netherlands. [7]Department of Epidemiology and Biostatistics, VU University Medical Center, Amsterdam, The Netherlands. [8]School of Health and Life Sciences, Glasgow Caledonian University, Glasgow, United Kingdom. [9]Delft University of Technology, Delft, The Netherlands. [10]Department of Psychiatry, VU University Medical Center, Amsterdam, The Netherlands.

References

1. Beaudreuil J, Bendaya S, Faucher M, Coudeyre E, Ribinik P, Revel M, Rannou F. Clinical practice guidelines for rest orthosis, knee sleeves, and unloading knee braces in knee osteoarthritis. Joint Bone Spine. 2009;76:629–36.
2. Bryk FF, Jesus JF, Fukuda TY, Moreira EG, Marcondes FB, Santos MG. Immediate effect of the elastic knee sleeve use on individuals with osteoarthritis. Rev Bras Reumatol. 2011;51:440–6.
3. Schween R, Gehring D, Gollhofer A. Immediate effects of an elastic knee sleeve on frontal plane gait biomechanics in knee osteoarthritis. PLoS One. 2015;10:e0115782.
4. Berry H, Black C, Fernandes L, Berstein RM, Whittington J. Controlled trial of a knee support ('Genutrain') in patients with osteoarthritis of the knee. Eur J Rheumatol Inflamm. 1992;12:30–4.
5. Callaghan MJ, Parkes MJ, Hutchinson CE, Gait AD, Forsythe LM, Marjanovic EJ, Lunt M, Felson DT. A randomised trial of a brace for patellofemoral osteoarthritis targeting knee pain and bone marrow lesions. Ann Rheum Dis. 2015;74:1164–70.
6. Cudejko T, van der Esch M, van der Leeden M, Roorda LD, Pallari J, Bennell KL, Lund H, Dekker J. Effect of soft braces on pain and physical function in patients with knee osteoarthritis: systematic review with meta-analyses. Arch Phys Med Rehabil. 2017; https://doi.org/10.1016/j.apmr.2017.04.029.
7. Hall JE. Somatic sensation: I. General organisation; the tactile and position senses. In: Guyton AC, editor. Textbook of medical physiology. Philadelphia: PA: Saunders; 1996. p. 595–607.
8. Schmitt LC, Fitzgerald GK, Reisman AS, Rudolph KS. Instability, laxity, and physical function in patients with medial knee osteoarthritis. Phys Ther. 2008;88:1506–16.
9. van der Esch M, Knoop J, van der Leeden M, Voorneman R, Gerritsen M, Reiding D, Romviel S, Knol DL, Lems WF, Dekker J, Roorda LD. Self-reported knee instability and activity limitations in patients with knee osteoarthritis: results of the Amsterdam osteoarthritis cohort. Clin Rheumatol. 2012;31: 1505–10.
10. Skou ST, Wrigley TV, Metcalf BR, Hinman RS, Bennell KL. Association of knee confidence with pain, knee instability, muscle strength, and dynamic varus-valgus joint motion in knee osteoarthritis. Arthritis Care Res (Hoboken). 2014;66:695–701.
11. van der Esch M, Steultjens M, Harlaar J, Knol D, Lems W, Dekker J. Joint proprioception, muscle strength, and functional ability in patients with osteoarthritis of the knee. Arthritis Rheum. 2007;57:787–93.
12. Bellamy N, Buchanan WW, Goldsmith CH, Campbell J, Stitt LW. Validation study of WOMAC: a health status instrument for measuring clinically important patient relevant outcomes to antirheumatic drug therapy in patients with osteoarthritis of the hip or knee. J Rheumatol. 1988;15: 1833–40.
13. Roorda LD, Jones CA, Waltz M, Lankhorst GJ, Bouter LM, van der Eijken JW, Willems WJ, Heyligers IC, Voaklander DC, Kelly KD, Suarez-Almazor ME. Satisfactory cross cultural equivalence of the Dutch WOMAC in patients with hip osteoarthritis waiting for arthroplasty. Ann Rheum Dis. 2004;63: 36–42.
14. Fitzgerald GK, Piva SR, Irrgang JJ. Reports of joint instability in knee osteoarthritis: its prevalence and relationship to physical function. Arthritis Rheum. 2004;51:941–6.
15. Hassan BS, Mockett S, Doherty M. Influence of elastic bandage on knee pain, proprioception, and postural sway in subjects with knee osteoarthritis. Ann Rheum Dis. 2002;61:24–8.
16. Altman R, Asch E, Bloch D, Bole G, Borenstein D, Brandt K, Christy W, Cooke TD, Greenwald R, Hochberg M. Development of criteria for the classification and reporting of osteoarthritis. Classification of osteoarthritis of the knee. Diagnostic and Therapeutic Criteria Committee of the American Rheumatism Association. Arthritis Rheum. 1986;29:1039–49.
17. Knoop J, Dekker J, van der Leeden M, van der Esch M, Thorstensson CA, Gerritsen M, Voorneman RE, Peter WF, de RM, Romviel S, Lems WF, Roorda LD, Steultjens MP. Knee joint stabilization therapy in patients with osteoarthritis of the knee: a randomized, controlled trial. Osteoarthritis Cartil. 2013;21:1025–34.
18. Cruz-Almeida Y, King CD, Goodin BR, Sibille KT, Glover TL, Riley JL, Sotolongo A, Herbert MS, Schmidt J, Fessler BJ, Redden DT, Staud R, Bradley LA, Fillingim RB. Psychological profiles and pain characteristics of older adults with knee osteoarthritis. Arthritis Care Res (Hoboken). 2013;65:1786–94.
19. Holla JF, Steultjens MP, Roorda LD, Heymans MW, Ten WS, Dekker J. Prognostic factors for the two-year course of activity limitations in early osteoarthritis of the hip and/or knee. Arthritis Care Res (Hoboken). 2010;62: 1415–25.
20. van der Esch M, van der Leeden M, Roorda LD, Lems WF, Dekker J. Predictors of self-reported knee instability among patients with knee osteoarthritis: results of the Amsterdam osteoarthritis cohort. Clin Rheumatol. 2016;35:3007–13.
21. Lin YC, Davey RC, Cochrane T. Tests for physical function of the elderly with knee and hip osteoarthritis. Scand J Med Sci Sports. 2001;11:280–6.
22. Piva SR, Fitzgerald GK, Irrgang JJ, Bouzubar F, Starz TW. Get up and go test in patients with knee osteoarthritis. Arch Phys Med Rehabil. 2004;85:284–9.
23. Hurley MV, Scott DL, Rees J, Newham DJ. Sensorimotor changes and functional performance in patients with knee osteoarthritis. Ann Rheum Dis. 1997;56:641–8.
24. Irrgang JJ, Snyder-Mackler L, Wainner RS, Fu FH, Harner CD. Development of a patient-reported measure of function of the knee. J Bone Joint Surg Am. 1998;80:1132–45.
25. Knoop J, van der Leeden M, van der Esch M, Thorstensson CA, Gerritsen M, Voorneman RE, Lems WF, Roorda LD, Dekker J, Steultjens MP. Association of lower muscle strength with self-reported knee instability in osteoarthritis of the knee: results from the Amsterdam Osteoarthritis cohort. Arthritis Care Res (Hoboken). 2012;64:38–45.
26. Roos EM, Roos HP, Lohmander LS, Ekdahl C, Beynnon BD. Knee Injury and Osteoarthritis Outcome Score (KOOS)–development of a self-administered outcome measure. J Orthop Sports Phys Ther. 1998;28:88–96.
27. Roos EM, Toksvig-Larsen S. Knee injury and Osteoarthritis Outcome Score (KOOS) - validation and comparison to the WOMAC in total knee replacement. Health Qual Life Outcomes. 2003;1:17.
28. de Groot IB, Favejee MM, Reijman M, Verhaar JA, Terwee CB. The Dutch version of the Knee Injury and Osteoarthritis Outcome Score: a validation study. Health Qual Life Outcomes. 2008;6:16.
29. Kellgren JH, Lawrence JS. Radiological assessment of osteo-arthrosis. Ann Rheum Dis. 1957;16:494–502.
30. Buckland-Wright JC, Macfarlane DG, Jasani MK, Lynch JA. Quantitative microfocal radiographic assessment of osteoarthritis of the knee from weight bearing tunnel and semiflexed standing views. J Rheumatol. 1994; 21:1734–41.
31. Hewitt C, Hahn S, Torgerson DJ, Watson J, Bland JM. Adequacy and reporting of allocation concealment: review of recent trials published in four general medical journals. BMJ. 2005;330:1057–8.
32. Seltman J. Experimental Design and Analysis. 2015. http://www.stat.cmu.edu/~hseltman/309/Book/Book.pdf. Accessed 15 Apr 2017.
33. Twisk JW. Applied longitudinal data analysis for epidemiology. Cambridge: England, Cambridge University Press; 2013.
34. Downs SH, Black N. The feasibility of creating a checklist for the assessment of the methodological quality both of randomised and non-randomised studies of health care interventions. J Epidemiol Community Health. 1998;52:377–84.
35. Salaffi F, Stancati A, Silvestri CA, Ciapetti A, Grassi W. Minimal clinically important changes in chronic musculoskeletal pain intensity measured on a numerical rating scale. Eur J Pain. 2004;8:283–91.
36. Sharma L, Chmiel JS, Almagor O, Moisio K, Chang AH, Belisle L, Zhang Y, Hayes KW. Knee instability and basic and advanced function decline in knee osteoarthritis. Arthritis Care Res (Hoboken). 2015;67:1095–102.
37. Kumar D, Swanik CB, Reisman DS, Rudolph KS. Individuals with medial knee osteoarthritis show neuromuscular adaptation when perturbed during walking despite functional and structural impairments. J Appl Physiol (1985). 2014;116:13–23.
38. Collins A, Blackburn JT, Olcott C, Yu B, Weinhold P. The impact of stochastic resonance electrical stimulation and knee sleeve on impulsive loading and muscle co-contraction during gait in knee osteoarthritis. Clin Biomech (Bristol, Avon). 2011;26:853–8.
39. Chuang SH, Huang MH, Chen TW, Weng MC, Liu CW, Chen CH. Effect of knee sleeve on static and dynamic balance in patients with knee osteoarthritis. Kaohsiung J Med Sci. 2007;23:405–11.
40 Mazzuca SA, Page MC, Meldrum RD, Brandt KD, Petty-Saphon S. Pilot study of the effects of a heat-retaining knee sleeve on joint pain, stiffness, and function in patients with knee osteoarthritis. Arthritis Rheum. 2004;51:716–21.
41 Brosseau L, Yonge KA, Robinson V, Marchand S, Judd M, Wells G, Tugwell P. Thermotherapy for treatment of osteoarthritis. Cochrane Database Syst Rev. 2003;4:CD004522.

Structural predictors of response to intra-articular steroid injection in symptomatic knee osteoarthritis

Nasimah Maricar[1,2,3], Matthew J. Parkes[1,2], Michael J. Callaghan[1,2,4], Charles E. Hutchinson[5], Andrew D. Gait[6], Richard Hodgson[6], David T. Felson[1,2,7†] and Terence W. O'Neill[1,2,8*†]

Abstract

Background: The aim was to examine if structural factors could affect response to intra-articular steroid injections (IASI) in knee osteoarthritis (OA).

Method: Persons with painful knee OA participated in an open-label trial of IASI where radiographic joint space narrowing (JSN) and Kellgren-Lawrence (KL) grade, whole-organ magnetic resonance imaging (MRI) scores (WORMS) and quantitative assessment of synovial tissue volume (STV) were assessed on baseline images. Participants completed the Knee Injury and Osteoarthritis Outcome Score (KOOS) and a question about knee pain with a visual analogue scale for pain during nominated activity (VAS_{NA}), and Outcome Measures in Rheumatology (OMERACT)-Osteoarthritis Research Society International (OARSI) criteria were used to assess responder status within 2 weeks (short term) and 6 months (longer term). Regression models were used to examine predictors of short and longer term response to IASI.

Results: Subjects ($n = 207$) attended and had IASI. Information on responder status was available on 199 participants. Of these, 188 subjects, mean age 63.2 years (standard deviation (SD) 10.3), 97 (51.6%) female, had x-rays and 120 had MRI scans available. Based on the OMERACT-OARSI criteria, 146 (73.4%) participants responded to therapy and 40 (20.1%) were longer term responders. A few factors were associated with a reduced KOOS-pain and VAS_{NA} response though none were associated with OMERACT-OARSI responder status in the short term. Higher MRI meniscal damage (odds ratio (OR) = 0.74; 95% CI 0.55 to 0.98), increasing KL maximal grade (OR = 0.43; 95% CI 0.23 to 0.82) and joint space narrowing (JSN) maximal score (OR = 0.60; 95% CI 0.36 to 0.99) were each associated with a lower odds of longer term responder status. Baseline synovitis was not associated with treatment response. The predicted probability of longer term response decreased from 38% to 12% as baseline maximal JSN increased from grade 0 to 3.

Conclusion: Compared with those who have mild structural damage, persons with more severe knee damage on either MRI or x-ray are less likely to respond to knee IASI.

Keywords: Knee osteoarthritis, Clinical trial, Intra-articular steroid injection, Predictors of response

* Correspondence: terence.o'neill@manchester.ac.uk
†Equal contributors
[1]Arthritis Research UK Centre for Epidemiology, Division of Musculoskeletal and Dermatological Sciences, Faculty of Biology, Medicine and Health, Manchester Academic Health Science Centre, University of Manchester, Manchester, UK
[2]NIHR Manchester Musculoskeletal Biomedical Research Unit, Central Manchester University Hospitals NHS Foundation Trust, Manchester Academic Health Sciences Centre, Manchester, UK
Full list of author information is available at the end of the article

Background

Intra-articular steroid injection (IASI) is an effective [1], widely used [2] and recommended treatment [3] for individuals with symptomatic osteoarthritis (OA) of the knee with short term pain relief lasting up to 3–4 weeks compared with placebo injection [1, 4–6], with some persons having longer term response up to 24 weeks [4, 7]. There are, however, significant variations in both the magnitude and duration of symptom relief following steroid injections [1, 4, 5, 8]. Such variation may be due to differences in the phenotypic expression, including severity of the disease; however, there are few published data on this issue and those studies that have examined structural factors predicting response have been small [6, 7, 9–14] and findings have been discrepant [6–8, 11, 13, 15]. Further, only radiographic [7, 9, 13, 15] and arthroscopic [7] predictor factors have been studied. Also in one trial factors predictive of IASIs were studied after combined treatment with arthroscopic lavage [7].

In our recent open-label study of IASI in knee OA [16], not all participants responded to the therapy in the short term (within 2 weeks). Of those who responded in the short term the majority, though not all, had a recurrence of pain within 6 months. As part of this study, we examined whether factors representing structural features of OA or of inflammation might identify persons who were likely to respond to IASI either in the short or longer term. Our study of IASI predictor of response was larger in scale and longer in follow up than prior studies, and also involved scoring of individual features through contrast-enhanced (CE)-magnetic resonance imaging (MRI), offering the opportunity to identify other OA features and synovial factors affecting response to IASI treatment. To optimize selection of persons for IASI treatment, it would be helpful to separate responders from non-responders.

We hypothesised that those with more severe joint damage would be less likely to respond, while those with an underlying "inflammatory" phenotype characterised by synovitis/effusion would be more likely to respond. Using data from our study, we looked at the impact of these "structural" factors based on radiographic and MRI on response to therapy in the short and longer term.

Methods

Participants

Men and women ($n = 209$) aged 40 years and over were recruited from primary and secondary care clinics for participation in an open-label study examining the efficacy of IASI in symptomatic knee OA (ISRCTN07329370). Subjects were included if they reported moderate knee pain for more than 48 hours in the previous 2 weeks on global rating or scored more than 7 out of 32 on the Knee Injury and Osteoarthritis Outcome Score (KOOS) [17], for questions P2–P9 (question P1 relates to frequency of knee pain, which is irrelevant given the inclusion criteria on pain frequency). Inclusion criteria included imaging confirmation of OA either radiologically in the index knee (in any compartment on anteroposterior (AP), skyline or lateral projection knee radiographs obtained within the previous 2 years) with a Kellgren-Lawrence (KL) score of 2 or more or, on MRI scan or at arthroscopy. For MRI and arthroscopy, we required typical changes of OA with at least evidence of cartilage loss. Exclusion criteria included gout, septic arthritis, inflammatory arthritis, hyaluronic acid or steroid injection within the previous 3 months, knee surgery within the previous 6 months, concurrent life threatening illnesses and any contraindication to MRI scanning.

Screening and baseline assessment

Subjects were assessed for eligibility at a screening visit [16]. For those in whom previous knee imaging within the previous 2 years was not available, radiographs of the index knee were performed at the screening assessment. Those who fulfilled the inclusion/exclusion criteria were invited to attend baseline assessments. Subjects completed a series of questionnaires including the KOOS-pain scale [17], a global Likert scale and visual analogue scale (VAS) for pain during an activity that a patient nominated as being most troublesome (VAS_{NA}). For those subjects who took part in the MRI sub-study, the MRI scans were undertaken immediately prior to IASI. Following the MRI scan the joint was injected with 80 mg methylprednisolone acetate (without local anaesthetic) with aspiration of synovial fluid in cases of clinical effusion. We treated and studied one knee per participant.

Follow up

Short term and longer term response was assessed using the Outcome Measures in Rheumatology-Osteoarthritis Research Society International (OMERACT-OARSI) responder criteria based on the KOOS-pain scale and global Likert scale [18]. A responder was defined as either (1) greater or equal to 20% change in KOOS-pain score and a "slightly" or "much better" score on the 5-point Likert scale for change in pain, or (2) greater or equal to 50% change in the KOOS-pain score; in both cases an absolute change of at least 3 units if the baseline KOOS score was 15 or less. Participants were seen usually within 2 weeks after the injection and we characterised their response then as short term response. Based on these criteria those who had not responded were not further followed up. Those who responded were followed with regular telephone calls during which the same KOOS-pain questions and global Likert scale were administered. Those whose pain rebounded to within 20% of the baseline KOOS-pain score were defined as having relapsed and were seen again for a final follow up. Those whose pain levels did not return to this level at 6 months of follow up were classified as "longer term responders".

Magnetic resonance imaging: acquisition and analysis

Using a 3-T Philips MRI scanner, sagittal post-contrast T1W FS (repetition time (TR) 550 ms, echo time (TE) 20 ms, field of view (FOV) 14 cm × 14 cm, size 320 × 320) and sagittal pre-contrast 3-D WATSC (TR 20 ms, TE 4.7 ms, FOV 15 cm × 15 cm, size 288 × 288) scans were obtained. Semi-quantitative assessment of the MRI images over 14 areas using the Whole-Organ Magnetic Resonance Imaging Score (WORMS) was used by an experienced musculoskeletal (MSK) radiologist to grade effusion, cartilage, bone attrition, bone marrow lesion (BML), synovitis, osteophytes, bone cyst, menisci and ligaments within the knee, using an approach previously described in which higher scores indicate greater severity of the feature [19]. Synovitis was scored 0–1–2–3 according to increasing synovial thickness [19]. Bone attrition, BML, effusion and cyst were scored 0–3, cartilage and menisci were scored 0–6 and osteophytes were scored 0–7 in each of the 14 areas [20]. For all MRI features, we used the maximal score, that is, the worst scoring in any region of the knee. Synovitis and effusion were scored using the sagittal contrast-enhanced (CE) MRI sequence [19, 20]. Intra-reader reliability was assessed by the same reader re-evaluating 19 films after an interval period, with weighted kappa scores of 0.71, 0.70, 0.63, 0.77, 0.88, 0.77 and 0.91 for cartilage, cysts, osteophytes, BMLs, menisci, synovitis and effusion, respectively. The CE images were then assessed quantitatively for synovial tissue volume (STV) [16]. To evaluate repeatability of assessment of synovial volumes, the segmenter was asked to segment 10 knees randomly selected (without replacement) from those that had been previously segmented with new identification numbers assigned [16]. The intra-class correlation coefficient (ICC) for intra-reader reliability of the manual segmentation was 0.94.

Radiographs

Knee radiographs were evaluated by an experienced MSK radiologist (CEH) who scored the KL and joint space narrowing (JSN) grades on skyline, weight-bearing AP and lateral projection radiographs of all participants for whom films were available. The KL and JSN grades were scored separately with KL scores 0–4 to denote the increasing level of joint degeneration [21], while JSN 0–3 indicated none, mild, moderate and severe reduction in joint space [22]. We looked also at anatomic mal-alignment. This was assessed on weight-bearing AP radiographs by one assessor (NM) using software installed within the hospital imaging system by calculating the angle from the intersection of the line from the midpoint of tibial spines bisecting the femoral shaft with the line from the midpoint of the tibial spines bisecting the tibial shaft [23]. The ICC was 0.99 for intra-rater reliability in the measurement of knee mal-alignment angle performed 3 months apart through random generated numbers of 50 images.

Statistical analysis

Subject characteristics were summarised using means and standard deviations (SD) for normally distributed variables and medians and interquartile ranges (IQR) for variables with a skewed distribution. We used the paired *t* test to look for change in pain, assessed using the KOOS and VAS_{NA} between baseline and the post-injection visit. We used a fixed-effects panel regression model to examine whether there was any association between the baseline structural factors and change in pain, a continuous outcome variable (assessed using both KOOS and VAS_{NA}) between baseline and initial follow up. For effusion, cartilage, bone attrition, BML, synovitis, osteophytes, bone cyst, menisci and ligaments we focused our analyses on the maximal WORMS for that feature and we included it in the model as a continuous variable; results were expressed as unstandardized b-coefficients and 95% confidence interval (CI). Logistic regression was used to determine whether baseline imaging parameters were associated with both short term and also longer term responder status (yes/no as outcome) to therapy. Results were expressed as odds ratios (OR) and 95% CI. Each factor of interest was investigated separately using a bivariate model, with either short term or longer term responder status as the outcome, and the factor of interest as the predictor variable. Data for short term and longer term response were analysed using a maximal case analysis using all available data for all variables. To examine the predictive probability of responder status (short/longer term), we extracted the predictive probabilities using the logistic regression model. Statistical analyses were undertaken using Stata version 13.1 (StataCorp, College Station, TX, USA).

Results

Participants

We recruited 209 participants. Two participants were withdrawn following recruitment and before treatment for receiving IASI from their General Practitioners (GPs) (see Fig. 1); 207 participants participated in the trial and received IASI. A further 8 subjects were later withdrawn for reasons listed in Fig. 1, with 199 participants remaining. Of these, 188 subjects had knee radiographs, mean age was 63.2 years (SD: 10.3 years) and 51.6% were female (see

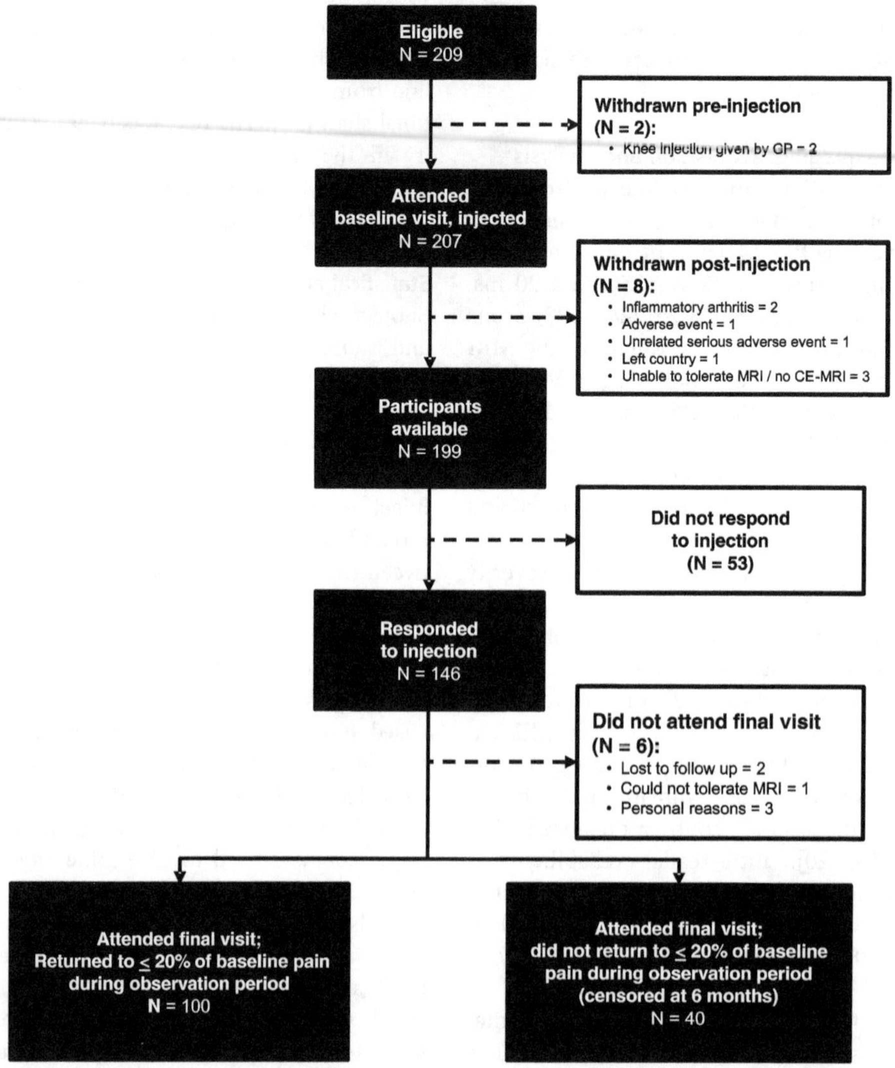

Fig. 1 Preferred reporting items for systematic reviews and meta-analyses (*PRISMA*) flow chart of participants for assessments of radiographs and magnetic resonance imaging (*MRI*) scans. *GP* General Practitioner, *CE* contrast-enhanced

Table 1). Median KOOS-pain score at baseline was 44.4 points (IQR: 36.1–55.6), and median VAS_{NA} was 7.0 cm on a 0–10 cm scale (IQR: 5.6–8.1). For all participants, the median time between baseline and post-injection follow up was 8 days (IQR: 7–14). Of the 120 participants who had MRI, it was possible to assess WORMS in 109 participants and synovial tissue volume in 111 participants.

Imaging characteristics

Of those with radiographs, 36.7% of participants had overall KL grade 2 at the knee, 53.7% had KL grade 3 and 9.6% had KL grade 4 (see Table 2). For JSN, we considered the scores in the medial tibiofemoral (TF), lateral TF and patellofemoral (PF) compartments and an overall JSN maximal score (any compartment). Overall 1.6% had a JSN maximal score of zero, 31.6% a JSN score of 1, 48.1% a JSN score of 2 and 18.7% a JSN score of 3. Table 2 shows the distribution of the maximal score for the MRI features including BML, meniscal damage, effusion, synovitis, cartilage, osteophytes and attrition.

Structural parameters and change in pain

At 2 weeks post injection, knee pain significantly improved when assessed by KOOS (+23.7 points; 95% CI: 20.9 to 26.5; $p < 0.001$) and VAS_{NA} (-3.3 cm; 95% CI: -3.8 to -2.9; $p < 0.001$). Among those with MRI scans, those with a higher maximal BML score (b coefficient = 0.76, 95% CI 0.16 to 1.36) and maximal meniscal damage score (b coefficient = 0.37, 95% CI 0.04 to 0.70) had less improvement in pain as determined by VAS_{NA} (see Table 3). Similarly, among those with radiographs, higher TF and PF KL scores, higher overall KL maximal score, higher PF

Table 1 Participant characteristics

Variable	MRI cohort	Radiograph cohort
Number	120[a]	188
Age (years), mean (SD)	62.3 (10.3)	63.2 (10.3)
Female, frequency (%)	62 (51.7)	97 (51.6)
Number of days to follow-up appointment, median (IQR)	8.0 (7.0–14.0)	8.0 (7.0–14.0)
KOOS-pain subscale score (0–100)[b], median (IQR)	44.4 (36.1–55.6)	44.4 (36.1–55.6)
Pain on nominated activity, VAS_{NA} (0–10 cm)[c], median (IQR)	7.0 (5.5–7.7)[d]	7.0 (5.6–8.1)[e]
Pain in last week, VAS (0–10 cm)[c], median (IQR)	6.5 (4.7–7.8)[d]	6.5 (4.9–8.0)[e]
Responders to injection, at follow-up visit, frequency, (%)	85 (70.8)	137 (72.9)

MRI magnetic resonance imaging, *SD* standard deviation, *IQR* interquartile range, *CI* confidence interval, *KOOS* Knee Injury and Osteoarthritis Outcome Score, *VAS* visual analogue scale, VAS_{NA} VAS for pain during nominated activity. [a]There were 109 baseline images available for assessment of Whole Organ Magnetic Resonance Imaging Score and 111 available for assessment of synovial tissue volume; [b]KOOS pain subscale is scored from 100 (no pain) to 0 (extreme pain); [c]VAS is scored from 0 cm (no pain) to 10 cm (pain as bad as you can imagine); [d]there were 5 and 3 patients who did not complete their VAS_{NA} and VAS for pain in the last week, respectively; [e]there were 8 and 4 patients who did not complete their VAS_{NA} and VAS for pain in last the week, respectively

JSN score and higher overall JSN maximal score were associated with less improvement in pain as assessed using VAS_{NA} (see Table 3). The presence of synovitis assessed using WORMS and also STV assessed quantitatively was not associated with change in pain. For pain assessed using KOOS, the results in relation to structural predictors were in the same direction though they were not statistically significant. Mal-alignment was not associated with response.

Predictors of responder status

Short term response

At short term follow up 146 (73.4%) of the 199 participants were OMERACT-OARSI responders. None of the MRI or radiographic variables was associated with OMERACT-OARSI responder status at short term follow up (see Table 4).

Longer term response

Of the 146 participants who were short term responders, 6 did not attend for a final visit. Of those who did, 100 had a recurrence of pain during the following 6 months, while 40 were longer term responders. Higher maximal score for meniscal damage, and higher radiographic TF KL score, overall KL maximal score and overall JSN maximal score were associated with decreased odds of being a longer term responder (see Table 4).

Predicted probability of response

Depending on the structural predictor, as disease severity increased there was a trend towards a reduced probability of being a responder to IASI. For instance, the probability of being a short term responder to IASI decreased from 82% (95% CI 69% to 95%) among those with an overall JSN maximal score of 0, to 66% (95% CI 53% to 79%) among those with a JSN maximal score of 3, though this difference was not statistically significant (see Table 5). In the longer term there was a significant threefold decrease in the chance of being a longer term responder to IASI when the overall JSN maximal scores increased from 0 (38%; 95% CI 16% to 60%) to 3 (12%; 95% CI 4% to 19%) and a fivefold decrease when the

Table 2 MRI and radiographic features at baseline

Maximal score	MRI features (WORMS)							Radiographic features	
	BML (*n*)	Menisci (*n*)	Effusion (*n*)	Synovitis (*n*)	Cartilage (*n*)	Osteophyte (*n*)	Attrition (*n*)	KL[a] (*n*)	JSN[a] (*n*)
0	5	35	22	0	5	0	3	0	3
1	30	0	46	2	5	1	19	0	59
2	26	9	32	18	9	10	49	69	90
2.5	-	-	-	-	10	-	-	-	-
3	48	24	9	89	8	19	38	101	35
4		41			26	25		18	
5		0			36	16			
6		0			10	33			
7						5			

MRI magnetic resonance imaging, *WORMS* Whole organ magnetic resonance imaging score, *BML* bone marrow lesion, *KL* Kellgren-Lawrence, *JSN* joint space narrowing. WORMS range of scores differs for each feature. [a]Maximal score in any region; 188 participants with available images for KL grading and 187 for JSN scoring

Table 3 Baseline imaging characteristics and their relation to change in pain at 2 weeks among persons treated with intra-articular steroids

Predictor variable in regression	KOOS pain score			Pain on nominated activity VAS		
	N	b coefficient (95% CI)[c]	*P* value	*N*	b coefficient (95% CI)[d]	*P* value
MRI (WORMS)						
Synovitis maximal score (0–3)	109	-1.94 (-11.15 to 7.26)	0.677	96	0.45 (-0.83 to 1.74)	0.487
Bone marrow lesion maximal score (0–3)	109	-3.48 (-7.76 to 0.80)	0.110	96	0.76 (0.16 to 1.36)*	0.013
Bone attrition maximal score (0–3)	109	-1.78 (-6.98 to 3.42)	0.498	96	-0.07 (-0.81 to 0.66)	0.846
Cartilage damage maximal score (0–6)	109	0.09 (-2.55 to 2.72)	0.948	96	0.16 (-0.20 to 0.53)	0.378
Cyst maximal score (0–3)	108	0.56 (-4.48 to 5.60)	0.827	95	0.27 (-0.48 to 1.01)	0.475
Menisci damage maximal score (0–6)	109	-2.12 (-4.49 to 0.25)	0.079	96	0.37 (0.04 to 0.70)*	0.027
Osteophyte maximal score (0–7)	109	0.56 (-2.23 to 3.36)	0.690	96	0.18 (-0.22 to 0.57)	0.377
Synovial effusion (0–3)	109	-1.22 (-5.90, 3.46)	0.608	96	0.17 (-0.49 to 0.83)	0.606
MRI (quantitative)						
Synovial tissue volume (1000 mm^3)	111	-0.05 (-0.67 to 0.57)	0.883	98	0.03 (-0.05 to 0.12)	0.408
Radiographs						
Tibiofemoral KL score (0–4)	186	-2.40 (-6.80 to 2.00)	0.284	170	0.66 (0.02 to 1.30)*	0.042
Patellofemoral KL score (0–4)	187	-0.001 (-3.16 to 3.16)	0.999	171	0.64 (0.18 to 1.10)*	0.006
Overall KL maximal score[a] (0–4)	187	-1.97 (-6.64 to 2.71)	0.408	171	0.94 (0.27 to 1.62)*	0.007
Lateral tibiofemoral JSN score (0–3)	185	-0.001 (-4.12 to 4.12)	1.000	169	0.05 (-0.56 to 0.67)	0.865
Medial tibiofemoral JSN score (0–3)	186	-1.26 (-5.17 to 2.65)	0.524	170	0.21 (-0.38 to 0.79)	0.486
Patellofemoral JSN score (0–3)	178	-0.52 (-3.60 to 2.56)	0.738	162	0.52 (0.06 to 0.98)*	0.026
Overall JSN maximal score[b] (0–3)	186	-1.34 (-5.26 to 2.57)	0.499	170	0.72 (0.14 to 1.29)*	0.015
Knee mal-alignment angle (per degree)	191	0.03 (-0.53 to 0.59)	0.924	173	-0.04 (-0.13 to 0.04)	0.291

KOOS Knee Injury and Osteoarthritis Outcome Score, *VAS* visual analogue scale, *MRI* magnetic resonance imaging, *WORMS* Whole Organ Magnetic Resonance Imaging Score, *KL* Kellgren-Lawrence, *JSN* joint space narrowing. Results shown are from fixed panel regression. [a]maximal KL grade of the tibiofemoral or patellofemoral joint; [b]maximal JSN score of the lateral or medial tibiofemoral or patellofemoral joint; [c]KOOS pain score ranges from 0–100 with lower scores representing more severe pain. Negative coefficients signify that more severe imaging findings were associated with less pain improvement; [d]pain on nominated activity ranged from 0 to 10 with higher values representing more severe pain. Positive coefficients signify that more severe imaging findings were associated with less pain improvement. *Represent results that are significant at $p < 0.05$

maximal meniscal score increased from 0 (28%; 95% CI 14% to 43%) to 6 (6%; 95% CI 0% to 13%).

Discussion

In this study, 73.4% of participants were short term responders after an IASI, while one in four was a longer term responder. Using OMERACT-OARSI criteria as our definition of response, we found no short term structural predictors of response. Increasing disease severity as determined by MRI and plain radiographs was associated with longer term non-responder status.

Radiographic markers of disease severity including higher KL and JSN scores were associated with poorer response to IASI in the short term as defined by a change in VAS_{NA}. Similarly, MRI features were also linked with response, with features suggestive of more structural damage being linked with a poorer short term response.

There are few studies that have looked at the influence of structural factors on response to IASI. In a systematic review we found a paucity of data on predictors of response to IASI and inconsistent results relating to disease severity [8]. The findings of the current study are consistent with two studies where increasing radiographic severity of OA was linked with reduced response [7, 15]. Smith et al. [7] in a study of 38 patients with knee OA who received 120 mg methylprednisolone acetate preceded by arthroscopy, found that severity was linked with reduced OARSI response at 4 weeks, while in a study of 79 participants with OA, higher radiographic grade was linked with less improvement in Western Ontario and McMaster Universities Osteoarthritis Index (WOMAC) pain score at 26 weeks ($p < 0.05$); however, the analysis was based on combined outcome of their steroid and lavage/tidal irrigation groups [15]. In contrast, two other studies did not find that radiographic OA grading predicted short term response ($\leq$6 weeks) to IASI in knee OA when VAS pain was used as the outcome [9, 13]. The small sample size of these studies (16–42 participants) might have contributed to low power to detect response [9, 13]. Another factor, which may have explained the potential discrepancy, is the dose

Table 4 Prediction of responder status at short term (2 weeks) and longer term (6 months) follow up, by baseline imaging characteristics

Predictor variable in regression	Short term responder at 2 weeks (yes/no)			Longer term responder at 6 months (yes/no)		
	N	Odds ratio (95% CI)	*P* value	*N*	Odds ratio (95% CI)	*P* value
MRI (WORMS)						
Synovitis maximal score (0–3)	109	0.82 (0.32 to 2.13)	0.689	109	0.43 (0.17 to 1.12)	0.084
Bone marrow lesion maximal score (0–3)	109	0.76 (0.49 to 1.19)	0.231	109	1.12 (0.66 to 1.92)	0.668
Bone attrition maximal score (0–3)	109	0.94 (0.56 to 1.57)	0.804	109	0.59 (0.32 to 1.10)	0.097
Cartilage damage maximal score (0–6)	109	0.98 (0.75 to 1.27)	0.869	109	1.03 (0.74 to 1.42)	0.873
Cyst maximal score (0–3)	108	0.74 (0.46 to 1.20)	0.222	108	1.27 (0.72 to 2.22)	0.408
Menisci damage maximal score (0–6)	109	0.95 (0.74 to 1.20)	0.647	109	0.74 (0.55 to 0.98)*	0.039
Osteophyte maximal score (0–7)	109	1.13 (0.86 to 1.49)	0.386	109	0.98 (0.70 to 1.38)	0.919
Synovial effusion (0–3)	109	0.83 (0.52 to 1.31)	0.420	109	0.79 (0.44 to 1.41)	0.421
MRI (quantitative)						
Synovial tissue volume (per 1000 mm^3)	111	1.00 (1.00 to 1.00)	0.612	111	0.96 (0.88 to 1.04)	0.327
Radiographs						
Tibiofemoral KL score (0–4)	187	0.79 (0.49 to 1.28)	0.341	187	0.52 (0.30 to 0.91)*	0.021
Patellofemoral KL score (0–4)	188	0.86 (0.60 to 1.22)	0.391	188	0.80 (0.54 to 1.19)	0.269
Overall KL maximal score[a] (0–4)	188	0.72 (0.43 to 1.20)	0.205	188	0.43 (0.23 to 0.82)*	0.010
Lateral tibiofemoral JSN score (0–3)	186	1.27 (0.79 to 2.03)	0.327	186	0.86 (0.51 to 1.45)	0.569
Medial tibiofemoral JSN score (0–3)	187	0.91 (0.59 to 1.40)	0.661	187	0.69 (0.42 to 1.15)	0.154
Patellofemoral JSN score (0–3)	179	0.83 (0.59 to 1.16)	0.265	179	0.85 (0.56 to 1.28)	0.425
Overall JSN maximal score[b] (0–3)	187	0.75 (0.49 to 1.16)	0.196	187	0.60 (0.36 to 0.99)*	0.047
Knee mal-alignment angle (per degree)	192	0.98 (0.92 to 1.04)	0.481	192	1.01 (0.94 to 1.08)	0.801

MRI magnetic resonance imaging, *WORMS* Whole Organ Magnetic Resonance Imaging Score, *KL* Kellgren-Lawrence, *JSN* joint space narrowing. Results presented are from logistic regression. [a]maximal KL grade of the tibiofemoral or patellofemoral joint; [b]maximal JSN score of the lateral or medial tibiofemoral or patellofemoral joint. *Represent results that are significant at $p < 0.05$

of steroid used. The two previous positive studies used either 40 mg of triamcinolone acetonide or 120 mg methylprednisolone acetate [7, 15], while the two that did not show any association of severity of disease with response used a smaller dose - 20 mg triamcinolone hexacetonide [9, 13]. Further, the focus of prior studies on short term outcomes may have also made it difficult for these studies to detect an association between disease severity and outcome, as the large majority of patients respond over the short term. Additionally no previous studies have examined both short term and longer term predictors of outcomes within the same trial. In our study we found no significant associations between structural damage and short term response as defined by

Table 5 Predictive probabilities of being a short term and longer term responder: radiographs and MRI features

	Probability						
Overall KL maximal grade[a]	0	1	2	3	4		
Short term predicted probability[b]	0.87[d]	0.83[d]	0.78	0.71	0.64		
Longer term predicted probability	0.69[d]	0.49[d]	0.29	0.15	0.07		
Overall JSN maximal score[c]	0	1	2	3			
Short term predicted probability[b]	0.82	0.77	0.72	0.66			
Longer term predicted probability	0.38	0.27	0.18	0.12			
Menisci maximal WORMS	0	1	2	3	4	5	6
Short term predicted probability	0.72	0.70	0.69	0.68	0.67	0.66	0.64
Longer term predicted probability	0.28	0.22	0.18	0.14	0.10	0.08	0.06

KL Kellgren-Lawrence, *JSN* joint space narrowing, *WORMS* Whole Organ Magnetic Resonance Imaging Score; [a]maximal KL grade of the tibiofemoral or patellofemoral joint; [b]trend not statistically significant; [c]maximal JSN score of the lateral or medial tibiofemoral or patellofemoral joint; [d]values based on modelling a change in KOOS; however, the direction of effect (suggesting a poorer response) was similar to that observed for the VAS_{NA}.

To our knowledge, this is also the first study to have looked at MRI predictors of response. The results are consistent with the radiographic findings, though perhaps because of smaller numbers in the responder analysis, not all MRI features attained statistical significance. The association between higher meniscal damage with a lesser reduction in pain in the short term, and also reduced odds of being a longer term responder, is consistent with greater meniscus damage being associated with greater severity of OA disease [24]. Larger BMLs were also associated with a lesser reduction in pain in the short term; previous studies have shown that increase in the size of BMLs is associated with increased severity of joint degeneration [25–27].

At the outset, we hypothesised that there would be a link between synovitis and response, with those with greater baseline synovitis being more likely to respond; however, we did not find this in the study. The mechanism of the therapeutic effect of corticosteroids in knee OA is unclear, though it has been thought likely related in part to their potent anti-inflammatory effect. We have already shown correlation between change in STV, which is a marker for synovitis, and change in pain, in a previous paper [16] and had expected to find a link between baseline synovitis and response. The most plausible explanation for the apparent discordant findings is that any within-person change in pain due to reduced synovitis is masked by other sources of between-person variations in levels of pain including structural factors. The null findings, though, are in keeping with observations made in previous studies that used either clinical or ultrasound assessment of synovial hypertrophy and power Doppler assessment of synovitis [6, 10, 11].

The presence of an effusion on MRI was not a predictor of response. Previous studies that correlated positive response to IASI with effusion had used clinical assessment to detect knee effusion [9, 15], though one other study that used clinical assessment of effusion found no such correlation [10]. Non-contrast ultrasound assessment of effusion has not been shown to predict response [6, 11].

In our study, the early-responder rate (73.4%) was similar to most though not all studies [1]. There are much fewer data on longer term response. We found 20% of participants maintained their improvement in pain for at least 6 months. This is consistent with Arden et al. [15] who reported that 29% of participants maintained improvement at their 6-month follow up. Smith et al. [7] reported a higher (42% or 16 participants) longer term responder rate at 6 months; it is possible this could be explained by the higher dose of steroid used (120 mg methylprednisolone acetate) and also by the fact that 30 out of their 38 participants received a second course of IASI at the time of relapse during the period of the study.

Using radiographic and MRI data, we derived a predictive table, though the short term radiographic prediction probabilities should be viewed with caution given their non-significant results and their wide CIs. Our predictive probabilities suggest people with advanced radiographic disease are unlikely to benefit from IASI in the longer term. Based on the degree of JSN observed on radiographs, the odds of having longer term response is increased from around 10% to almost 40% as the disease becomes less severe.

Our study is the largest yet performed looking at response to IASI. There are some limitations to be considered in interpreting the analysis. The study included individuals who received steroid injections only and it is likely that the overall response to the injection is at least in part due to a "placebo" effect. It seems, however, very unlikely that this can explain our findings relating to factors identified as predicting response. As noted previously, earlier studies of intra-articular steroids without a control group have not reported an association between structural severity and response, and while structural severity has been linked to a worse pain trajectory in some studies [28], other longitudinal studies have reported no association between baseline structural severity and the trajectory of pain [29, 30]. In relation to limb mal-alignment we used conventional non-standardised images to estimate the angle and did not use a full-limb weight-bearing radiograph, which is a gold standard for measuring knee mal-alignment; it is possible that misclassification may have resulted in a bias of the results towards the null. There is, however, evidence of strong correlation between the femur-tibia angle measured from knee radiographs with hip-knee-ankle angle measured from full-limb radiographs ($r = 0.86$; 95% CI: 0.81 to 0.90) [23].

Our MRI sequences were optimised for the detection of BMLs, which may have contributed to our negative findings with the other knee structures. Further, radiographs in the study could have been taken up to 24 months prior to the IASI and it is possible that progression of disease may have led to some misclassification of radiographic disease severity with underestimation of OA severity in a small proportion of subjects. Based on data from the MOST study we estimate that over a 24-month period up to 20% of subjects would have KL progression; however, for most subjects in our study the time interval was significantly shorter [31]. It is possible, however, that this may have had a small impact on the predictive probabilities observed. Some subjects did not complete the pain questions at baseline and follow up. We have repeated the analysis using complete case analysis based on data from participants with complete data on all variables with similar results to the maximal case analysis.

Conclusion

Over two thirds of people with painful knee OA respond significantly in the short term to IASI and one in four have persisting benefit beyond 6 months. Those with more severe knee joint damage are less likely to respond to knee IASI in the longer term. In contrast, the presence of synovitis/effusion does not appear to predict successful response to steroid injection therapy.

Abbreviations

AP: Antero-posterior; BML: Bone marrow lesion; CE: Contrast-enhanced; GP: General Practitioner; IASI: Intra-articular steroid injection; ICC: Intra-class correlation coefficient; IQR: Interquartile range; JSN: Joint space narrowing; KL: Kellgren-Lawrence; KOOS: Knee injury and osteoarthritis outcome score; MRI: Magnetic resonance imaging; MSK: musculoskeletal; OA: Osteoarthritis; OARSI: Osteoarthritis Research Society International; OMERACT: Outcome Measures in Rheumatology; OR: Odds ratio; PF: Patellofemoral; STV: Synovial tissue volume; TF: Tibiofemoral; VAS: Visual analogue scale; VAS_{NA}: Visual analogue scale for pain during nominated activity; WORMS: Whole organ magnetic resonance imaging score

Acknowledgements

We appreciate the expert assistance of Laura Heathers, Laura Forsythe and the assistance of the rest of the Research in Osteoarthritis Manchester (ROAM) team. The authors are thankful for the generous contributions of time and energy of study subjects. The authors would like to acknowledge the equipment and facilities provided by the Salford Royal NHS Foundation Trust.

Funding

This research was funded by Arthritis Research UK grant 18676. The funding agency had no role in any of the following: design and conduct of the study; collection, management, analysis, and interpretation of the data; and preparation, review, or approval of the manuscript; and decision to submit the manuscript for publication. This report includes independent research supported by the National Institute for Health Research Biomedical Research Unit Funding Scheme. The views expressed in this publication are those of the author (s) and not necessarily those of the NHS, the National Institute for Health Research or the Department of Health. The ROAM group is supported by the Manchester Academic Health Sciences Centre (MAHSC). Prof. Felson is supported by NIH AR4778. Nasimah Maricar is supported by an NIHR Allied Health Professional Clinical Doctoral Fellowship. The authors would like to acknowledge the equipment and facilities provided by Salford Royal NHS Foundation Trust.

Authors' contributions

NM was involved in the acquisition, analysis and interpretation of data, and also drafting and revising the manuscript. MJP performed the statistical analysis and helped revise the manuscript. MJC contributed to the analysis and interpretation of data and helped revise the manuscript. CEH designed the imaging protocol, was involved in acquisition and interpretation of imaging data and helped to revise the manuscript. ADG contributed to the analysis and interpretation of the MRI data and helped revise the manuscript. RH was involved in the analysis and interpretation of the radiographic data, and helped revise the manuscript. DTF was involved in the study conception and design, analysis and interpretation of data and helped to draft the manuscript. TWON contributed to the study design, data analysis and interpretation and drafting of the manuscript. The corresponding author (TWON) had full access to all the data in the study and takes responsibility for the integrity of the data and the accuracy of the data analysis. All authors read and approved the final manuscript.

Competing interests

DTF reported that he serves as a consultant for Zimmer, Knee Creations. None of the other authors report any competing interests in the manuscript.

Author details

[1]Arthritis Research UK Centre for Epidemiology, Division of Musculoskeletal and Dermatological Sciences, Faculty of Biology, Medicine and Health, Manchester Academic Health Science Centre, University of Manchester, Manchester, UK. [2]NIHR Manchester Musculoskeletal Biomedical Research Unit, Central Manchester University Hospitals NHS Foundation Trust, Manchester Academic Health Sciences Centre, Manchester, UK. [3]Department of Physiotherapy, Salford Royal Hospital NHS Foundation Trust, Manchester, UK. [4]Department of Health Professions, Manchester Metropolitan University, Manchester, UK. [5]Imaging Sciences, University of Warwick, Warwick Medical School, Coventry, UK. [6]Centre for Imaging Sciences, Institute of Population Health, The University of Manchester, Manchester, UK. [7]Clinical Epidemiology Unit, Boston University School of Medicine, Boston, MA, USA. [8]Department of Rheumatology, Salford Royal Hospital NHS Foundation Trust, Manchester, UK.

References

1. Bellamy N, Campbell J, Welch V, Gee TL, Bourne R, Wells GA. Intraarticular corticosteroid for treatment of osteoarthritis of the knee. Cochrane Database of Syst Rev. 2006(2):CD005328. doi:10.1002/14651858.CD005328.pub2.
2. Dhawan A, Mather III RC, Karas V, et al. An epidemiologic analysis of clinical practice guidelines for non-arthroplasty treatment of osteoarthritis of the knee. Arthroscopy. 2014;30:65–71.
3. McAlindon TE, Bannuru RR, Sullivan MC, et al. OARSI guidelines for the non-surgical management of knee osteoarthritis. Osteoarthr Cartil. 2014;22:363–88.
4. Arroll B, Goodyear-Smith F. Corticosteroid injections for osteoarthritis of the knee: meta-analysis. BMJ. 2004;328:869–73.
5. Bjordal JM, Klovning A, Ljunggren AE, Slordal L. Short term efficacy of pharmacotherapeutic interventions in osteoarthritic knee pain: a meta-analysis of randomised placebo-controlled trials. Eur J Pain. 2007;11:125–38.
6. Chao J, Wu C, Sun B, et al. Inflammatory characteristics on ultrasound predict poorer longterm response to intraarticular corticosteroid injections in knee osteoarthritis. J Rheumatol. 2010;37:650–5.
7. Smith MD, Wetherall M, Darby T, et al. A randomized placebo-controlled trial of arthroscopic lavage versus lavage plus intra-articular corticosteroids in the management of symptomatic osteoarthritis of the knee. Rheumatology (Oxford). 2003;42:1477–85.
8. Maricar N, Callaghan MJ, Felson DT, O'Neill TW. Predictors of response to intra-articular steroid injections in knee osteoarthritis - a systematic review. Rheumatology (Oxford). 2013;52:1022–32.
9. Gaffney K, Ledingham J, Perry JD. Intra-articular triamcinolone hexacetonide in knee osteoarthritis: factors influencing the clinical response. Ann Rheum Dis. 1995;54:379–81.
10. Jones A, Doherty M. Intra-articular corticosteroids are effective in osteoarthritis but there are no clinical predictors of response. Ann Rheum Dis. 1996;55:829–32.
11. Pendleton A, Millar A, O'Kane D, Wright GD, Taggart AJ. Can sonography be used to predict the response to intra-articular corticosteroid injection in primary osteoarthritis of the knee? Scand J Rheumatol. 2008;37:395–7.
12. Shah KD, Wright V. Intra-articular hydrocortisone in osteo-arthrosis. Ann Rheum Dis. 1967;26:316–8.
13. Dieppe PA, Sathapatayavongs B, Jones HE, Bacon PA, Ring EF. Intra-articular steroids in osteoarthritis. Rheumatol Rehab. 1980;19:212–7.
14. Pyne D, Ioannou Y, Mootoo R, Bhanji A. Intra-articular steroids in knee osteoarthritis: a comparative study of triamcinolone hexacetonide and methylprednisolone acetate. Clin Rheumatol. 2004;23:116–20.
15. Arden NK, Reading IC, Jordan KM, et al. A randomised controlled trial of tidal irrigation vs corticosteroid injection in knee osteoarthritis: the KIVIS Study. Osteoarthr Cartil. 2008;16:733–9.
16. O'Neill TW, Parkes MJ, Maricar N, et al. Synovial tissue volume: a treatment target in knee osteoarthritis (OA). Ann Rheum Dis. 2015;75(1):84–90.
17. Roos EM, Roos HP, Lohmander LS, Ekdahl C, Beynnon BD. Knee Injury and Osteoarthritis Outcome Score (KOOS)–development of a self-administered outcome measure. J Orthop Sports Phys Ther. 1998;28:88–96.

18. Pham T, van der Heijde D, Altman RD, et al. OMERACT-OARSI initiative: Osteoarthritis Research Society International set of responder criteria for osteoarthritis clinical trials revisited. Osteoarthr Cartil. 2004;12:389–99.
19. Roemer FW, Kassim JM, Guermazi A, et al. Anatomical distribution of synovitis in knee osteoarthritis and its association with joint effusion assessed on non-enhanced and contrast-enhanced MRI. Osteoarthr Cartil. 2010;18:1269–74.
20. Peterfy CG, Guermazi A, Zaim S, et al. Whole-Organ Magnetic Resonance Imaging Score (WORMS) of the knee in osteoarthritis. Osteoarthr Cartil. 2004;12:177–90.
21. Schiphof D, Boers M, Bierma-Zeinstra SMA. Differences in descriptions of Kellgren and Lawrence grades of knee osteoarthritis. Ann Rheum Dis. 2008;67:1034–6.
22. Altman RD, Gold GE. Atlas of individual radiographic features in osteoarthritis, revised. Osteoarthr Cartil. 2007;15(Suppl A):A1–56.
23. Issa SN, Dunlop D, Chang A, et al. Full-limb and knee radiography assessments of varus-valgus alignment and their relationship to osteoarthritis disease features by magnetic resonance imaging. Arthritis Rheum. 2007; 57:398–406.
24. Cotofana S, Buck R, Wirth W, et al. Cartilage thickening in early radiographic knee osteoarthritis: a within-person, between-knee comparison. Arthritis Rheum. 2012;64:1681–90.
25. Felson DT, McLaughlin S, Goggins J, et al. Bone marrow edema and its relation to progression of knee osteoarthritis. Ann Intern Med. 2003;139:330–6.
26. Hunter DJ, Zhang Y, Niu J, et al. Increase in bone marrow lesions associated with cartilage loss: a longitudinal magnetic resonance imaging study of knee osteoarthritis. Arthritis Rheum. 2006;54:1529–35.
27. Roemer FW, Guermazi A, Javaid MK, et al. Change in MRI-detected subchondral bone marrow lesions is associated with cartilage loss: the MOST Study. A longitudinal multicentre study of knee osteoarthritis. Ann Rheum Dis. 2009;68:1461–5.
28. Oak SR, Ghodadra A, Winalski CS, Miniaci A, Jones MH. Radiographic joint space width is correlated with 4-year clinical outcomes in patients with knee osteoarthritis: data from the osteoarthritis initiative. Osteoarthr Cartil. 2013;21:1185–90.
29. Johnson SR, Archibald A, Davis AM, Badley E, Wright JG, Hawker GA. Is self-reported improvement in osteoarthritis pain and disability reflected in objective measures? J Rheumatol. 2007;34:159–64.
30. Thomas E, Peat G, Mallen C, et al. Predicting the course of functional limitation among older adults with knee pain: do local signs, symptoms and radiographs add anything to general indicators? Ann Rheum Dis. 2008;67:1390–8.
31. Felson DT, Nevitt MC, Yang M, et al. A new approach yields high rates of radiographic progression in knee osteoarthritis. J Rheumatol. 2008;35:2047–54.

14

Protein oxidation, nitration and glycation biomarkers for early-stage diagnosis of osteoarthritis of the knee and typing and progression of arthritic disease

Usman Ahmed[1], Attia Anwar[1], Richard S. Savage[2], Paul J. Thornalley[1,2] and Naila Rabbani[1,2*]

Abstract

Background: There is currently no blood-based test for detection of early-stage osteoarthritis (OA) and the anti-cyclic citrullinated peptide (CCP) antibody test for rheumatoid arthritis (RA) has relatively low sensitivity for early-stage disease. Morbidity in arthritis could be markedly decreased if early-stage arthritis could be routinely detected and classified by clinical chemistry test. We hypothesised that damage to proteins of the joint by oxidation, nitration and glycation, and with signatures released in plasma as oxidized, nitrated and glycated amino acids may facilitate early-stage diagnosis and typing of arthritis.

Methods: Patients with knee joint early-stage and advanced OA and RA or other inflammatory joint disease (non-RA) and healthy subjects with good skeletal health were recruited for the study (n = 225). Plasma/serum and synovial fluid was analysed for oxidized, nitrated and glycated proteins and amino acids by quantitative liquid chromatography-tandem mass spectrometry. Data-driven machine learning methods were employed to explore diagnostic utility of the measurements for detection and classifying early-stage OA and RA, non-RA and good skeletal health with training set and independent test set cohorts.

Results: Glycated, oxidized and nitrated proteins and amino acids were detected in synovial fluid and plasma of arthritic patients with characteristic patterns found in early and advanced OA and RA, and non-RA, with respect to healthy controls. In early-stage disease, two algorithms for consecutive use in diagnosis were developed: (1) disease versus healthy control, and (2) classification as OA, RA and non-RA. The algorithms featured 10 damaged amino acids in plasma, hydroxyproline and anti-CCP antibody status. Sensitivities/specificities were: (1) good skeletal health, 0.92/0.91; (2) early-stage OA, 0.92/0.90; early-stage RA, 0.80/0.78; and non-RA, 0.70/0.65 (training set). These were confirmed in independent test set validation. Damaged amino acids increased further in severe and advanced OA and RA.

Conclusions: Oxidized, nitrated and glycated amino acids combined with hydroxyproline and anti-CCP antibody status provided a plasma-based biochemical test of relatively high sensitivity and specificity for early-stage diagnosis and typing of arthritic disease.

Keywords: Osteoarthritis, Rheumatoid arthritis, Machine learning, Oxidative stress, 3-nitrotyrosine, Glycation

* Correspondence: n.rabbani@warwick.ac.uk
[1]Warwick Medical School, Clinical Sciences Research Laboratories, University of Warwick, University Hospital, Coventry CV2 2DX, UK
[2]Warwick Systems Biology Centre, Senate House, University of Warwick, Coventry CV4 7AL, UK

Background

Oxidation, nitration and glycation of proteins are non-enzymatic processes in tissues and body fluids that produce some of the most quantitatively and functionally important spontaneous post-translational modifications of proteins in clinical disease. Reaction of reactive oxygen species (ROS) with proteins produces a characteristic profile of oxidative damage: trace level oxidized amino acid residues in proteins such as methionine sulfoxide (MetSO), dityrosine (DT), N-formylkynurenine (NFK) and others. Reaction of proteins with reactive nitrogen species (RNS) such as peroxynitrite characteristically forms 3-nitrotyrosine (3-NT). Protein glycation occurs at N-terminal and lysine residue sidechain amino groups to form N_ε-(1-deoxyfructosyl)lysine (FL) and other fructosamine derivatives, which degrade slowly to form end-stage stable adducts collectively called advanced glycation endproducts (AGEs). Reactive dicarbonyl metabolites such as glyoxal, methylglyoxal (MG) and 3-deoxyglucosone (3-DG) are also important physiological glycating agents and react mainly with arginine residues of proteins to form AGEs. Clinical measurement of protein oxidation, nitration and glycation adducts was recently reviewed [1] (see Additional file 1: Figure S1).

One of the first examples of involvement of oxidative damage in clinical disease was modification of cartilage and other proteins of the joint during development of rheumatoid arthritis (RA) [2, 3]. Increased oxidative damage and nitration to proteins in RA likely arises as a consequence of increased ROS and RNS formed in the respiratory burst of neutrophils and macrophages migrating into the arthritic joint [4]. Osteoarthritis (OA) is also driven by inflammation, at least in the early stages, and may involve increased ROS and RNS exposure [5]. Increased ROS also originates from mitochondrial dysfunction of chondrocytes and other cells implicated in both RA and OA development [6, 7]. Protein glycation has also been implicated in the development of arthritis, which may arise through oxidative stress-driven glycation or "glycoxidation" in RA [8, 9] and through age-related accumulation of AGEs in cartilage, facilitating development of OA [10]. Oxidative damage, nitration and glycation of cartilage is associated with misfolding and aggregation of the proteoglycan–collagen network surrounding chondrocytes and matrix degradation. These damaging modifications are thought to compromise structural integrity and viscoelasticity of cartilage, impairing its ability to sustain mechanical pressures and joint function [11].

In principle, measurement of protein oxidation, nitration and glycation adducts could provide multiple mechanistic biomarkers of arthritic disease to aid in clinical-chemistry-based diagnosis and progression of disease. This is particularly important for detection of early-stage disease. In the detection of early-stage RA (eRA), use of disease-modifying anti-rheumatic drugs (DMARDs) has produced the prospect of a therapeutic cure for RA [12]. Severe life impairment by development of OA may likely be prevented if arthritic disease is identified and treated in the early stages [13].

Currently, magnetic resonance imaging techniques have been developed for evaluation of cartilage damage in early-stage OA (eOA). These imaging techniques have approximately 70 % sensitivity and 90 % specificity compared to reference diagnosis by arthroscopy. They require expensive instrumentation, time and facilities [14]. They cannot be used in patients with implanted pacemakers or aneurysm coils.

Detection of RA by clinical chemistry assessments has been improved by introduction of the anti-cyclic citrullinated peptide (CCP) antibody test, which has 68 % sensitivity and 98 % specificity in established disease [15]. The presumed antigen is citrullinated protein (CP), which we recently identified as increased in both eRA and eOA, with only dominant immunogenicity in the former [16]. The anti-CCP antibody test is now considered state-of-the-art in RA diagnosis. It has relatively low sensitivity for eRA of 61 % and hence, improvement is desirable [15].

In searching for biomarkers for clinical diagnosis, analysis of proteins is often considered and preferred over analysis of amino acids, because proteins are typically longer-lived than amino acids and may be linked functionally to the mechanism of the target disease. Restricted access to samples of affected tissues often precludes measurement of target tissue-based proteins. Proteins damaged by oxidation, nitration and glycation undergo proteolysis to release oxidized, nitrated and glycated amino acids - also called oxidation, nitration and glycation free adducts [1]. Increase in such trace-level damaged amino acids in synovial fluid equilibrates rapidly with plasma. Amino acids may be detected with high analytical specificity and sensitivity and robustly quantified by stable isotopic dilution analysis liquid chromatography-tandem mass spectrometry (LC-MS/MS) [17]. Plasma levels of oxidized, nitrated and glycated amino acids may thereby provide signatures of protein damage, dysfunction and disease progression in the joint in early and advanced stage arthritis. In combination with the biomarker of bone turnover and resorption - hydroxyproline (Hyp) - and anti-CCP antibody status, the signature may be made specific for arthritic disease [15, 16, 18].

In this study we explored changes in the level of oxidized, nitrated and glycated proteins and related trace-level oxidized, nitrated and glycated amino acids in plasma and synovial fluid from subjects with early-stage and advanced or severe OA and RA or non-RA and healthy controls with good skeletal health.

Methods

Patients, healthy subjects and sampling

Patient recruitment, characteristics and sampling was as previously described [16]. The recruited study groups are illustrated in Fig. 1a and b. Briefly, patients with eOA (n = 46), eRA (n = 45) and inflammatory arthritis other than RA (non-RA (n = 42)), and patients with longstanding severe, advanced OA, aOA (n = 17), and advanced RA, aRA (n = 22), were recruited at multiple sites: Orthopaedic Clinics, University Hospital Coventry & Warwickshire (UHCW), Coventry, UK; Department of Rheumatology, Ipswich Hospital NHS Trust, UK; Department of Rheumatology, Royal Devon and Exeter NHS Foundation Trust, Exeter, UK; and Rapid Access Rheumatology Clinic, City Hospital, Birmingham, UK.

Criteria for eOA were: subjects presenting with new-onset knee pain, normal radiographs of the symptomatic knee and routine exploratory arthroscopy with macroscopic findings classified as grade I/II on the Outerbridge scale; recruited at UHCW, Coventry, UK. Patients with eRA and non-RA were recruited within 5 months of the onset of symptoms of inflammatory arthritis at the Rapid Access Rheumatology Clinic, City Hospital, Birmingham, UK. Synovial fluid and peripheral venous blood samples were collected on initial presentation and diagnostic outcomes were determined at follow up. A diagnosis of early rheumatoid arthritis (eRA) was made

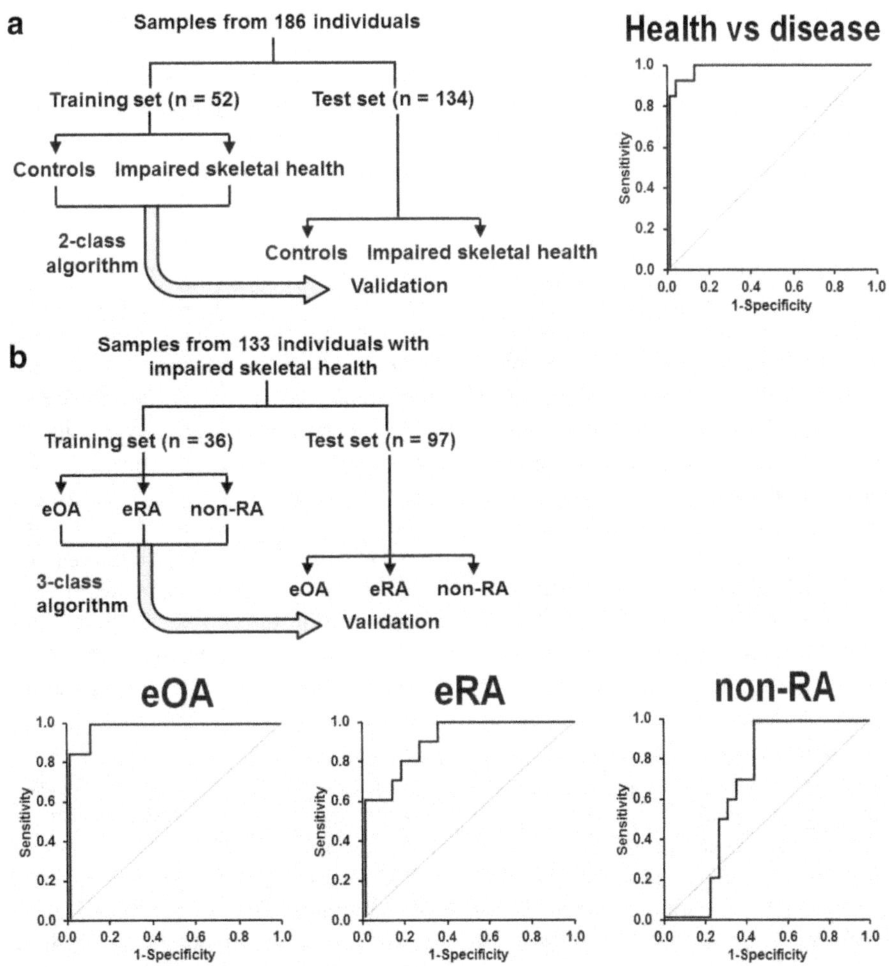

Fig. 1 Training and validation of two-stage diagnostic algorithms for detection of impaired skeletal health and discrimination of early-stage osteoarthritis (*eOA*), rheumatoid arthritis (*RA*) and other inflammatory joint disease. **a** Training set and test set study groups for detection of impaired skeletal health. A receiver operating characteristic (ROC) curve is given for the training set. The area under the ROC curve (AUROC) was 0.99 (95 % confidence interval 0.97–1.00). Comparators were eOA + early RA (*eRA*) + non-RA versus healthy controls. A random outcome is 0.50. **b** Training set and test set study groups for discrimination of eOA, eRA and non-RA. ROC curves are given for the training set with AUROC and confidence intervals: eOA, 0.98 (0.96–1.00); eRA, 0.91 (0.81–1.00); and non-RA, 0.68 (0.50–0.86). Comparators were eOA, eRA or non-RA versus other early-stage arthritic diseases combined. A random outcome is 0.33

according to the 1987 American Rheumatoid Association criteria [19]. A diagnosis of non-RA was made where alternative rheumatological diagnoses explained the inflammatory arthritis, as described [20]. For example, training-set non-RA subjects had reactive arthritis (n = 6), pseudogout (n = 1), and unclassified (n = 3). Criteria for aOA were: longstanding or established severe symptoms of OA (≥2 years duration of disease) with corresponding radiographic changes (Kellgren-Lawrence grade IV changes on radiographs) and undergoing therapeutic knee aspiration and corticosteroid instillation or total knee replacement; and recruited at UHCW, Coventry, UK and Ipswich Hospital NHS Trust, Ipswich, UK. Criteria for aRA were: joint stiffness in the mornings of at least one hour duration; symmetrical swelling in three or more joints; radiographic evidence of bone erosions; rheumatoid nodules with increased serum rheumatoid factor (RF); and symptoms of ≥2 years duration [19]. Patients with aRA were recruited at Ipswich Hospital NHS Trust, UK and Royal Devon and Exeter NHS Foundation Trust, Exeter, UK. Criteria for these clinical classifications are similar to those suggested in consensus position and best practice statements [21, 22].

Healthy controls were recruited at participating clinical centres (n = 53). For healthy control subjects the inclusion criteria were no history of joint symptoms, arthritic disease or other morbidity. Exclusion criteria were: history of injury or pain in either knee; taking medication excepting oral contraceptives and vitamins; and any abnormality identified on physical examination of the knee. Control subjects and patients with early-stage disease were recruited as two independent cohorts for a training set and independent test set for data analysis in machine learning methods as explained subsequently.

Peripheral venous blood samples from healthy subjects and patients with eOA were collected after overnight fasting with EDTA anti-coagulant. Synovial fluid from the eOA study group was collected concurrently. Venous blood and synovial fluid samples for eRA, non-RA, aOA and aRA study groups were collected in the non-fasted state. For analytes studied herein, diurnal variation in serum Hyp from healthy subjects was 20 % and for other amino acids up to 13–25 %, depending on the analyte [23, 24]. Diurnal variation in plasma protein glycation and oxidative stress in healthy subjects was <15 %, as judged by plasma fructosamine and plasma cysteine, respectively [25, 26]. Synovial fluid was collected from patients with aOA and aRA and eOA, eRA and with non-RA recruited for the training set cohort. Synovial fluid was not collected from patients with eOA, eRA or non-RA in the test set cohort in which analytes were determined only in plasma/serum.

Blood and synovial fluid were centrifuged (2000 g, 10 minutes) and the plasma and synovial fluid supernatant were removed and stored at −80 °C until analysis. Samples were centrifuged within one hour of collection. A critical time-limiting feature for sample processing is the rate of sample oxidation, as judged by loss of reduced glutathione (GSH) and other thiols, which leads to subsequent increase in protein oxidation adducts (see subsequent text). This prompt sample processing maintains >70 % GSH and thereby avoids artefactual increase in protein oxidation adducts in sample collection [27, 28]. Repeated freeze thawing was avoided as this increases estimates of the protein oxidation adduct, methionine sulfoxide [29].

Serum was available for the eRA and non-RA study groups and plasma was available for all others. Serum is comparable to plasma as a sample matrix where the major protein lost during clotting (fibrinogen) does not affect median glycation, oxidation and nitration adduct residue content normalised to amino-acid-modified and related free adduct and Hyp concentrations [1, 16].

Analysis of oxidized, nitrated and glycated protein and oxidation, nitration and glycation free adducts in plasma/serum and synovial fluid

The contents of oxidation, nitration and glycation adduct residues in plasma/serum and synovial proteins were quantified in exhaustive enzymatic digests by stable isotopic dilution analysis LC-MS/MS, with correction for autohydrolysis of hydrolytic enzymes as described [17]. Oxidation, nitration and glycation free adducts were determined in the ultrafiltrates of the same samples. Ultrafiltrate of plasma/serum or synovial fluid (100 μl) was collected by microspin ultrafiltration (10 kDa cutoff) at 4 °C. Retained protein was diluted with water to 500 μl and washed by four cycles of concentration to 50 μl and dilution to 500 μl with water over the microspin ultrafilter at 4 °C. The final washed protein (100 μl) was delipidated and hydrolysed enzymatically as described [16, 17].

Protein hydrolysate (25 μl, 32 μg protein equivalent) or ultrafiltrate was mixed with stable isotopic standard analytes (for amounts see Additional file 1: Table S1) and analysed by LC-MS/MS using an Acquity™ UPLC system with a Quattro Premier tandem mass spectrometer (Waters, Manchester, U.K.) [17]. Samples are maintained at 4 °C in the autosampler during batch analysis. The columns were: 2.1 × 50 mm and 2.1 mm × 250 mm, 5 μm particle size Hypercarb™ (Thermo Scientific), in series with programmed switching, at 30 °C. Chromatographic retention is necessary to resolve oxidized analytes from their amino acid precursors to avoid interference from partial oxidation of the latter in the electrospray ionization source of the mass spectrometric detector. Analytes were detected by electrospray positive ionization and mass spectrometry multiple reaction monitoring (MRM) mode where analyte detection response is specific for mass/charge ratio of the analyte molecular ion and major fragment ion generated by collision-induced dissociation in the mass spectrometer collision cell. The ionization source and desolvation gas temperatures were 120 °C and 350 °C, respectively, cone gas and desolvation gas flow rates were 99 and 900 l/h and the capillary voltage was 0.60 kV. Argon gas (5.0×10^{-3} mbar) was in the collision cell.

For MRM detection, molecular ion and fragment ion masses and collision energies optimized to ± 0.1 Da and ± 1 eV, respectively, were programmed (Additional file 1: Table S1). Analytes determined were: oxidation adducts - MetSO, DT and NFK; nitration adduct –3-NT; and glycation adducts - FL, and advanced glycation endproducts (AGEs), N_ε-carboxymethyl-lysine (CML), N_ε-(1-carboxyethyl)lysine (CEL), N_ω-carboxymethylarginine (CMA), hydroimidazolones derived from glyoxal, methylglyoxal and 3-deoxyglucosone (G-H1, MG-H1 and 3DG-H), respectively), pentosidine and methylglyoxal-derived lysine dimer (MOLD); and others - Hyp and amino acids - arg, lys, tyr, trp, met and val (Additional file 1: Figure S1). Valine is determined in protein hydrolysates for the protease autohydrolysis correction [17]. Oxidation, nitration and glycation adduct residues are normalised to their amino acid residue precursors and given as mmol/mol amino acid modified; and related free adducts are given in nM. Chemical structures and biochemical and clinical significance of these analytes have been described elsewhere [1, 16].

Other assessments

Anti-CCP antibody positivity was assessed by automated enzymatic immunoassay (EliA CCP; Phadia, Uppsala, Sweden).

Machine learning analysis

The objective was to distinguish between the following four groups: healthy control, eOA, eRA and non-RA. In all cases, the diagnostic algorithms were trained on the training data set, before being used to predict the disease class for each sample in the test data set (Fig. 1a and b). A two-stage approach was taken: (1) to distinguish between disease and healthy control; and (2) to distinguish between eOA, eRA and non-RA. The outcome was to assign, for each test set sample, a set of probabilities corresponding to each of the disease/control groups - the group assignment being that for which the probability is highest. Test data were held separate from algorithm training; algorithm settings were not adjusted once we began to analyse the test set data, thereby guarding against overfitting and hence providing a rigorous estimate of predictive performance. We also performed fivefold cross-validation separately on each of the training, test data sets, to assess predictive performance internally for each data set. Four algorithm types were tested for performance using random forests, multi-class logistic regression, multi-class sparse logistic regression, and support vector machines [30–32]. In the training set cross-validations, we use a panel of 15 plasma biomarkers: RF, anti-CCP antibody positivity, Hyp and MetSO, DT, NFK, 3-NT, FL, CML, CEL, CMA, G-H1, MG-H1, 3DG-H and pentosidine free adducts. Methylglyoxal-derived lysine dimer (MOLD) was omitted as levels were close to the limit of detection.

We used the area under the curve of the receiver operating characteristic (ROC) plot (AUROC) statistic as our measure of performance [33], with the 95 % CI determined via bootstrap analysis using the R package pROC [34]. In the training-set test set cross-validation we used the minimum set of features giving the maximum AUROC. This minimum feature set was used in the test set validation. We produced sensitivity/specificity values from the ROC curves using an automated procedure that finds where the sensitivity/specificity values are most similar. Where we consider three classes, we consider a set of one-versus-all ROC curves (one per class). Fivefold cross-validation was carried out on the training set data to give an initial estimate of predictive performance, and to identify the best-performing machine learning method. We then trained the algorithm on the entire training set, before making predictions for the test data set. We also performed fivefold cross-validation on the test set data. Data were analysed using R version 3.1.3.

Statistical analyses

Non-normally distributed variables are summarized as median (lower to upper quartile), two groups were compared using the Mann–Whitney *U* test and four groups were compared using the Kruskal-Wallis test for independent samples and Wilcoxon's signed ranks test for two-group, paired samples (plasma and synovial fluid from the same donor). Correlation analysis was performed using the Spearman method. Data were analysed using SPSS, version 22.0. A Bonferroni correction of 13 was applied for testing of multiple protein oxidation, nitration and glycation adduct levels, assuming a null hypothesis that any of the 13 adducts measured may have levels that are significantly changed in the arthritic disease study groups. Data were considered significantly different when the *P* value was $<0.05/13$ or <0.0038. This report adheres to the guidelines for transparent reporting of a multivariable prediction model for individual prognosis or diagnosis (TRIPOD statement) [35].

Results

Summary description of protein oxidation, nitration and glycation adduct changes in the plasma and synovial fluid and inter-compartment correlations in patients with early and advanced arthritis

Changes in protein oxidation, nitration and glycation status in plasma and synovial fluid in patients with eOA, aOA, eRA, aRA and non-RA with respect to plasma levels in healthy controls are summarised in a heat map (Fig. 2). Data and detailed descriptions of the changes are given in Additional file 1: Supplementary information and Tables S2–S7, including a description of the effects of drug therapy in aRA. The heat map indicates there were changes in protein oxidation, nitration and glycation adduct levels in both adduct contents of protein and free adduct concentrations in plasma and synovial fluid. The different patterns of adduct levels provides the basis to detect and distinguish the presence and type of arthritis at the early stage of clinical development, and in advanced-stage disease.

In plasma for healthy controls and early-stage disease (eOA, eRA and non-RA), there were changes in oxidation, nitration and glycation adduct contents of protein (MetSO, DT, 3-NT, FL, MG-H1, CMA and pentosidine) and oxidation and glycation free adduct concentrations (MetSO, NFK, DT, CMA and MOLD; $P < 0.05$, Kruskal-Wallis), indicating disrupted proteostasis in protein glycation, oxidation and nitration in the plasma compartment and tissue release into plasma of free adducts from proteolysis of oxidized and glycated proteins. Similar analysis for early-stage and advanced disease of the same type showed the following changes in plasma: for aOA versus eOA, increased NFK, DT, 3-NT, CML and 3DG-H adducts of protein and increased MetSO, NFK, DT, 3-NT, CEL and CMA free adducts; and for aRA versus eRA, increased DT, 3-NT, FL, CML, G-H1, MG-H1 and CMA adducts of protein and increased MetSO, DT and pentosidine free adducts.

To assess if changes of analyte in the synovial fluid are reflected by similar increases in plasma we computed inter-compartment homotypic correlation (correlation between levels of a marker in plasma and synovial fluid from the same subject) (Table 1). For eOA and eRA combined, in early-stage disease there were 10 homotypic correlations between synovial fluid and plasma for oxidized, nitrated and glycated amino acids and only 5 homotypic correlations for oxidation nitration and glycation adducts of protein. For aOA and aRA combined, in advanced disease there were 9 homotypic correlations between synovial fluid and plasma for oxidized, nitrated and glycated amino acids and 13 homotypic correlations for oxidation nitration and glycation adducts of protein: in non-RA there were 3 homotypic correlations for amino acids (3 glycated amino acids) and one homotypic correlation for protein (glycated protein). This suggests that oxidized, nitrated and glycated amino acids equilibrate readily between synovial fluid and plasma compartments in early-stage arthritis and both oxidized, nitrated and glycated amino acids and proteins equilibrate between synovial fluid and plasma compartments in advanced-stage arthritis.

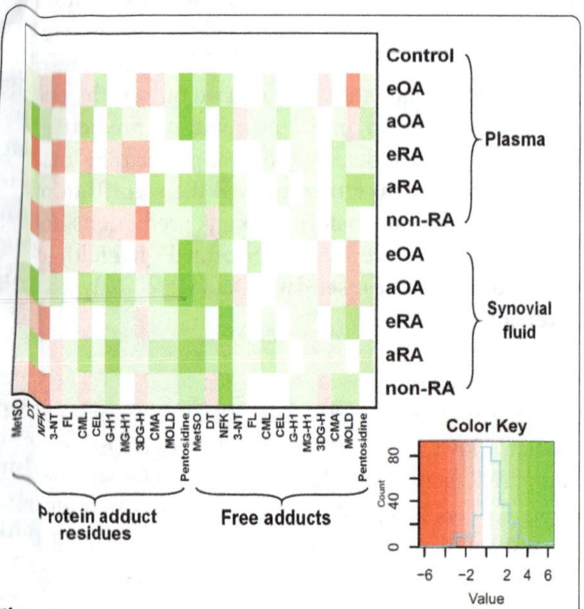

Fig. 2 Heat map of changes in glycated, oxidized and nitrated proteins and amino acids in plasma and synovial fluid from patients with early and advanced arthritis. Data are given in Additional file 1: Tables S2–S7. Heat map values are on a $\log_2$ scale, normalised to levels in plasma from healthy control subjects, with the key and frequency of changes (*light blue line*) given (*inset*). *eOA* early osteoarthritis, *aOA* advanced osteoarthritis, *eRA* early rheumatoid arthritis, *aRA* advanced rheumatoid arthritis *CML* N_ε-carboxymethyl-lysine, *CEL* N_ε-(1- carboxyethyl) -lysine, *MetSO* methionine sulfoxide, *DT* dityrosine, *FL* N_ε-fructosyl-lysine, *MG-H1* methylglyoxal-derived hydroimidazolone, *3DG-H* 3-deoxyglucosone-derived hydroimidazolone isomers, *NFK* N-formylkynurenine, *3-NT* 3-nitrotyrosine, *G-H1* glyoxal-derived hydroimidazolone, *CMA* N_ω-carboxymethylarginine, *MOLD* methylglyoxal-derived lysine dimer

Machine learning analysis

To explore the diagnostic utility of protein damage measurements we analysed plasma amino acid analyte data by a machine learning approach. Random forests was the best-performing method. Application of two algorithms consecutively gave the best diagnostic outcome. First, with algorithm 1 we discriminated between healthy control and early-stage arthritis. Second, with algorithm 2 we identified types of arthritis - eOA, eRA and non-RA. Algorithms were trained with a training set subject group and validated independently in a different test set subject group (Fig. 1). Training set data are in Additional file 1: Tables S3, S6 and S7 and test set data are in Additional file 1: Tables S8–S10. Algorithm features for maximum AUROC were:

Table 1 Homotypic correlation of protein oxidation, nitration and glycation adducts in synovial fluid and plasma compartments

Study group	Protein adduct residue	Free adduct
eOA	CML ($r = 0.60$, $P < 0.05$), CEL ($r = 0.82$, $P < 0.001$), MetSO ($r = 0.61$, $P < 0.05$), DT ($r = 0.53$, $P < 0.05$)	CEL ($r = 0.59$, $P < 0.05$), 3DG-H ($r = 0.62$, $P < 0.05$), pentosidine (r r = 0.71)
aOA	FL ($r = 0.58$, $P < 0.05$), MG-H1 ($r = 0.80$, $P < 0.001$) 3DG-H ($r = 0.72$, $P < 0.01$), MetSO ($r = 0.63$, $P < 0.05$)	FL ($r = 0.75$, $P < 0.01$), CEL ($r = 0.63$, $P < 0.05$), G-H1 ($r = 0.71$, $P < 0.01$), MG-H1 (r = 0.91, P < 0.001), NFK (r = 0.73, P < 0.05)
eRA	Pentosidine ($r = 0.82$, $P < 0.01$)	FL ($r = 0.87$, $P < 0.01$), CML ($r = 0.67$, $P < 0.05$), CEL ($r = 0.81$, $P < 0.01$), MG-H1 ($r = 0.92$, $P < 0.001$), 3DG-H ($r = 0.83$, $P < 0.01$), CMA (0.72, $P < 0.05$), pentosidine ($r = 0.78$, $P < 0.01$)
aRA	CML ($r = 0.56$, $P < 0.05$), CEL ($r = 0.70$, $P < 0.01$), G-H1 ($r = 0.52$, $P < 0.05$), MG-H1 ($r = 0.86$, $P < 0.001$), 3DG-H ($r = 0.86$, $P < 0.001$), CMA (0.50, $P < 0.05$), pentosidine ($r = 0.83$, $P < 0.01$), NFK ($r = 0.56$, $P < 0.05$), DT ($r = 0.64$, $P < 0.01$)	G-H1 ($r = 0.53$, $P < 0.05$), MG-H1 ($r = 0.87$, $P < 0.001$) 3DG-H ($r = 0.73$, $P < 0.01$), 3-NT (0.67, $P < 0.01$)
Non-RA	Pentosidine ($r = 0.76$, $P < 0.05$)	CEL ($r = 0.73$, $P < 0.05$), MG-H1 ($r = 0.76$, $P < 0.05$), MOLD ($r = 0.81$, $P < 0.01$)

eOA early osteoarthritis, *aOA* advanced osteoarthritis, *eRA* early rheumatoid arthritis, *aRA* advanced rheumatoid arthritis, *CML* N_ε-carboxymethyl-lysine, *CEL* N_ε-(1-carboxyethyl)-lysine, *MetSO* methionine sulfoxide, *DT* dityrosine, *FL* N_ε-fructosyl-lysine, *MG-H1* methylglyoxal-derived hydroimidazolone, *3DG-H* 3-deoxyglucosone-derived hydroimidazolone isomers, *NFK* N-formylkynurenine, *3-NT* 3-nitrotyrosine, *G-H1* glyoxal-derived hydroimidazolone, *CMA* N_ω-carboxymethylarginine

(1) Disease (eOA, eRA and non-RA) versus healthy control: Hyp, MetSO, DT, NFK, 3-NT, CEL, CMA, G-H1, MG-H1, 3DG-H and pentosidine free adducts. The AUROC value was 0.99, 0.96 and 0.77, for the training set and test set cross-validations and test set validation, respectively. A random outcome is 0.50. Related sensitivity/specificity was 0.92/0.91, 0.89/0.90 and 0.73/0.72, respectively (Fig. 1a, Table 2 (algorithm feature) and Table 3 (confusion matrices)).
(2) Typing of eOA, eRA and non-RA: anti-CCP antibody positivity, MetSO, DT, 3-NT, FL, CML, CEL, CMA, MG-H1, 3DG-H and pentosidine free adducts.

For eOA, eRA and non-RA, AUROC values were in the range 0.68–0.98, 0.77–0.93 and 0.62–0.91 for training set and test set cross-validations and test set validation, respectively. A random outcome is 0.33 (three disease classes). Omission of anti-CCP antibody positivity assessment decreased the AUROC by 0.0023. Related sensitivities/specificities for eOA, eRA and non-RA were: 0.92/0.90, 0.80/0.78 and 0.70/0.65; 0.83/0.84, 0.77/0.76 and 0.72/0.71; and 0.83/0.84, 0.60/0.61 and 0.81/0.80 (Fig. 1b and Table 2 (algorithm feature) and Table 3 (confusion matrices)).

Discussion

Increased protein oxidation, nitration and glycation of cartilage have long been implicated as damaging modifications in the joint, mediating development of arthritic disease [2, 3, 8]. There have been few studies on protein damage in early-stage disease. Experimental studies of gene deletion and pharmacological activation of nuclear factor erythroid 2-related factor 2 (Nrf2), a transcription factor that coordinates basal and inducible expression of enzymes protective against oxidative stress and dicarbonyl glycation [36, 37], supports a role of oxidative damage and dicarbonyl glycation in the development of OA and RA [38, 39]. Trace-level oxidation, nitration and glycation free adducts potentially indicate the presence of this in plasma.

Early-stage detection of arthritic disease and effective lifestyle and/or pharmaceutical interventions could markedly decrease morbidity in OA, achieve a cure for RA and improve outcomes for other arthritic disease [12, 13]. Development of drugs to suppress oxidative damage and glycation damage to collagen in arthritis will be facilitated by availability of companion diagnostic tests based on related biomarkers [40]. There is no established method to detect eOA. Radiography remains the method of choice for later staging of aOA but shows little or no change in eOA. The anti-CCP antibody test is now a clinical standard biochemical test for RA and diagnosis is often confirmed before damage to the joint occurs. Even for eRA, however, the anti-CPP antibody test has relatively low sensitivity [15]; indeed, we observed sensitivity of 56 % herein with patients recruited within 5 months of the onset of symptoms [16]. Hitherto, biomarkers of protein oxidation, nitration and glycation have not been developed for clinical diagnostic application in arthritis, excepting studies on plasma 3-NT [41]; the trace-level of these biomarkers leads to them often being overlooked in untargeted approaches to biomarkers in arthritis [42].

Herein we comprehensively and quantitatively measured protein glycation, oxidation and nitration adducts in plasma and synovial fluid in arthritis. Analysis for diagnostic application suggests a rapid plasma-based test derived for diagnosis of presence and typing of early-stage arthritis suitable for skeletal health screening based on plasma oxidized, nitrated and glycated amino acids in combination

Table 2 Predictive algorithm outcomes using the random forest algorithm diagnostic characteristics

	Algorithm 1	Algorithm 2		
Features	Hyp and MetSO, DT, NFK, 3-NT, CEL, CMA, G-H1, MG-H1, 3DG-H and pentosidine	anti-CCP antibody positivity and MetSO, DT, 3-NT, FL, CML, CEL, CMA, MG-H1, 3DG-H and pentosidine		
Comparators	Disease versus control	eOA	eRA	non-RA
Training set cross-validation				
Correct, *n*	44/46	13/13	6/8	8/12
Sensitivity	0.92 (0.64–1.00)	0.92 (0.64–1.00)	0.80 (0.44 - 0.97)	0.70 (0.35 - 0.93)
Specificity	0.91 (0.76–0.98)	0.90 (0.68–0.99)	0.78 (0.56–0.93)	0.65 (0.43–0.84)
AUROC	0.99 (0.97–1.00)	0.98 (0.96–1.00)	0.91 (0.82–1.00)	0.68 (0.49–0.86)
Positive predictive value	1.0	1.0	0.60	0.80
Negative predictive value	0.85	1.0	0.84	0.83
Positive likelihood ratio	10.2	9.2	3.6	2.0
Negative likelihood ratio	0.09	0.09	0.26	0.46
Test set cross-validation				
Correct, *n*	119/134	30/31	22/27	27/39
Sensitivity	0.89 (0.75–0.97)	0.83 (0.65–0.94)	0.77 (0.6–0.9)	0.72 (0.53–0.86)
Specificity	0.90 (0.82–0.95)	0.84 (0.73–0.92)	0.76 (0.63–0.86)	0.71 (0.58–0.81)
AUROC	0.96 (0.93–0.99)	0.93 (0.88–0.98)	0.87 (0.8–0.94)	0.77 (0.68–0.86)
Positive predictive value	0.96	0.97	0.81	0.69
Negative predictive value	0.75	1.0	0.81	0.91
Positive likelihood ratio	8.9	5.2	3.2	2.5
Negative likelihood ratio	0.12	0.20	0.30	0.39
Test set validation				
Correct, *n*	63/134	18/19	8/35	31/32
Sensitivity	0.73 (0.56–0.86)	0.83 (0.65–0.94)	0.60 (0.42–0.76)	0.81 (0.64–0.93)
Specificity	0.72 (0.62–0.81)	0.84 (0.73–0.92)	0.61 (0.46–0.72)	0.80 (0.68–0.89)
AUROC	0.77 (0.69–0.85)	0.91 (0.84–0.99)	0.62 (0.5–0.75)	0.84 (0.77–0.92)
Positive predictive value	0.62	0.60	0.23	0.97
Negative predictive value	0.05	0.99	0.97	0.43
Positive likelihood ratio	2.6	5.2	1.5	4.1
Negative likelihood ratio	0.38	0.20	0.67	0.24

The 95 % CI for sensitivity and specificity are given in brackets. *eOA* early osteoarthritis, *aOA* advanced osteoarthritis, *eRA* early rheumatoid arthritis, *aRA* advanced rheumatoid arthritis, *CML* N_ε-carboxymethyl-lysine, *CEL* N_ε-carboxyethyl-lysine, *MetSO* methionine sulfoxide, *DT* dityrosine, *FL* Nε-fructosyl-lysine, *MG-H1* methylglyoxal-derived hydroimidazolone, *3DG-H* 3-deoxyglucosone-derived hydroimidazolone isomers, *NFK* N-formylkynurenine, *3-NT* 3-nitrotyrosine, *G-H1* glyoxal-derived hydroimidazolone, *CMA*N_ω-carboxymethylarginine

with Hyp and the anti-CCP antibody test is available and suitable for further validation and development.

In developing an improved test for detection and typing of early-stage arthritis we focussed on the trace glycated, oxidized and nitrated amino acids in plasma as reporters of damaging modifications of proteins in joints. Plasma is readily accessed, ultrafiltrate easily prepared and analytes rapidly and robustly quantifiable by stable isotopic dilution analysis LC-MS/MS [1]. This technology is available in most clinical chemistry laboratories; it is the most stable mass spectrometry platform and relatively inexpensive to implement, with analyte interference-free multiplexing and low cost. A rapid escape rate of amino acids in synovial fluid to plasma [43, 44] suggested that plasma/serum is a suitable surrogate sample for synovial fluid. The findings of similar levels of analytes in synovial fluid and plasma in patients and positive correlation between plasma and synovial fluid levels of analytes for the different study groups support this.

Basing our diagnostic algorithm test on oxidized, nitrated and glycated amino acids rather than oxidized, nitrated and glycated proteins provided for simple and rapid pre-analytic processing; *cf.* 4 days for enzymatic hydrolysis of proteins [17]. Changes in normal, undamaged amino acids of plasma in advanced arthritis were studied previously but had limited diagnostic utility [45, 46]; the damaging

Table 3 Predictive algorithm outcomes using the random forest: confusion matrices

Algorithm 1			Algorithm 2			
Clinical class	Predicted class		Clinical class	Predicted class		
	Control	Disease		eOA	eRA	Non-RA
Training set cross-validation						
Control	11	2	eOA	13	0	0
Disease	0	33	eRA	0	6	4
			Non-RA	0	2	8
Test set cross-validation						
Control	33	4	eOA	30	0	0
Disease	11	86	eRA	1	22	12
			Non-RA	0	5	27
Test set validation						
Control	2	35	eOA	18	2	10
Disease	36	61	eRA	0	8	27
			Non-RA	1	0	31

eOA early osteoarthritis, *aOA* advanced osteoarthritis, *eRA* early rheumatoid arthritis, *aRA* advanced rheumatoid arthritis, *CML* N_ε-carboxymethyl-lysine, *CEL* N_ε-(1- carboxyethyl)-lysine, *MetSO* methionine sulfoxide, *DT* dityrosine, *FL* Nε-fructosyl-lysine, *MG-H1* methylglyoxal-derived hydroimidazolone, *3DG-H* 3-deoxyglucosone-derived hydroimidazolone isomers, *NFK* N-formylkynurenine, *3-NT* 3-nitrotyrosine, *G-H1* glyoxal-derived hydroimidazolone, *CMA* N_ω-carboxymethylarginine

modifications of oxidation, nitration and glycation provide a mechanistic link to arthritic disease and thereby diagnostic significance. Oxidized, nitrated and glycated amino acids are changed in other disease conditions [47–49]; combination of the responses with Hyp, however, make for specific detection of arthritic disease [16].

Surprisingly, there was evidence of decreased oxidation, nitration and glycation adducts in proteins of early-stage disease in eOA, eRA and non-RA. This may relate to increased capillary permeability and increased transcapillary escape rate (TER) of albumin in early-stage disease [50]. Albumin thereby has shorter residence time in plasma and longer residence time in interstitial fluid in the peripheral tissues at a lower concentration and likely in the presence of lower concentrations of oxidizing, nitrating and glycating agents. It will thereby have an overall decreased rate of oxidation, nitration and glycation. Increased capillary permeability has been observed in RA [51]. This effect is lost when marked increase in protein glycation, oxidation and nitration in the joints in advanced disease outweighs the effects of increased protein residence time at interstitial sites. Albumin TER has been described previously as a confounding factor in the diagnostic use of plasma protein glycation [52].

In the two-step algorithm-based diagnosis, feature selection by the data-driven machine learning process produced algorithms with multiple oxidation, nitration and glycation adducts, suggesting estimates of these adducts contribute to the diagnostic power to discriminate both disease versus control and also typing of early-stage disease. Hyp was important in discriminating disease versus control but not for typing of early-stage arthritis. This is likely because increased Hyp was common to all types of early-stage arthritis [16]. Similarly, anti-CCP antibody status was important in discriminating types of arthritis and hence was a feature only in the second algorithm. This analysis builds on the wealth of experience and diagnostic value of anti-CCP antibody positivity in the detection of RA [15].

AUROC values were very high (0.99 for skeletal health versus disease, and 0.98 for eOA), indicating a high probability of correctly identifying early-stage OA. Omission of the anti-CCP antibody positivity assessment gave only a minor improvement in AUROC for arthritis typing and so may be omitted with minor loss of performance. These were observed particularly for cross-validations in both training set and test set data and were lower in independent test set validation. Further validation is required in independent patient cohorts and study of the association of the diagnostic response to clinical symptoms and radiographic changes. There is also potential for monitoring of disease progression.

There have been no similar machine learning studies excepting our previous study with plasma Hyp and CP [16]. AUROC values herein were markedly improved for detection of healthy controls, eOA and non-RA, and slightly decreased for eRA (0.93 versus 0.98). Addition of plasma CP estimates from our previous study [16] in the algorithm optimisation herein did not improve diagnostic performance. Other studies have developed algorithms based on measurement of cytokines but for advanced OA and RA [53]. Clinical detection of early-stage arthritis herein is potentially advantageous. Other serum markers for eOA detection have been suggested - disintegrin and metalloproteinase with thrombospondin motifs (ADAMTS)-4, ADAMTS-5, matrix metalloproteinase (MMP)-1 and MMP-3 - but sensitivity and specificity was not reported [54]. The diagnostic performance of the two-step algorithm herein improves significantly on other current candidate biomarkers proposed for early-stage arthritis [16, 55, 56].

Conclusions

There were characteristic profiles of protein oxidation, nitration and glycation adducts in protein from synovial fluid and plasma, and related oxidized, nitrated and glycated amino acids, in good skeletal health and arthritis disease, with changes in the latter associated with classification and severity of disease. Combination of estimates of oxidized, nitrated and glycated amino acids with hydroxyproline and anti-CCP antibody status in plasma provided a biochemical test of relatively high sensitivity and specificity for early-stage diagnosis and typing of arthritic disease.

Abbreviations

3-DG: 3-deoxyglucosone; 3DG-H: 3-deoxyglucosone-derived hydroimidazolone isomers; 3-NT: 3-nitrotyrosine; ADAMTS: a disintegrin and metalloproteinase with thrombospondin motifs; AGE: advanced glycation endproduct; aOA: advanced osteoarthritis; aRA: advanced rheumatoid arthritis; AUROC: area under the curve of the receiver operating characteristic plot; CCP: cyclic citrullinated peptide; CEL: N_ε-(1-carboxyethyl)lysine; CMA: N_ω-carboxymethylarginine; CML: N_ε-carboxymethyl-lysine; CP: citrullinated proteins; DMARD: disease-modifying anti-rheumatic drug; DT: dityrosine; EDTA: ethylenediaminetetra-acetic acid; eOA: early-stage osteoarthritis; eRA: early-stage rheumatoid arthritis; FL: N_ε-fructosyl-lysine; G-H1: glyoxal-derived hydroimidazolone; Hyp: hydroxyproline; LC-MS/MS: liquid chromatography-tandem mass spectrometry; MetSO: methionine sulfoxide; MG: methylglyoxal; MG-H1: methylglyoxal-derived hydroimidazolone; MMP: matrix metalloproteinase; MOLD: methylglyoxal-derived lysine dimer; NFK: N-formylkynurenine; non-RA: inflammatory joint disease other than rheumatoid arthritis (often self-resolving); OA: osteoarthritis; RA: rheumatoid arthritis; RF: rheumatoid factor; RNS: reactive nitrogen species; ROC: receiver operating characteristic; ROS: reactive oxygen species; TER: transcapillary escape rate; TROPID: transparent reporting of a multivariable prediction model for individual prognosis or diagnosis; UPLC: ultra high performance liquid chromatography

Acknowledgements

We thank Matthew L. Costa (Warwick Medical School, Clinical Sciences Research Laboratories, University of Warwick, University Hospital, Coventry, UK), Andrew Filer and Karim Raza (Sandwell and West Birmingham Hospital NHS Trust, Dudley Road, Birmingham, West Midlands, UK), Richard A. Watts (Ipswich Hospital NHS Trust, Ipswich, Suffolk, UK), and Paul G. Winyard, Joanna Tarr and Richard C. Haigh (University of Exeter Medical School, St Luke's Campus, Exeter EX1 2 LU, UK) for assistance with patient and heathy subject recruitment and clinical sample collection.

Funding

This study was supported by grants from the University of Warwick Impact Fund to NR and from the Wellcome Trust equipment grant to PJT.

Authors' contributions

UA, PJT and NR contributed to conception and design. UA, AA, PJT and NR collected and assembled the data. UA, RSS, PJT and NR analysed and interpreted the data. UA, RSS, PJT and NR drafted the report and all authors reviewed and revised it critically and approved the final version to be published. PJT provided statistical expertise and UA, PJT and NR obtained funding.

Authors' information

Not applicable.

Competing interests

The authors declare that they have no competing interests.

References

1. Thornalley PJ, Rabbani N. Detection of oxidized and glycated proteins in clinical samples using mass spectrometry - a user's perspective. Biochim Biophys Acta. 2014;1840(2):818–29.
2. McCord JM. Free Radicals and Inflammation: Protection of synovial fluid by superoxide dismutase. Science. 1974;185(4150):529–31.
3. Kaur H, Halliwell B. Evidence for nitric oxide-mediated oxidative damage in chronic inflammation. Nitrotyrosine in serum and synovial fluid from rheumatoid patients. FEBS Lett. 1994;350(1):9–12.
4. Wright HL, Moots RJ, Bucknall RC, Edwards SW. Neutrophil function in inflammation and inflammatory diseases. Rheumatology. 2010;49(9):1618–31.
5. Sellam J, Berenbaum F. The role of synovitis in pathophysiology and clinical symptoms of osteoarthritis. Nat Rev Rheumatol. 2010;6(11):625–35.
6. Fearon U, Canavan M, Biniecka M, Veale DJ. Hypoxia, mitochondrial dysfunction and synovial invasiveness in rheumatoid arthritis. Nat Rev Rheumatol. 2016;12(7):385–97.
7. Blanco FJ, Rego I, Ruiz-Romero C. The role of mitochondria in osteoarthritis. Nat Rev Rheumatol. 2011;7(3):161–9.
8. Miyata T, Ishiguro N, Yasuda Y, Ito T, Nangaku M, Iwata H, Kurokawa K. Increased pentosidine, an advanced glycation end product, in plasma and synovial fluid from patients with rheumatoid arthritis and its relation with inflammatory markers. Biochem Biophys Res Comm. 1998;244:45–9.
9. Drinda S, Franke S, Canet CC, Petrow P, Brauer R, Huttich C, Stein G, Hein G. Identification of the advanced glycation end products Nε-carboxymethyllysine in the synovial tissue of patients with rheumatoid arthritis. Ann Rheum Dis. 2002;61(6):488–92.
10. DeGroot J, Verzijl N, Wenting-van Wijk MJG, Jacobs KMG, Van El B, Van Roermund PM, Bank RA, Bijlsma JWJ, TeKoppele JM, Lafeber F. Accumulation of advanced glycation end products as a molecular mechanism for aging as a risk factor in osteoarthritis. Arthritis Rheum. 2004; 50(4):1207–15.
11. Hardin JA, Cobelli N, Santambrogio L. Consequences of metabolic and oxidative modifications of cartilage tissue. Nat Rev Rheumatol. 2015;11(9):521–9.
12. Isaacs JD. The changing face of rheumatoid arthritis: sustained remission for all? Nature Rev Immunol. 2010;10(8):605–11.
13. Roos EM, Arden NK. Strategies for the prevention of knee osteoarthritis. Nat Rev Rheumatol. 2016;12(2):92–101.
14. Menashe L, Hirko K, Losina E, Kloppenburg M, Zhang W, Li L, Hunter DJ. The diagnostic performance of MRI in osteoarthritis: a systematic review and meta-analysis. Osteoarthr Cartil. 2012;20(1):13–21.
15. Van Venrooij WJ, van Beers JJBC, Pruijn GJM. Anti-CCP antibodies: the past, the present and the future. Nat Rev Rheumatol. 2011;7(7):391–8.
16. Ahmed U, Anwar A, Savage RS, Costa ML, Mackay N, Filer A, Raza K, Watts RA, Winyard PG, Tarr J, et al. Biomarkers of early stage osteoarthritis, rheumatoid arthritis and musculoskeletal health. Sci Rep. 2015;5:9259. 9251-9257.
17. Rabbani N, Shaheen F, Anwar A, Masania J, Thornalley PJ. Assay of methylglyoxal-derived protein and nucleotide AGEs. Biochem Soc Trans. 2014;42(2):511–7.
18. Seibel MJ. Biochemical markers of bone turnover: part I: biochemistry and variability. Clin Biochem Rev. 2005;26(4):97–122.
19. Arnett FC, Edworthy SM, Bloch DA, McShane DJ, Fries JF, Cooper NS, Healey LA, Kaplan SR, Liang MH, Luthra HS, et al. American Rheumatism Association 1987 revised criteria for the classification of rheumatoid arthritis. Arthritis Rheum. 1988;31(3):315–24.
20. Raza K, Falciani F, Curnow SJ, Ross EJ, Lee C-Y, Akbar AN, Lord JM, Gordon C, Buckley CD, Salmon M. Early rheumatoid arthritis is characterized by a distinct and transient synovial fluid cytokine profile of T cell and stromal cell origin. Arthritis Res Ther. 2005;7(4):1–12.
21. Ryd L, Brittberg M, Eriksson K, Jurvelin JS, Lindahl A, Marlovits S, Möller P, Richardson JB, Steinwachs M, Zenobi-Wong M. Pre-osteoarthritis: definition and diagnosis of an elusive clinical entity. Cartilage. 2015;6(3):156–65.
22. Raza K, Buckley CE, Salmon M, Buckley CD. Treating very early rheumatoid arthritis. Best Pract Res Clin Rheumatol. 2006;20(5):849–63.
23. Gasser AB, Wootton R, Beyeler S, Celada A, Depierre D. Biological variation in free serum hydroxyproline concentration. Clin Chim Acta. 1980;106(1):39–43.
24. Thompson DK, Sloane R, Bain JR, Stevens RD, Newgard CB, Pieper CF, Kraus VB. Daily variation of serum acylcarnitines and amino acids. Metabolomics. 2012;8(4):556–65.
25. Brunnbauer M, Kuenburg E, Winter F, Muller MM, Prager R. Diurnal variations of fructosamine in patients with type II diabetes mellitus. Wien Klin Wochenschr. 1990;180:72–3.
26. Blanco RA, Ziegler TR, Carlson BA, Cheng P-Y, Park Y, Cotsonis GA, Accardi CJ, Jones DP. Diurnal variation in glutathione and cysteine redox states in human plasma. Am J Clin Nutr. 2007;86(4):1016–23.
27. McLellan AC, Thornalley PJ, Benn J, Sonksen PH. The glyoxalase system in clinical diabetes mellitus and correlation with diabetic complications. ClinSci. 1994;87(1):21–9.
28. Kleinman WA, Richie Jr JP. Status of glutathione and other thiols and disulfides in human plasma. Biochem Pharmacol. 2000;60(1):19–29.
29. Breier M, Wahl S, Prehn C, Fugmann M, Ferrari U, Weise M, Banning F, Seissler J, Grallert H, Adamski J, et al. Targeted metabolomics identifies reliable and stable metabolites in human serum and plasma samples. PLoS ONE. 2014;9(2):e89728.
30. Breiman L. Random forests. Mach Learn. 2001;45(1):5–32.
31. Friedman J, Hastie T, Tibshirani R. Regularization paths for generalized linear models via coordinate descent. J Stat Software. 2010;33(1):1–22.

32. Sajda P. Machine learning for detection and diagnosis of disease. Annu Rev Biomed Eng. 2006;8(1):537–65.
33. Fawcett T. An introduction to ROC analysis. Pattern Recogn Lett. 2006; 27(8):861–74.
34. Robin X, Turck N, Hainard A, Tiberti N, Lisacek F, Sanchez JC, Muller M. pROC: an open-source package for R and S plus to analyze and compare ROC curves. BMC Bioinformatics. 2011;12:77–85.
35. Collins GS, Reitsma JB, Altman DG, Moons KGM. Transparent reporting of a multivariable prediction model for individual prognosis or diagnosis (TRIPOD): the TRIPOD Statement. Ann Intern Med. 2015;162(1):55–63.
36. Kobayashi M, Li L, Iwamoto N, Nakajima-Takagi Y, Kaneko H, Nakayama Y, Eguchi M, Wada Y, Kumagai Y, Yamamoto M. The antioxidant defense system Keap1-Nrf2 comprises a multiple sensing mechanism for responding to a wide range of chemical compounds. Molec Cell Biol. 2009;29(2):493–502.
37. Xue M, Rabbani N, Momiji H, Imbasi P, Anwar MM, Kitteringham NR, Park BK, Souma T, Moriguchi T, Yamamoto M, et al. Transcriptional control of glyoxalase 1 by Nrf2 provides a stress responsive defence against dicarbonyl glycation. Biochem J. 2012;443(1):213–22.
38. Wruck CJ, Fragoulis A, Gurzynski A, Brandenburg L-O, Kan YW, Chan K, Hassenpflug J, Freitag-Wolf S, Varoga D, Lippross S, et al. Role of oxidative stress in rheumatoid arthritis: insights from the Nrf2-knockout mice. Ann Rheum Dis. 2011;70:844–50.
39. Davidson RK, Jupp O, de Ferrars R, Kay CD, Culley KL, Norton R, Driscoll C, Vincent TL, Donell ST, Bao Y, et al. Sulforaphane represses matrix-degrading proteases and protects cartilage from destruction in vitro and in vivo. Arthritis Rheum. 2013;65(12):3130–40.
40. Gibson DS, Bustard MJ, McGeough CM, Murray HA, Crockard MA, McDowell A, Blayney JK, Gardiner PV, Bjourson AJ. Current and future trends in biomarker discovery and development of companion diagnostics for arthritis. Expert Rev Mol Diagn. 2015;15(2):219–34.
41. Misko TP, Radabaugh MR, Highkin M, Abrams M, Friese O, Gallavan R, Bramson C, Le Graverand MPH, Lohmander LS, Roman D. Characterization of nitrotyrosine as a biomarker for arthritis and joint injury. Osteoarthr Cartil. 2013;21(1):151–6.
42. Guma M, Tiziani S, Firestein GS. Metabolomics in rheumatic diseases: desperately seeking biomarkers. Nat Rev Rheumatol. 2016;12(5):269–81.
43. Simkin PA, Bassett JE. Pathways of microvascular permeability in the synovium of normal and diseased human knees. J Rheumatol. 2011; 38(12):2635–42.
44. Levick JR. A method for estimating macromolecular reflection by human synovium, using measurements of intra-articular half lives. Ann Rheum Dis. 1998;57(6):339–44.
45. Zabek A, Swierkot J, Malak A, Zawadzka I, Deja S, Bogunia-Kubik K, Mlynarz P. Application of 1H NMR-based serum metabolomic studies for monitoring female patients with rheumatoid arthritis. J Pharm Biomed Anal. 2016;117:544–50.
46. Zhai G, Wang-Sattler R, Hart DJ, Arden NK, Hakim AJ, Illig T, Spector TD. Serum branched-chain amino acid to histidine ratio: a novel metabolomic biomarker of knee osteoarthritis. Ann Rheum Dis. 2010;69(6):1227–31.
47. Agalou S, Ahmed N, Babaei-Jadidi R, Dawnay A, Thornalley PJ. Profound mishandling of protein glycation degradation products in uremia and dialysis. J Amer Soc Nephrol. 2005;16(5):1471–85.
48. Ahmed N, Babaei-Jadidi R, Howell SK, Beisswenger PJ, Thornalley PJ. Degradation products of proteins damaged by glycation, oxidation and nitration in clinical type 1 diabetes. Diabetologia. 2005;48(8):1590–603.
49. Ahmed N, Thornalley PJ, Luthen R, Haussinger D, Sebekova K, Schinzel R, Voelker W, Heidland A. Processing of protein glycation, oxidation and nitrosation adducts in the liver and the effect of cirrhosis. J Hepatol. 2004;41:913–9.
50. Margarson MP, Soni N. Serum albumin: touchstone or totem? Anaesthesia. 1998;53(8):789–803.
51. Hachulla E, Perezcousin M, Flipo RM, Houvenagel E, Cardon T, Catteau MH, Duquesnoy B, Devulder B. Increased capillary-permeability in systemic rheumatoid vasculitis - detection by dynamic fluorescence nailfold videomicroscopy. J Rheumatol. 1994;21(7):1197–202.
52. Masania J, Malczewska-Malec M, Razny U, Goralska J, Zdzienicka A, Kiec-Wilk B, Gruca A, Stancel-Mozwillo J, Dembinska-Kiec A, Rabbani N, et al. Dicarbonyl stress in clinical obesity. Glycoconj J. 2016;33:581–9.
53. Heard BJ, Rosvold JM, Fritzler MJ, El-Gabalawy H, Wiley JP, Krawetz RJ. A computational method to differentiate normal individuals, osteoarthritis

45. Zabek A, Swierkot J, Malak A, Zawadzka I, Deja S, Bogunia-Kubik K, Mlynarz P. Application of 1H NMR-based serum metabolomic studies for monitoring female patients with rheumatoid arthritis. J Pharm Biomed Anal. 2016;117:544–50.
46. Zhai G, Wang-Sattler R, Hart DJ, Arden NK, Hakim AJ, Illig T, Spector TD. Serum branched-chain amino acid to histidine ratio: a novel metabolomic biomarker of knee osteoarthritis. Ann Rheum Dis. 2010;69(6):1227–31.
47. Agalou S, Ahmed N, Babaei-Jadidi R, Dawnay A, Thornalley PJ. Profound mishandling of protein glycation degradation products in uremia and dialysis. J Amer Soc Nephrol. 2005;16(5):1471–85.
48. Ahmed N, Babaei-Jadidi R, Howell SK, Beisswenger PJ, Thornalley PJ. Degradation products of proteins damaged by glycation, oxidation and nitration in clinical type 1 diabetes. Diabetologia. 2005;48(8):1590–603.
49. Ahmed N, Thornalley PJ, Luthen R, Haussinger D, Sebekova K, Schinzel R, Voelker W, Heidland A. Processing of protein glycation, oxidation and nitrosation adducts in the liver and the effect of cirrhosis. J Hepatol. 2004;41:913–9.
50. Margarson MP, Soni N. Serum albumin: touchstone or totem? Anaesthesia. 1998;53(8):789–803.
51. Hachulla E, Perezcousin M, Flipo RM, Houvenagel E, Cardon T, Catteau MH, Duquesnoy B, Devulder B. Increased capillary-permeability in systemic rheumatoid vasculitis - detection by dynamic fluorescence nailfold videomicroscopy. J Rheumatol. 1994;21(7):1197–202.
52. Masania J, Malczewska-Malec M, Razny U, Goralska J, Zdzienicka A, Kiec-Wilk B, Gruca A, Stancel-Mozwillo J, Dembinska-Kiec A, Rabbani N, et al. Dicarbonyl stress in clinical obesity. Glycoconj J. 2016;33:581–9.
53. Heard BJ, Rosvold JM, Fritzler MJ, El-Gabalawy H, Wiley JP, Krawetz RJ. A computational method to differentiate normal individuals, osteoarthritis

15

Serum levels of interleukin-17 and adiponectin are associated with infrapatellar fat pad volume and signal intensity alteration in patients with knee osteoarthritis

Kang Wang[1,2], Jianhua Xu[1], Jingyu Cai[1], Shuang Zheng[1], Weiyu Han[2], Benny Antony[2] and Changhai Ding[1,2*]

Abstract

Background: In the present study, we sought to generate hypotheses regarding the associations of serum levels of interleukin (IL)-17, adiponectin, and resistin with magnetic resonance imaging-measured infrapatellar fat pad (IPFP) size and signal intensity alterations in patients with knee osteoarthritis (OA).

Methods: A total of 170 subjects with symptomatic knee OA (mean age 55.4 years, range 34–74, 88.2 % females) were included. IPFP volume was measured on T1-weighted spoiled gradient-recalled acquisition in the steady state images and was computed by using a software program. IPFP high signal intensity (grades 0–3) was assessed on T2-weighted fast spin echo images. Serum IL-17, adiponectin, and resistin levels were measured using an enzyme-linked immunosorbent assay.

Results: In multivariable analyses, serum IL-17 was negatively associated with IPFP volume ($\beta = -0.185$, 95 % CI −0.337 to −0.034) but positively associated with the severity of IPFP signal intensity alteration (OR 1.23, 95 % CI 1.06–1.42) after adjustment for age, sex, weight, and height. Serum adiponectin was positively associated with IPFP volume ($\beta = 0.016$, 95 % CI 0.001–0.032) but negatively associated with IPFP signal intensity alteration (OR 0.99, 95 % CI 0.98–1.00) after adjustment for covariates. Resistin was positively associated with IPFP signal intensity alteration (OR 1.13, 95 % CI 1.04–1.23) but not with IPFP volume. The significant associations of adiponectin or resistin disappeared after further adjustment for IL-17; in contrast, the significant associations of IL-17 remained after further adjustment for adiponectin.

Conclusions: While serum IL-17 and resistin were associated with reduced IPFP volume and/or increased abnormal signal intensity alteration, serum adiponectin had opposite associations that were largely through IL-17. These findings suggest that serum adipocytokines may have a role to play in IPFP changes of knee OA.

Keywords: Osteoarthritis, Infrapatellar fat pad, Adipokines, Cytokines, Cartilage, Epidemiology

Abbreviations: BMI, Body Mass Index; IL, Interleukin; ELISA, Enzyme-linked Immunosorbent Assay; IPFP, Infrapatellar Fat Pad; JSN, Joint Space Narrowing; K-L, Kellgren-Lawrence; MMP, Matrix Metalloproteinase; MRI, Magnetic Resonance Imaging; OA, Osteoarthritis; ROA, Radiographic Osteoarthritis; SPGR, Spoiled Gradient-recalled Acquisition in the Steady State; TNF, Tumor Necrosis Factor; VEGF, Vascular Endothelial Growth Factor

* Correspondence: changhai.ding@utas.edu.au
[1]Department of Rheumatology and Immunology, Arthritis Research Institute, the First Affiliated Hospital of Anhui Medical University, 218 Jixi Street, Hefei, China
[2]Menzies Institute for Medical Research, University of Tasmania, Private Bag 23, Hobart, Tasmania 7000, Australia

Background

Osteoarthritis (OA) is a common joint disease with multiple pathogenetic mechanisms, affecting the whole joint. Obesity is considered one of the potent risk factors for developing OA [1]. Although the pathogenesis of OA is not well known, recent studies indicate that obesity-related proinflammatory and metabolic factors contribute to OA progression [2]. Infrapatellar fat pad (IPFP), a local adipose tissue in knee joints with an abundance of adipocytes, immune cells, vessels, and nerve fibers, may be an active joint tissue involved in the initiation and progression of knee OA [3].

IPFP, also known as Hoffa's fat pad, is an intracapsular and extrasynovial structure [4]. It is thought to have primarily a biomechanical function of absorbing forces generated in the knee [5], and thus to have a protective effect physiologically. Indeed, in two recent studies, researchers reported that larger IPFP size was associated with reduced knee abnormal structural changes and symptoms [5, 6]. On the contrary, IPFP signal intensity alteration assessed using magnetic resonance imaging (MRI) was positively associated with the prevalence and/or incidence of knee pain, cartilage defects, bone marrow lesions, and radiographic osteoarthritis (ROA) in older adults [7], and thus it may have a detrimental effect. IPFP has been considered an important source of cytokines and adipokines (i.e., adipocytokines) in OA [8]. IPFP tissues acquired from patients with knee OA can produce cytokines such as interleukin (IL)-1β, tumor necrosis factor (TNF)-α, IL-6, IL-8, IL-17, basic fibroblast growth factor, and vascular endothelial growth factor (VEGF) [8–10]. It can also produce various adipokines such as leptin, resistin, and adiponectin [11]. Researchers in an *in vitro* study reported that conditioned media from cultured white adipose tissue from OA IPFP that contained leptin could induce cartilage collagen release and increase matrix metalloproteinase (MMP)-1 and MMP-13 expression in chondrocytes, and thus had catabolic effects on cartilage [12].

Although the local inflammatory profile of IPFP tissue has been investigated *in vitro*, the associations between serum adipocytokines and IPFP changes have not been examined in epidemiological or clinical studies. Osteoarthritic IPFP explants can release high protein levels of IL-17, resistin, and adiponectin [10]. While serum IL-17 and resistin (proinflammatory adipocytokines) concentrations were significantly higher in patients with knee OA than in control subjects [13], serum levels of adiponectin (an anti-inflammatory adipocytokine) were associated with decreased disease severity of knee OA [14]. It is unknown if IPFP measures such as size and signal intensity alteration are associated with increased or decreased release of systemic IL-17, resistin, and adiponectin in knee OA. We expected that IPFP size would be associated with decreased levels of serum IL-17 and resistin and an increased level of serum adiponectin, but IPFP high signal intensity would be associated with increased levels of serum IL-17 and resistin and a decreased level of serum adiponectin in patients with knee OA. The aim of this study was therefore to generate hypotheses regarding the associations between serum levels of IL-17, adiponectin, and resistin and the volume and signal intensity alteration of IPFP measured using MRI in patients with symptomatic knee OA.

Methods

Study design and patients

We consecutively enrolled into the Anhui Osteoarthritis Study 205 patients with OA who fulfilled the American College of Rheumatology criteria for the classification of clinical knee OA at the Outpatient Clinics, Department of Rheumatology, First Affiliated Hospital of Anhui Medical University, from January 2012 to November 2013. We excluded institutionalized persons, patients with rheumatoid arthritis or other inflammatory diseases, patients with severe knee OA who were planning to have knee arthroplasty in 2 years (this study was ongoing with 2 years of follow-up), and patients with contraindications to MRI (including metal sutures, presence of shrapnel, iron filings in the eye, and claustrophobia). The study was approved by the First Affiliated Hospital of Anhui Medical University Ethics Committee, and all participants signed the informed consent forms.

Anthropometrics

Weight was measured to the nearest 0.1 kg (with shoes, socks, and bulky clothing removed) using a single pair of electronic scales (RGZ-120; Jiangsu Province, China) that were calibrated using a known weight at the beginning of each clinic. Height was measured to the nearest 0.1 cm by using a stadiometer with shoes, socks, and headgear removed. Body mass index (BMI) (weight [kg]/height [m^2]) was calculated.

Radiographic OA assessment

All patients underwent knee radiography. The 15-degree flexion, standing, anteroposterior view image was taken in the symptomatic knees (the severer one if both knees were affected; the right one if both knees were equally painful). Radiographic assessment was performed by a radiology specialist using the Kellgren-Lawrence (K-L) grading system (grades 0–4): grade 0, normal; grade 1, no joint space narrowing (JSN), suspicious osteophytes; grade 2, suspicious JSN, mild osteophytes; grade 3, definite JSN, moderate osteophytes, and/or subchondral bone sclerosis; and grade 4, marked JSN, large osteophytes, and/or severe subchondral bone sclerosis [15]. Radiographic OA was defined as a K-L grade ≥2.

Assessments of IPFP volume and signal intensity changes

MRI of the selected knee was performed with a 3.0-T whole-body magnetic resonance imaging unit (Signa HDxT 3.0T; GE Healthcare, Little Chalfont, UK), using a commercial transmit/receive extremity coil. The following sequence and parameters were used:

1. A T1-weighted fat saturation three-dimensional spoiled gradient-recalled acquisition in the steady state (SPGR), flip angle 30 degrees; repetition time 31 milliseconds; echo time 6.71 milliseconds; field of view 16 cm; 60 partitions; 512 × 512-pixel matrix; acquisition time 11 minutes, 56 milliseconds; and 1 acquisition (Sagittal images were obtained at a partition thickness of 1.5 mm and an in-plane resolution of 0.31 × 0.31 [512 × 512 pixels].)
2. A T2-weighted fat saturation two-dimensional fast spin echo, flip angle 90 degrees, repetition time 3067 milliseconds, echo time 112 milliseconds, field of view 16 cm, 15 partitions, 256 × 256-pixel matrix (Sagittal images were obtained at a slice thickness of 4 mm with an interslice gap of 1.0 mm. Images were checked for image noise and structural abnormalities interfering with segmentation.)

IPFP area was measured by manually drawing disarticulation contours around the IPFP boundaries on T1-weighted SPGR MRI scans using OsiriX software (Pixmeo Sàrl, Bernex, Switzerland). IPFP volume was computed by using the software program. IPFP signal intensity alteration on T2-weighted MRI studies was recorded if hyperintense signal alterations were observed within the IPFP. Signal intensity alteration, defined as discrete areas of increased signal within the IPFP, was graded as follows: grade 0, none; grade 1, <10 % of the region; grade 2, 10–20 % of the region; and grade 3, >20 % of the region [16]. All images were grouped together and read in randomized order by two readers, with the reader blinded to subjects' information. Intraobserver reliability was measured in 30 subjects, with an intraclass correlation coefficient of 0.95 (95 % CI 0.89–0.97). Interobserver reliability was 0.94 (95 % CI 0.85–0.97).

Serum adipocytokine measurements

Morning fasting blood samples were collected from patients. Serum was separated, aliquoted into plastic storage tubes, and stored at −80 °C until analysis. Serum levels of IL-17, adiponectin, and resistin were measured by enzyme-linked immunosorbent assay (ELISA) (eBioscience, San Diego, CA, USA) kits according to the manufacturer's instructions. The optical density was measured at 450 nm using an automatic ELISA reader (Sunrise; Tecan, Männedorf, Switzerland). The limits of detection for IL-17, adiponectin, and resistin were 0.5 pg/ml, 0.01 ng/ml, and 3.1 pg/ml, respectively, and the coefficients of variation were 7.1 %, 4.2 %, and 5.1 %, respectively.

Data analysis

Student's *t* test, the χ^2 test, and the Mann-Whitney *U* test was used to compare means, proportions, and medians, respectively. Pearson's correlations or Spearman's analyses were used to analyze the correlations of serum levels of IL-17 (log-transformed) with serum levels of adiponectin and resistin (log-transformed) or K-L grading. Linear regression analyses were used to examine the associations between IL-17, adiponectin, or resistin and IPFP volume (the dependent variable that was normally distributed) before and after adjustment for covariates including age, sex, weight, and height. Ordinal regression analyses were used to examine the associations between IL-17, adiponectin, or resistin and IPFP signal intensity alteration (the dependent variable). Standard diagnostic checks of model fit and residuals were routinely done, and data points with large residuals and/or high influence were investigated for data errors. A p value <0.05 (two-tailed) or a 95 % CI not including the null point was regarded as statistically significant. All statistical analyses were performed using SPSS 13.0 for Windows (SPSS, Chicago, IL, USA).

Results

A total of 170 subjects (88.2 % females) aged between 34 and 74 years (mean 55.4 years) were included in the analyses, and another 35 subjects were excluded from the study because of incomplete data. There were no significant differences in demographic factors between those included and excluded (data not shown). The median IL-17 level was 2.00 pg/ml, the mean IPFP volume was 20.46 ml (range 12.39–42.90 ml), and the IPFP signal intensity alteration mean value was 0.78 (range 0–3). There were 73 % patients who had established ROA.

Characteristics of the subjects based on the median value of IL-17 are presented in Table 1. Patients with higher and lower levels of IL-17 were similar in terms of sex, BMI, height, weight, knee OA, IPFP signal intensity alteration, IPFP volume, and resistin level. However, patients with higher levels of IL-17 were older and had lower adiponectin levels. Serum levels of IL-17 were significantly associated with serum levels of adiponectin ($r = -0.234$, $p = 0.002$) and resistin ($r = 0.165$, $p = 0.032$). Serum IL-17 and resistin were not associated with K-L grade, but adiponectin was negatively correlated with K-L grade ($\rho = -0.211$, $p = 0.006$).

Serum level of IL-17 was significantly and negatively associated with IPFP volume after adjustment for age, sex, weight, and height (Table 2, Fig. 1), and this association remained unchanged after further adjustment for

Table 1 Characteristics of participants (split by median level of interleukin 17)

	Total ($n = 170$)	IL-17 ≤ median ($n = 85$)	IL-17 > median ($n = 85$)	p Values
Age, years[a]	55.45 (8.25)	54.07 (8.17)	56.66 (8.39)	**0.044**
Female sex, %[b]	88.2	89	87	0.634
Height, cm[a]	159.00 (6.89)	159.09 (7.01)	158.58 (6.88)	0.638
Weight, kg[a]	64.83 (10.56)	64.23 (9.62)	65.09 (10.70)	0.591
BMI, kg/m^2[a]	25.64 (3.85)	25.35 (3.20)	25.87 (3.88)	0.341
K-L grade, %[b]				0.268
1	27.9	25.7	28.6	
2	41.9	50.0	35.1	
3	25.7	20.3	31.2	
4	4.5	4.1	5.2	
Knee ROA, %[b]	72.1	74.3	71.4	0.689
IPFP signal intensity alteration, %[b]	43.1	44.2	40	0.298
IPFP volume, mm^3[a]	20.46 (5.01)	20.57 (5.53)	20.42 (4.88)	0.855
Adiponectin, pg/ml[c]	18.67 (3.94–53.07)	35.08 (11.36–71.26)	12.82 (3.00–46.94)	**0.001**
Resistin, ng/ml[c]	2.37 (1.40–5.57)	2.18 (1.45–4.86)	2.81 (1.32–5.78)	0.532

Abbreviations: BMI body mass index, *K-L* Kellgren-Lawrence, *IL* interleukin, *ROA* radiographic osteoarthritis, *IPFP* infrapatellar fat pad

ROA was defined as a K-L grade ≥2. IL-17 median level 2.00 pg/ml (interquartile range 1.56–2.82). Data in bold denote statistically significant results

[a] *t* tests were used for mean (SD)

[b] χ^2 tests were used for the proportions

[c] Mann-Whitney *U* tests were used for median (interquartile range)

adiponectin (Table 2). Serum level of adiponectin was significantly and positively associated with IPFP volume after adjustment for age, sex, weight, and height, but this became nonsignificant after further adjustment for IL-17 (Table 2). There was no significant association between resistin and IPFP volume before or after adjustment for potential confounders.

Serum levels of IL-17 were significantly and positively associated with severity of IPFP signal intensity alteration before and after adjustment for age, sex, weight, and height, and this association remained significant after further adjustment for adiponectin (Fig. 2, Table 3). Adiponectin had a negatively significant and resistin a positively significant association with IPFP signal intensity alteration before and after adjustment for age, sex, weight, and height, but these associations became nonsignificant after further adjustment for IL-17 (Table 3).

The significant associations of IL-17 and resistin remained significant, but associations of adiponectin became nonsignificant, after adjustment for K-L grade (data not shown).

Discussion

To our knowledge, this is the first epidemiological study to illustrate the relationship between serum levels of adipocytokines and IPFP volume and signal intensity alteration in patients with knee OA. After adjustment for age, sex, weight, and height, we found that higher serum IL-17 level was associated with lower IPFP volume and increased IPFP signal intensity alteration (indicating poorer IPFP quality). Higher adiponectin level was associated with higher IPFP volume and better IPFP quality, but higher serum resistin level was associated only with poorer IPFP quality. These suggest that serum levels of adipocytokines are associated with IPFP pathophysiology in knee OA.

The role of IPFP in OA progression is inconclusive. In our previous studies, we have reported that IPFP size may have a protective role in knee OA structural

Table 2 Association between adipocytokines and infrapatellar fat pad volume

Adipocytokines	Multivariable[a] β (95 % CI)	p Value	Multivariable β (95 % CI)	p Value
IL-17	**−0.19 (−0.34 to −0.03)**	**0.017**	**−0.16 (−0.32 to −0.01)**[b]	**0.047**
Adiponectin	**0.02 (0.01 to 0.03)**	**0.039**	0.01 (−0.01 to 0.03)[c]	0.190
Resistin	−0.07 (−0.20 to 0.06)	0.303	0.02 (−0.01 to 0.18)[c]	0.773

IL interleukin

Dependent variable: infrapatellar fat pad volume. Independent variable: cytokines. Data in bold denote statistically significant results

[a] Adjusted for age, sex, weight and height

[b] Further adjustment for adiponectin

[c] Further adjustment for IL-17

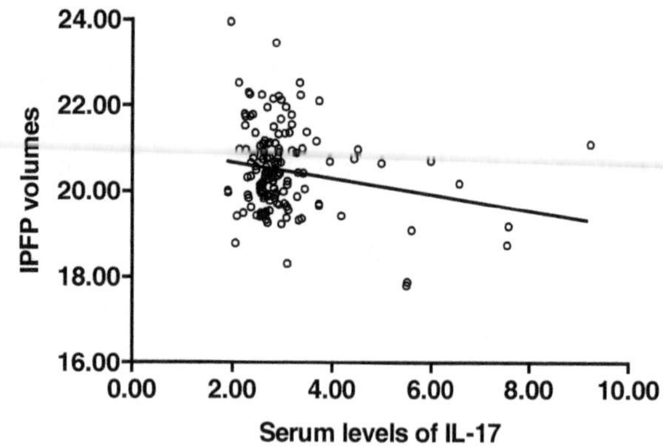

Fig. 1 Association between serum IL-17 and infrapatellar fat pad volume in patients with knee osteoarthritis. $r = -0.199$, $p = 0.015$ after adjustment for age, sex, height and weight. *IL* interleukin, *IPFP* infrapatellar fat pad

changes: Greater IPFP maximal area is associated with greater cartilage volume and lesser cartilage defects, bone marrow lesions, and R OA cross-sectionally and/or longitudinally in older adults [5, 6]. Although researchers in one study reported that IPFP volume was correlated only with age in patients with knee OA and might not be related to the progression of OA [17], we recently reported that, in patients with knee OA, IPFP volume was associated with greater cartilage volume and fewer cartilage defects, bone marrow lesions, and osteophytes [18]. The signal intensity changes in IPFP were positively associated with the prevalence and/or incidence of knee pain, cartilage defects, bone marrow lesions, and R OA in older adults [7], suggesting that abnormal quality of IPFP is detrimental for knee symptoms and structures. This is supported by a recent study demonstrating that synovitis

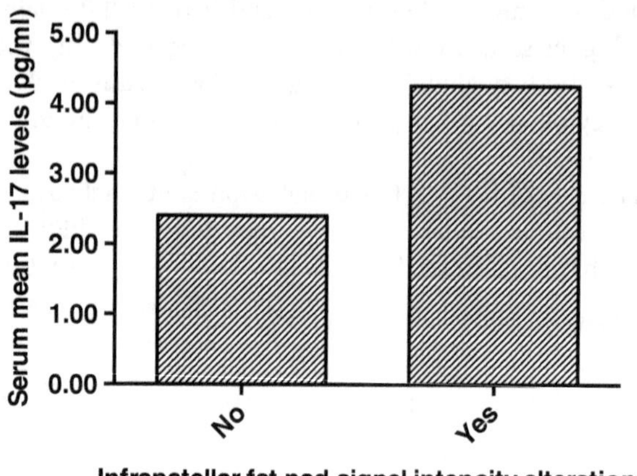

Fig. 2 Association between serum IL-17 and infrapatellar fat pad signal intensity alteration in patients with knee osteoarthritis. Serum IL-17 levels were higher in those with signal intensity alteration ($p = 0.001$)

measured using IPFP signal intensity change (Hoffa's synovitis) is associated with the development of radiographic knee OA [19]. The severity of inflammation in IPFP measured by dynamic contrast-enhanced MRI was associated with the severity of pain in knee OA [20].

Animal or *in vitro* studies have indicated a potentially important role of IPFP in mediating knee intra-articular inflammation. IPFP produced an elevated level of inflammatory cytokines, growth factors, and adipokines in a high-fat diet-induced murine OA model, and the expression levels of the adipokines were significantly correlated with expression of TNF-α, VEGF, and transforming growth factor β [21]. Rates of IL-6 expression and secretion were higher in IPFP tissue than in subcutaneous adipose tissue, indicating that the IPFP cytokine profile could play a role in paracrine inflammation via the local production of IL-6 and contribute to damage in adjacent cartilage in patients with OA [8]. IPFP explants from patients with OA could produce a variety of cytokines, and the production was increased by local cytokine stimulation [9].

Preliminary evidence has shown that adipocytokines such as IL-17 may have roles to play in knee OA. A significant proportion (up to 20 %) of chondrocytes in cartilage samples from patients with OA expressed IL-17R [22]. An in vitro study suggested that IL-17 induced the release of chemokines by chondrocytes and synovial fibroblasts, contributing to cartilage breakdown and synovial infiltration in OA [23]. Researchers in a cross-sectional study reported that serum IL-17 concentrations were significantly higher in patients with knee OA than in control subjects, and synovial IL-17 concentrations were positively correlated with K-L grade and Lequesne index in patients with knee OA [24]. So far, there have been no studies illustrating the relationship between serum IL-17 levels and IPFP changes in patients with knee OA. We found that serum level of IL-17 was negatively associated with IPFP volume and positively with IPFP high signal intensity in patients with knee OA. According to the biopsies from the infrapatellar region in knee OA, chronic low-grade inflammation was detected as signal changes on fluid-sensitive MRI sequences [25]. Our results suggest that serum IL-17 is associated with IPFP pathophysiology, but it is unknown if IL-17 contributes to IPFP inflammation or if abnormal IPFP may produce IL-17, which could play a role in OA pathogenesis. The causal relationship needs to be confirmed in future longitudinal studies.

The role of adiponectin in OA is largely unclear. In vitro findings suggested that adiponectin increased nitric oxide and MMP production in human OA chondrocytes mainly via the AMP-activated protein kinase/c-Jun N-terminal kinase pathway, which would lead to accelerated degradation of OA cartilage matrix ex vivo [26]. Adiponectin can also induce IL-6 secretion in a cultured

Table 3 Association between adipocytokines and infrapatellar fat pad signal intensity alteration

Adipocytokines	Multivariable[a] OR (95 % CI)	*p* Value	Multivariable OR (95 % CI)	*p* Value
IL-17	**1.23 (1.06–1.42)**	**0.007**	**1.20 (1.03–1.38)**[b]	**0.017**
Adiponectin	**0.99 (0.98–1.00)**	**0.042**	0.99 (0.98–1.00)[c]	0.177
Resistin	**1.13 (1.04–1.23)**	**0.004**	1.11 (1.00–1.23)[c]	0.054

IL interleukin
Dependent variables: IPFP signal intensity alteration (0–3). Independent variable: adipocytokines. Data in bold denote statistically significant results
[a]Adjusted for age, sex, weight, and height
[b]Further adjustment for adiponectin
[c]Further adjustment for IL-17

chondrogenic cell line [27]. In contrast, adiponectin levels in both plasma and synovial fluid decreased significantly as the severity of OA (evaluated by K-L grading) increased in humans [28]. Serum adiponectin levels were negatively associated with radiographic progression in patients with hand OA [29, 30]. Furthermore, adiponectin expression in IPFP was higher than in subcutaneous adipose tissue in patients with knee OA [8] and was higher in patients with OA in end stage than in early stage [31]. In our present study, the serum levels of adiponectin were positively associated with IPFP volume and negatively with IPFP signal intensity alteration, indicating that adiponectin may have a role in IPFP of knee OA. This association was dependent on IL-17 and K-L grade, suggesting that this may be mediated largely by IL-17 or ROA.

The biological effects of resistin in OA remain controversial. Recently, researchers in one study reported that resistin could upregulate the expression of multiple chemokines, cytokines, and matrix-degrading genes that are involved in OA pathobiology [32]. Researchers in a cross-sectional study reported that serum resistin levels in patients with hand ROA were higher than in patients with nonradiographic hand OA and control subjects, and were associated with radiographic bone erosion in hand OA [33]. In the present study, we did not find a significant association between resistin and IPFP volume, but we found a significantly positive association between resistin and IPFP signal intensity alteration, suggesting a potential role of resistin in abnormal IPFP changes of knee OA.

The present study has some limitations. First, it was a cross-sectional study designed to generate hypotheses, and the causal relationship cannot be interpreted. Second, the subjects were recruited from the clinics consecutively rather than from the community randomly, so the results may not generalizable to patients with general knee OA. Third, the signal intensity alteration of IPFP was assessed by unenhanced MRI, which was nonspecific, and its pathology is largely unclear [34]. Last, the levels of adipocytokines were measured in serum rather than in synovial fluid, so their local effects are unknown.

Conclusions

While serum IL-17 and resistin were associated with reduced IPFP volume and/or increased abnormal signal intensity alteration, serum adiponectin had opposite associations, which were largely through IL-17. These results suggest that serum levels of adipocytokines may have a role to play in IPFP changes of knee OA.

Acknowledgements
Special thanks go to the subjects who made this study possible. We also thank Hui Zhang for technical support.

Funding
This study was supported by the National Natural Science Foundation of China (81172865).

Authors' contributions
KW had full access to all the study and took responsibility for the integrity of the data and accuracy of the statistical analyses. CD, JX, and KW designed the study. KW, JX, JC, SZ, WH, and BA acquired data. KW and CD interpretation data. KW, JX, JC, SZ, WH, BA, and CD prepared and approved the manuscript.

Authors' information
CD's research interests center on epidemiological and clinical investigation of osteoarthritis using modern techniques such as magnetic resonance imaging. He is looking at the inflammatory and metabolic mechanisms of osteoarthritis and osteoporosis, and he is interested in evaluating new therapies for osteoarthritis and other inflammatory diseases. He has received grants from competitive sources totaling more than $4 million, and he has published over 150 manuscripts in international peer-reviewed journals with an *h*-index of 35.

Competing interests
The authors declare that they have no competing interests.

References

1. Grotle M, Hagen KB, Natvig B, Dahl FA, Kvien TK. Obesity and osteoarthritis in knee, hip and/or hand: an epidemiological study in the general population with 10 years follow-up. BMC Musculoskel Dis. 2008;9:132.
2. Wang X, Hunter D, Xu J, Ding C. Metabolic triggered inflammation in osteoarthritis. Osteoarthritis Cartilage. 2015;23:22–30.
3. Clockaerts S, Bastiaansen-Jenniskens YM, Runhaar J, Van Osch GJ, Van Offel JF, Verhaar JA, et al. The infrapatellar fat pad should be considered as an active osteoarthritic joint tissue: a narrative review. Osteoarthritis Cartilage. 2010;18:876–82.

4. Saddik D, McNally EG, Richardson M. MRI of Hoffa's fat pad. Skeletal Radiol. 2004;33:433–44.
5. Han W, Cai S, Liu Z, Jin X, Wang X, Antony B, et al. Infrapatellar fat pad in the knee: is local fat good or bad for knee osteoarthritis? Arthritis Res Ther. 2014;16:R145.
6. Pan F, Han W, Wang X, Liu Z, Jin X, Antony B, et al. A longitudinal study of the association between infrapatellar fat pad maximal area and changes in knee symptoms and structure in older adults. Ann Rheum Dis. 2015;74:1818–24.
7. Han W, Aitken D, Zhu Z, Halliday A, Wang X, Antony B, et al. Signal intensity alteration in the infrapatellar fat pad at baseline for the prediction of knee symptoms and structure in older adults: a cohort study. Ann Rheum Dis. 2015. doi:10.1136/annrheumdis-2015-208360.
8. Klein-Wieringa IR, Kloppenburg M, Bastiaansen-Jenniskens YM, Yusuf E, Kwekkeboom JC, El-Bannoudi H, et al. The infrapatellar fat pad of patients with osteoarthritis has an inflammatory phenotype. Ann Rheum Dis. 2011; 70:851–7.
9. Distel E, Cadoudal T, Durant S, Poignard A, Chevalier X, Benelli C. The infrapatellar fat pad in knee osteoarthritis: an important source of interleukin-6 and its soluble receptor. Arthritis Rheum. 2009;60:3374–7.
10. Clockaerts S, Bastiaansen-Jenniskens YM, Feijt C, De Clerck L, Verhaar JA, Zuurmond AM, et al. Cytokine production by infrapatellar fat pad can be stimulated by interleukin 1β and inhibited by peroxisome proliferator activated receptor α agonist. Ann Rheum Dis. 2012;71:1012–8.
11. Eymard F, Pigenet A, Citadelle D, Flouzat-Lachaniette CH, Poignard A, Benelli C, et al. Induction of an inflammatory and prodegradative phenotype in autologous fibroblast-like synoviocytes by the infrapatellar fat pad from patients with knee osteoarthritis. Arthritis Rheumatol. 2014; 66:2165–74.
12. Hui W, Litherland GJ, Elias MS, Kitson GI, Cawston TE, Rowan AD, et al. Leptin produced by joint white adipose tissue induces cartilage degradation via upregulation and activation of matrix metalloproteinases. Ann Rheumatic Dis. 2012;71:455–62.
13. de Boer TN, van Spil WE, Huisman AM, Polak AA, Bijlsma JW, Lafeber FP, et al. Serum adipokines in osteoarthritis; comparison with controls and relationship with local parameters of synovial inflammation and cartilage damage. Osteoarthritis Cartilage. 2012;20:846–53.
14. Zheng S, Xu J, Xu S, Zhang M, Huang S, He F, et al. Association between circulating adipokines, radiographic changes, and knee cartilage volume in patients with knee osteoarthritis. Scand J Rheumatol. 2016;45:224–9.
15. Kellgren JH, Lawrence JS. Radiological assessment of osteoarthrosis. Ann Rheum Dis. 1957;16:494–502.
16. Hunter DJ, Guermazi A, Lo GH, Grainger AJ, Conaghan PG, Boudreau RM, et al. Evolution of semi-quantitative whole joint assessment of knee OA: MOAKS (MRI Osteoarthritis Knee Score). Osteoarthritis Cartilage. 2011;19:990–1002.
17. Chuckpaiwong B, Charles HC, Kraus VB, Guilak F, Nunley JA. Age-associated increases in the size of the infrapatellar fat pad in knee osteoarthritis as measured by 3 T MRI. J Orthop Res. 2010;28:1149–54.
18. Cai J, Xu J, Wang K, Zheng S, He F, Huan S, et al. Association between infrapatellar fat pad volume and knee structural changes in patients with knee osteoarthritis. J Rheumatol. 2015;42:1878–84.
19. Roemer FW, Kwoh CK, Hannon MJ, Hunter DJ, Eckstein F, Fujii T, et al. What comes first? Multitissue involvement leading to radiographic osteoarthritis: magnetic resonance imaging–based trajectory analysis over four years in the Osteoarthritis Initiative. Arthritis Rheumatol. 2015;67:2085–96.
20. Ballegaard C, Riis RG, Bliddal H, Christensen R, Henriksen M, Bartels EM, et al. Knee pain and inflammation in the infrapatellar fat pad estimated by conventional and dynamic contrast-enhanced magnetic resonance imaging in obese patients with osteoarthritis: a cross-sectional study. Osteoarthritis Cartilage. 2014;22:933–40.
21. Iwata M, Ochi H, Hara Y, Tagawa M, Koga D, Okawa A, et al. Initial responses of articular tissues in a murine high-fat diet-induced osteoarthritis model: pivotal role of the IPFP as a cytokine fountain. PLoS One. 2013;8:e60706.
22. Honorati MC, Meliconi R, Pulsatelli L, Canè S, Frizziero L, Facchini A. High in vivo expression of interleukin-17 receptor in synovial endothelial cells and chondrocytes from arthritis patients. Rheumatology. 2001;40:522–7.
23. Honorati MC, Bovara M, Cattini L, Piacentini A, Facchini A. Contribution of interleukin 17 to human cartilage degradation and synovial inflammation in osteoarthritis. Osteoarthritis Cartilage. 2002;10:799–807.
24. Chen B, Deng Y, Tan Y, Qin J, Chen LB. Association between severity of knee osteoarthritis and serum and synovial fluid interleukin 17 concentrations. J Int Med Res. 2014;42:138–44.
25. Fernandez-Madrid F, Karvonen RL, Teitge RA, Miller PR, An T, Negendank WG. Synovial thickening detected by MR imaging in osteoarthritis of the knee confirmed by biopsy as synovitis. Magn Reson Imaging. 1995;13:177–83.
26. Kang EH, Lee YJ, Kim TK, Chang CB, Chung JH, Shin K, et al. Adiponectin is a potential catabolic mediator in osteoarthritis cartilage. Arthritis Res Ther. 2010;12:R231.
27. Lago R, Gomez R, Otero M, Lago F, Gallego R, Dieguez C, et al. A new player in cartilage homeostasis: adiponectin induces nitric oxide synthase type II and pro-inflammatory cytokines in chondrocytes. Osteoarthritis Cartilage. 2008;16:1101–9.
28. Honsawek S, Chayanupatkul M. Correlation of plasma and synovial fluid adiponectin with knee osteoarthritis severity. Arch Med Res. 2010;41:593–8.
29. Klein-Wieringa IR, Andersen SN, Herb-van Toorn L, Kwekkeboom JC, van der Helm-van Mil AHM, Meulenbelt I, et al. Are baseline high molecular weight adiponectin levels associated with radiographic progression in rheumatoid arthritis and osteoarthritis? J Rheumatol. 2014;41:853–7.
30. Yusuf E, Ioan-Facsinay A, Bijsterbosch J, Klein-Wieringa I, Kwekkeboom J, Slagboom PE, et al. Association between leptin, adiponectin and resistin and long-term progression of hand osteoarthritis. Ann Rheum Dis. 2011;70: 1282–4.
31. Gandhi R, Takahashi M, Virtanen C, Syed K, Davey JR, Mahomed NN. Microarray analysis of the infrapatellar fat pad in knee osteoarthritis: relationship with joint inflammation. J Rheumatol. 2011;38:1966–72.
32. Zhang Z, Xing X, Hensley G, Chang LW, Liao W, Abu-Amer Y, et al. Resistin induces expression of proinflammatory cytokines and chemokines in human articular chondrocytes via transcription and messenger RNA stabilization. Arthritis Rheum. 2010;62:1993–2003.
33. Choe JY, Bae J, Jung HY, Park SH, Lee HJ, Kim SK. Serum resistin level is associated with radiographic changes in hand osteoarthritis: cross-sectional study. Joint Bone Spine. 2012;79:160–5.
34. Roemer FW, Guermazi A, Zhang Y, Yang M, Hunter DJ, Crema MD, et al. Hoffa's fat pad: evaluation on unenhanced MR images as a measure of patellofemoral synovitis in osteoarthritis. AJR Am J Roentgenol. 2009;192: 1696–700.

16

Evaluation of a quantitative measurement of suprapatellar effusion by ultrasonography and its association with symptoms of radiographic knee osteoarthritis

Daisuke Chiba[1,2*], Eiichi Tsuda[1], Shugo Maeda[1], Eiji Sasaki[1], Ippei Takahashi[2], Shigeyuki Nakaji[2] and Yasuyuki Ishibashi[1]

Abstract

Background: Quantitative measurement of knee joint effusion by ultrasonography has not been well established; however, a categorical measurement (e.g., a ≥4-mm-deep suprapatellar pouch) is recommended. Therefore, the current study aimed to elucidate the association between symptoms of knee osteoarthritis (OA) and the quantitative measurement of suprapatellar effusion by ultrasonography.

Methods: One hundred twenty-seven volunteers participated (31 men and 96 women; mean age: 68.3 ± 9.8 years; body mass index: 23.2 ± 3.0 kg/m^2). The Kellgren-Lawrence grades (KLGs) of both knees were assessed; all subjects had definitive osteoarthritic change (KLG ≥2) in both knee joints. Joint effusion was evaluated using an ultrasound probe, which was placed longitudinally on the suprapatellar pouch, and we determined the area (mm^2) of the echo-free space. Then we summed the effusion area of both knees. All subjects answered the knee injury and osteoarthritis outcome scale (KOOS) questionnaire. Multiple linear regression analysis was conducted to elucidate the association between the summed value of the knee effusion area and the KOOS subscales, which were adjusted by age, sex, body mass index, and KLG.

Results: Of 254 knees, 180 were KLG 2, 57 were KLG 3, and 17 were KLG 4. The multiple regression models showed that the quantitative knee effusion area significantly correlated with the following KOOS subscales: pain ($B = -0.057$; $\beta = -0.253$; $P = 0.002$), symptom ($B = -0.053$; $\beta = -0.251$; $P = 0.002$), sport and recreation ($B = -0.069$; $\beta = -0.205$; $P = 0.007$), and quality of life ($B = -0.083$; $\beta = -0.276$; $P = 0.001$).

Conclusion: In this cross-sectional study, the quantitative measurement of suprapatellar effusion by ultrasonography was associated with symptoms of radiographic knee OA.

Keywords: Knee osteoarthritis, Ultrasonography, Suprapatellar effusion, Knee symptoms

* Correspondence: dachiba@hirosaki-u.ac.jp
[1]Department of Orthopaedic Surgery, Hirosaki University Graduate School of Medicine, Hirosaki, Japan
[2]Department of Social Medicine, Hirosaki University Graduate School of Medicine, Hirosaki, Japan

Background

Knee osteoarthritis (OA) is a common joint disease that causes knee pain and stiffness, especially in the aging population. In our large-scale, domestic cohort, the prevalence rates of knee OA, which were estimated to be high in individuals aged ≥40 years, were 42.6 % in men and 62.4 % in women [1]. In this aging population, knee OA has a significant effect on general health. Knee pain secondary to OA impairs daily living activities [2] and leads to structural deterioration of the knee joint cartilage [3]. Thus, it is important to control and estimate the pain status of patients with knee OA.

Knee synovitis is accompanied by knee symptoms and cartilage destruction, and it induces synovial hypertrophy and the development of effusion in the joint cavity [4]. To determine the severity of synovitis, many researchers have used magnetic resonance imaging (MRI) (non-contrast or contrast-enhanced) [5, 6] and serum biomarkers [7–9]. Several previous studies have shown that it is possible to detect synovial hypertrophy and knee joint effusion using ultrasonography [10, 11]. However, most previous studies have only described the effect of knee effusion based on categorical evaluations such as the whole-organ magnetic resonance imaging score (WORMS) [12] using MRI or the European League Against Rheumatism recommendation [10] to determine whether the depth of the suprapatellar pouch is ≥4 mm or deeper on ultrasonography. Nevertheless, it is still unclear whether the quantitative evaluation of knee effusion has any effect in determining the patient's pain status. Although there are numerous previous MRI studies on the diagnosis of knee synovitis, few studies have confirmed an association between knee synovitis and knee symptoms detected using ultrasonography. Therefore, the present study aimed to (1) establish a novel method for quantitatively measuring suprapatellar effusion on an ultrasonographic image by tracing the border of effusion and calculating its area, and (2) elucidate the association between the quantitative evaluation of suprapatellar effusion and pain status in Japanese patients.

Methods

The Iwaki Health Promotion Project

The Iwaki Health Promotion Project is a community-based program that promotes improvement of the average life span. This 10-year program was initiated in 2005. Approximately 1000 adults aged ≥20 years who live in the Iwaki area of Hirosaki City, Japan (the western Aomori prefecture) participate in this program annually. In addition to an orthopedic specialist, physicians, general surgeons, gynecologists, urologists, psychiatrists, dermatologists, and dentists are involved in this project. Our department collects biochemical and biomechanical data related to knee OA, including that of the spine, hip, and other joints.

Subjects

Overall, 1167 participants underwent the health checkup in 2014. They answered questionnaires about their past and present medical history, lifestyle, occupation, family history, health-related quality of life, and disease-specific information such as knee symptoms. Of those who completed their questionnaire and underwent a radiographic examination, we randomly selected 500 participants to undergo a knee examination by ultrasonography because the number of eligible participants was limited. Finally, 127 volunteers who had radiographic OA of both knees were included in the current study. According to their responses, no participants had a history of hepatic or renal disease, malignancy, or rheumatoid arthritis. Subjects were also excluded if they had any history of severe knee trauma or knee surgery, or were taking any analgesic medications (e.g., non-steroidal anti-inflammatory drugs, acetaminophen, or tramadol) prescribed only by a medical institution. The Ethics Committee of the Hirosaki University Graduate School of Medicine approved the present study, and all subjects provided written informed consent before participation.

Assessment of the radiographic data and knee symptoms

Radiographs of both knees were obtainerd in the standing position, and the knees were categorized based on the Kellgren-Lawrence grade (KLG) by one orthopedist (ES, who has 7 years of experience) [13]. In accordance with the KLGs, the severity of OA in knees with higher KLGs was defined on an individual basis. As aforementioned, all subjects had radiographic OA in both knees. Therefore, their knees were graded at least KLG 2 or more, and they had definitive marginal osteophytes or joint space narrowing. All participants completed the knee injury and osteoarthritis outcome scale (KOOS) questionnaire by themselves; staff members of our department assisted elderly subjects with this questionnaire. The KOOS is a 42-item, knee-specific, self-administered questionnaire with five subscales: pain, symptom, activities of daily living (ADL), sport and recreation (sports), and knee-related quality of life (QOL). All items were scored 0–4 and then summed. Then the raw scores were transformed to a 0–100 scale, in which 100 represents the best result and 0 represents the worst result. A separate score was calculated for each of the five subscales. The KOOS score is a sufficiently reliable, valid, and responsive tool for assessing pain or stiffness and other symptoms, including ADL, function in sport and recreation, and QOL associated with many types of knee disorders [14, 15].

Ultrasonographic evaluation of suprapatellar effusion

To reduce bias, we performed ultrasonography after all participants had completed the questionnaire on knee pain. All ultrasound scans were evaluated by two examiners (DC, who has 5 years of experience in musculoskeletal ultrasonographic evaluation and SM, who has 8 years of experience). The subjects were examined lying in the supine position with both knees semi-flexed and their feet in the neutral position. The semi-flexed knee position was maintained by placing a pillow in both popliteal areas; in our preliminary data from 57 individuals, the knee flexion angle with this pillow was 20.0 ± 3.0°. Longitudinal ultrasound scans of the suprapatellar region were obtained; a linear transducer (12-MHz, Viamo^{TM}; Toshiba Medical Systems Corp., Otawara, Japan) was gently placed over the same area at the center and proximal poles of the patella. On these images, echo-free space represented a suprapatellar effusion. While the margins of these echo-free spaces were traced, the area (mm^2) of suprapatellar effusion was calculated automatically (Fig. 1). Finally, we summed the value of the effusion area in both knees to evaluate it effect on knee pain. During the examination, the transducers were placed as gently as possible, because pressure on the skin through the transducers should be avoided, as it can affect the acquired effusion area. For determining and calculating the knee effusion area in the suprapatellar pouch, the inter-rater reliability, intraclass/interclass correlation coefficient (ICC) (2,1) means the validation of evaluating effusion area, when two examiners test one subject, was 0.825 (95 % confidence interval (CI) 0.526, 0.935), and the intra-rater reliabilities, ICC (1,1) means the validation when one examiner test one subject, for examiners DC and SM were 0.991 (95 % CI 0.977, 0.997) and 0.988 (95 % CI 0.969, 0.995), respectively.

Statistical analysis

The data were statistically analyzed using SPSS, version 22.0 J software (SPSS Inc., Chicago, IL, USA). First, we conducted analysis of variance (Tukey post-hoc test) to compare the mean values of the suprapatellar effusion area, age, body mass index (BMI), and KOOS subscales according to the KLG. Second, correlation between the suprapatellar effusion area and age, sex, BMI, KLG, or

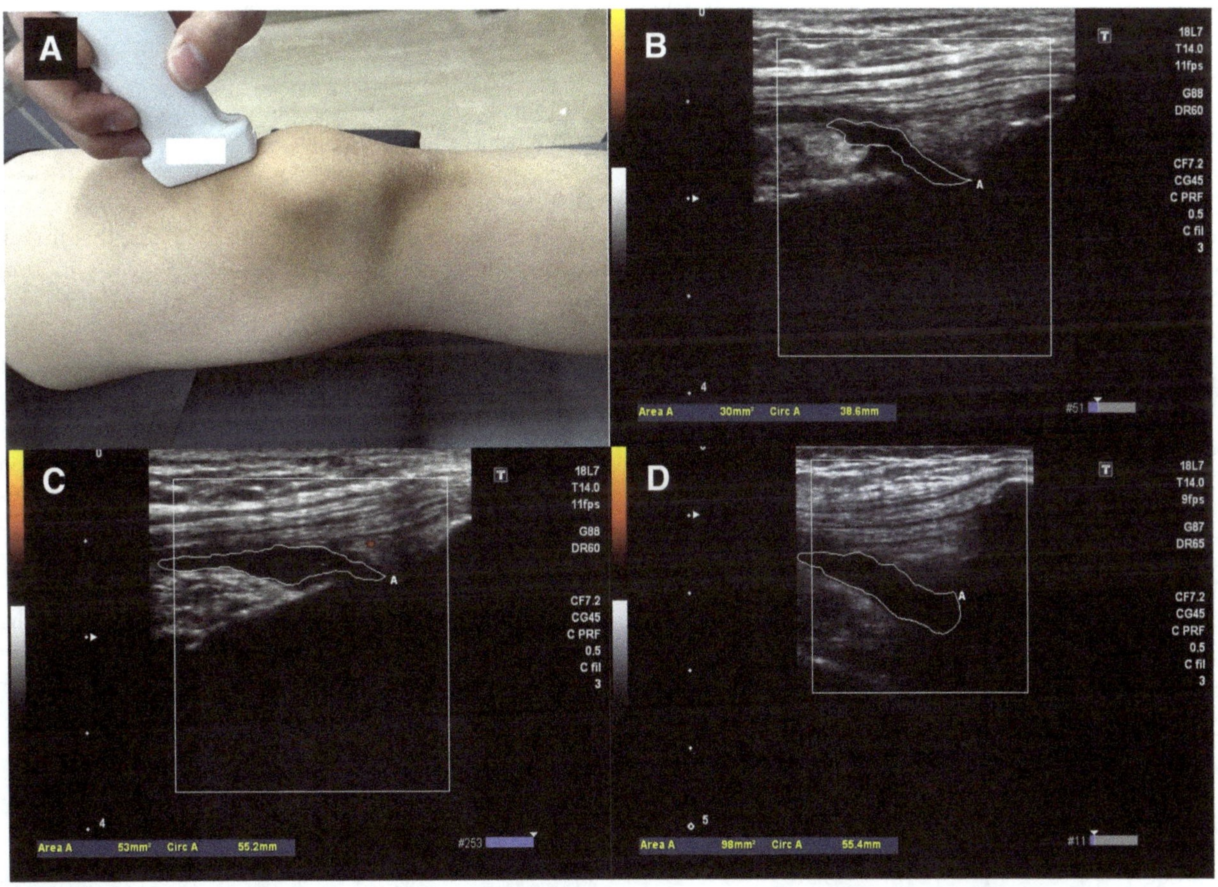

Fig. 1 Representative images of the suprapatellar effusion area. **a** Ultrasound scan image of the suprapatellar effusion acquired by placing a linear probe longitudinally on the suprapatellar pouch. The effusion area was calculated by tracing the margin of the echo-free space that corresponds with the suprapatellar pouch. During the examination, the transducers should be placed on the subject as gently as possible to avoid distorting the acquired area. Representative images of the suprapatellar effusion area: 30 mm^2 (**b**); 50 mm^2 (**c**); and 100 mm^2 (**d**)

the KOOS subscales were determined by calculating the Spearman rank correlation coefficient. Third, to evaluate crude association between variables, single linear regression analysis was conducted with each KOOS subscale as the dependent variable and the suprapatellar effusion area as the independent variable. Finally, to evaluate the adjusted association between variables, multiple linear regression analysis was conducted with each KOOS subscale as the dependent variable and the suprapatellar effusion area as the independent variable, including age, sex, BMI, and KLG as the co-variables. A P value ≤0.05 was considered statistically significant.

Results

Comparison of the suprapatellar effusion area identified on ultrasonography, demographic data, and KOOS subscales among the KLGs

Of 254 knees (127 subjects), 180 (70.9 %) were KLG 2, 57 (22.4 %) were KLG 3, and 17 (6.7 %) were KLG 4. Among all the subjects, 81 (63.8 %) were KLG 2, 33 (26.0 %) were KLG 3, and 13 (10.2 %) were KLG 4. The mean age was significantly higher in subjects with KLGs 3 and 4 than in those with KLG 2. Additionally, the mean BMI was higher in subjects with KLG 4 than in those with KLGs 2 and 3. The mean scores of the KOOS subscales were significantly lower in subjects with KLGs 3 and 4 than in those with KLG 2 (Table 1).

In 254 knees, the mean values of the suprapatellar effusion area identified on ultrasonography were 39.2 ± 40.2 mm^2 in those with KLG 2, 69.5 ± 59.3 mm^2 in those with KLG 3, and 93.0 ± 91.3 mm^2 in those with KLG 4. The suprapatellar effusion area increased with the progression of the KLG; the mean effusion area was significantly higher in those with KLGs 3 or 4 than in those with KLG 2 (Table 2).

Table 1 Comparison of the demographic values in subjects grouped by severity of knee osteoarthritis identified by radiography

	Total n = 127	KLG 2 n = 81	KLG 3 n = 33	KLG 4 n = 13
Age	68.3 ± 9.8	65.8 ± 9.8	71.5 ± 7.4^a	75.4 ± 9.3^a
Body mass index	23.2 ± 3.0	22.6 ± 2.7	23.6 ± 2.7	26.3 ± 3.7^{ab}
Kellgren-Lawrence grade	4.7 ± 1.1	4.0 ± 0	5.5 ± 0.5^a	7.3 ± 0.5^{ab}
Effusion area	99.2 ± 89.7	73.9 ± 65.8	139.3 ± 94.8^a	155.3 ± 139.8^a
KOOS pain	83.6 ± 20.3	91.3 ± 12.2	73.1 ± 24.3^a	62.8 ± 23.7^a
KOOS symptom	84.5 ± 19.0	91.3 ± 13.3	75.9 ± 20.4^a	64.3 ± 23.5^a
KOOS ADL	88.8 ± 16.6	94.7 ± 10.0	80.4 ± 19.9^a	74.0 ± 22.2^a
KOOS sport	72.8 ± 30.1	85.1 ± 21.1	55.8 ± 29.3^a	40.0 ± 36.1^a
KOOS QOL	70.3 ± 27.1	82.4 ± 17.1	49.6 ± 28.3^a	47.1 ± 29.6^a

Statistical analysis by analysis of variance (Tukey post-hoc test); $^aP \leq 0.01$ compared to Kellgren-Lawrence grade (KLG) 2; $^bP \leq 0.01$ compared to KLG 3. The effusion area and KLG values are the sum of these values for both knees. *KOOS* knee injury and osteoarthritis outcome scale, *ADL* activities of daily living, *QOL* quality of life

Correlation between the knee effusion and knee symptoms

According to Spearman correlation coefficient analysis, the suprapatellar effusion area assessed by ultrasonography had a significantly negative correlation with each KOOS subscale (Table 3). Results of single regression analysis also showed that the suprapatellar effusion area was inversely correlated with the following KOOS subscales: pain ($B = -0.093$; $\beta = -0.413$; $P < 0.001$), symptom ($B = -0.085$; $\beta = -0.403$; $P < 0.001$), ADL ($B = -0.056$; $\beta = -0.301$; $P = 0.001$), sports ($B = -0.127$; $\beta = -0.419$; $P < 0.001$), and QOL ($B = -0.135$; $\beta = -0.400$; $P < 0.001$) (Fig. 2). In the multiple regression model, the suprapatellar effusion area was consistently negatively correlated with the following KOOS subscales: pain ($B = -0.057$; $\beta = -0.253$; $P = 0.002$), symptom ($B = -0.053$; $\beta = -0.251$; $P = 0.002$), sports ($B = -0.069$; $\beta = -0.205$; $P = 0.007$), and QOL ($B = -0.083$; $\beta = -0.276$; $P = 0.001$). However, only the KOOS ADL subscale was insignificantly correlated with the suprapatellar effusion area ($B = -0.024$; $\beta = -0.132$; $P = 0.109$) when adjusted by age, sex, BMI, and KLG (Table 4).

Discussion

To our knowledge, the current study is the first to report on the association between knee symptoms and the quantitative suprapatellar effusion area assessed using ultrasonography. The larger the quantitative effusion area, the lower the KOOS subscale scores. In this cross-sectional study, the suprapatellar effusion area significantly negatively affected knee symptoms in the population with radiographic evidence of knee OA, even after adjusting for age, sex, BMI, and severity of radiographic knee OA.

Several previous studies that used MRI and ultrasonography have reported that knee effusion worsens symptoms [16–19]. In a longitudinal study, Zhang et al. reported that knee effusion worsens patients' pain status (Western Ontario and McMaster Universities osteoarthritis index

Table 2 Comparison of the effusion area identified by ultrasonography according to the severity of knee osteoarthritis identified by radiography

Effusion area (mm^2)	Total $N = 254$	KLG 2 $N = 180$	KLG 3 $N = 57$	KLG 4 $N = 17$
Average value	49.6 ± 52.4	39.2 ± 40.2	69.5 ± 59.3*	93.0 ± 91.3*
95 % CI	43.1, 56.1	33.3, 45.1	53.8, 85.3	46.0, 140.0

Statistical analysis was by analysis of variance (Tukey post-hoc test); $^*P \leq 0.01$ compared to Kellgren-Lawrence grade (KLG) 2. The effusion area of each knee joint was measured (n = 254 knees). *CI* confidence interval

Table 3 Correlation between the effusion area identified on ultrasonography, demographic data, and KOOS subscales

	Age	Sex	BMI	KLG	K-pain	K-sym	K-ADL	K-sports	K-QOL
Effusion area	0.187*	−0.158	0.142	0.422**	−0.382**	−0.370**	−0.373**	−0.441**	−0.433**
Age		0.076	0.135	0.353**	−0.143	−0.175*	−0.304**	−0.346**	−0.179*
Sex			−0.016	0.203*	−0.095	−0.160	−0.112	−0.039	−0.153
BMI				0.293**	−0.306**	−0.247**	−0.266**	−0.310**	−0.211*
KLG					−0.473**	−0.468**	−0.472**	−0.555**	−0.536**
K-pain						0.819**	0.843**	0.791**	0.877**
K-sym							0.754**	0.743**	0.789**
K-ADL								0.902**	0.798**
K-sports									0.755**

Statistical analysis was by Spearman rank correlation coefficient; *$P \leq 0.05$; **$P \leq 0.01$. The effusion area and KLG values are the sum of these values for both knees. *KLG* Kellgren-Lawrence grade, *K-pain* knee injury and osteoarthritis outcome scale (KOOS) pain subscale, *K-sym* KOOS symptom subscale, *K-ADL* KOOS activity of daily living subscale, *K-sports* KOOS sport and recreation subscale, *K-QOL* KOOS quality of life subscale

pain scale) according to the whole organ magnetic resonance imaging score (WORMS) using MRI [16]. Another previous study demonstrated that in middle-aged women, knee effusion worsened pain and deteriorated their physical performance in activities such as timed walking and stair climbing [18]. Lo et al. performed a more detailed study in which effusion affected weight-bearing pain more than non-weight-bearing pain [19]. D'Agostino et al. performed ultrasonographic evaluations in a large symptomatic population and reported a high prevalence of suprapatellar effusion, which correlated with the development of sudden pain [10]. Similarly, Naredo et al. reported that the rest and motion pain scale scores were higher in those with suprapatellar effusion (≥4 mm deep) than in those with a lesser degree of effusion [20]. In a detailed review of knee synovitis, the most typical method used for determining the degree of synovitis is to evaluate the area of the joint cavity that is enlarged on imaging studies, because knee synovitis and effusion are associated with each other [4, 5]. This evidence supports the evaluation of knee effusion as an effective method for determining the pain status of an individual.

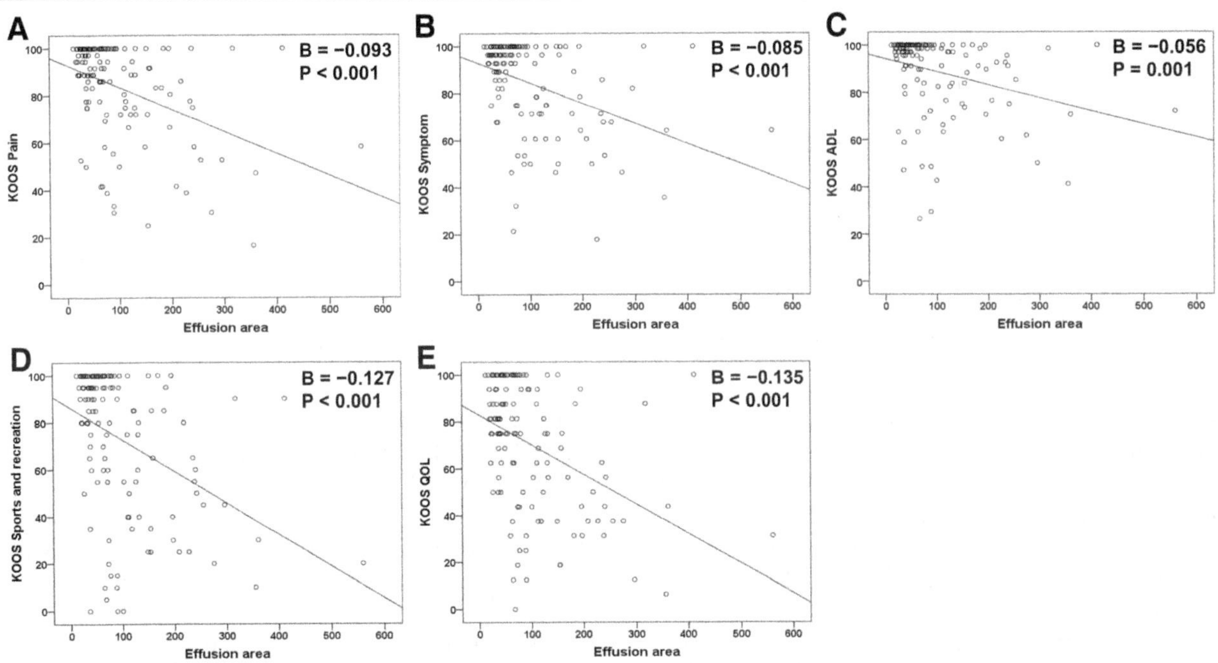

Fig. 2 Scattergram of the suprapatellar effusion area and knee injury and osteoarthritis outcome scale (*KOOS*) subscales. The *y-axis* corresponds with each KOOS subscale, and the *x-axis* corresponds with the summed area (mm^2) of suprapatellar effusion evaluated by ultrasonography (Fig. 1). The summed value of the effusion area was calculated by adding the value for the effusion areas of the right and left knees. **a** KOOS pain subscale; **b** KOOS symptom subscale; **c** KOOS activities of daily living (*ADL*) subscale; **d** KOOS sport and recreation subscale; **e** KOOS quality of life (*QOL*) subscale

Table 4 Multivariate analysis of the factors associated with knee pain

Dependent variable	R^2 (adjusted)	Independent variables	*B*	*β*	*P* value	95 % CI
KOOS pain	0.375	Intercept	162.510	-	<0.001	132.506 to 192.514
		Age	−0.043	−0.021	0.780	−0.351 to 0.264
		Sex	−0.617	−0.013	0.859	−7.462 to 6.228
		BMI	−1.663	−0.247	0.001	−2.658 to −0.667
		KLG	−6.469	−0.358	<0.001	−9.565 to −3.374
		Effusion area	−0.057	−0.253	0.002	−0.092 to −0.022
KOOS symptom	0.344	Intercept	159.128	-	<0.001	130.282 to 187.974
		Age	−0.137	−0.070	0.361	−0.433 to 0.159
		Sex	2.378	−0.054	0.476	−8.959 to 4.203
		BMI	−1.226	−0.194	0.012	−2.184 to −0.269
		KLG	−5.788	−0.341	<0.001	−8.764 to −2.811
		Effusion area	−0.053	−0.251	0.002	−0.087 to −0.020
KOOS ADL	0.319	Intercept	165.423	-	<0.001	139.804 to 191.043
		Age	−0.312	−0.184	0.020	−0.575 to −0.050
		Sex	−0.189	−0.005	0.949	−6.034 to 5.656
		BMI	−1.333	−0.242	0.002	−2.184 to −0.483
		KLG	−4.561	−0.308	0.001	−7.204 to −1.918
		Effusion area	−0.024	−0.132	0.109	−0.054 to 0.006
KOOS sports	0.424	Intercept	212.530	-	<0.001	169.674 to 255.386
		Age	−0.510	−0.165	0.023	−0.950 to −0.070
		Sex	1.477	0.021	0.765	−8.300 to 11.255
		BMI	−2.241	−0.224	0.002	−3.664 to −0.819
		KLG	−10.292	−0.382	<0.001	−14.714 to −5.871
		Effusion area	−0.069	−0.205	0.007	−0.119 to −0.019
KOOS QOL	0.358	Intercept	169.047	-	<0.001	128.343 to 209.751
		Age	−0.133	−0.048	0.529	−0.551 to 0.284
		Sex	−7.883	−0.125	0.095	−17.170 to 1.403
		BMI	−1.102	−0.122	0.109	−2.453 to 0.249
		KLG	−8.894	−0.367	<0.001	−13.093 to −4.694
		Effusion area	−0.083	−0.276	0.001	−0.131 to −0.036

Statistical analysis was by multiple linear regression analysis using each knee injury and osteoarthritis outcome score (KOOS) subscale as the dependent variable; age, sex, body mass index (BMI), Kellgren-Lawrence grade (KLG), and the suprapatellar effusion area were used as the independent variables. The effusion area and KLG values are the sum of these values for both knees. R^2 coefficient of determination, *B* regression coefficients, *β* standardized regression coefficients, *sports* sport and recreation, *ADL* activities of daily living, *QOL* quality of life, *CI* confidence interval

Conversely, recent reports have mentioned that knee effusion detected using ultrasonography was not correlated with patients' pain status [21, 22]. Bevers et al. reported that there was no significant correlation between suprapatellar effusion and knee pain; they included subjects who were on analgesic medications [21], so the result of this study should be interpreted with caution, as certain nonsteroidal anti-inflammatory drugs compromise knee pain and synovitis [23]. Hall et al. reported that the association between suprapatellar effusion and the pain scale score was significant but weak; thus, they concluded that knee effusion is simply a phenomenon caused by the constructive degeneration of knee OA such as the decrease in lymph vessels of the synovium [22]. In the current study, we used the multiple regression model and included the severity of radiographic knee OA to adjust for the inter-relationship of constructive knee OA severity; even when adjusted, quantitative measurement of knee effusion had a significant effect on the pain status as assessed using the KOOS subscales patients with definitive radiographic evidence of knee OA. Although we agree that structural degeneration is one of the significant factors associated with the development of effusion in osteoarthritic knees, it is still difficult to determine which of the two, structural degradation or synovitis, is a more important factor that affects the development of effusion, especially in patients with radiographic knee OA. Further studies are needed to clarify the mechanism.

There are several limitations to the present study. First, this was a cross-sectional study; thus, future longitudinal studies are needed to clarify the association between knee symptoms and suprapatellar effusion. Second, we only examined the suprapatellar pouch. Thus, it is still unclear whether other quantitative measurements are associated with knee synovitis, such as synovial hypertrophy, and that of other sites with knee effusion, such as the medial or lateral recess. Additionally, we only examined one sagittal image of the suprapatellar pouch and only one image with the knee in the semi-flexed position. Third, the number of subjects with higher KLGs was small, because this was primarily a study of healthy individuals, as there were only a few subjects with severe OA. Although most subjects had any osteoarthritic knees, the present data are meaningful, because we surveyed these individuals in the pre-hospitalized state and all subjects on medications were excluded. Moreover, we originally performed a quantitative evaluation to estimate the suprapatellar effusion area, and this quantitative knee effusion value represented the pain status of the population with radiographic knee OA. There are recent reports that knee effusion as identified on MRI is more likely to destroy the joint surface and lead to the development of radiographic evidence of knee OA, as seen in longitudinal cohort studies [24–26]. Longitudinal data is little showing that knee effusion identified by ultrasonography causes cartilage destruction or structural degenaration. However, ultrasound evaluation of knee effusion has been directly correlated with a catabolic biomarker and the serum cartilage oligomeric matrix protein level, and inversely correlated with an anabolic biomarker, the N-terminal propeptide of type II collagen [27]. Further investigation is warranted to clarify the pathological correlation between knee effusion identified by ultrasonography and the degree of knee pain or structural damage in patients with knee OA.

Conclusions

We quantitatively measured the sagittal area of knee effusion in the suprapatellar pouch by using ultrasonography and tracing the border of effusion on the ultrasound image, which is a novel method. An increase in the suprapatellar effusion area corresponded with worsened KOOS subscales in the population with radiographic evidence of knee OA. The current data support the finding that knee effusion can indicate the pain status of patients with knee OA.

Abbreviations

ADL, activities of daily living; BMI, body mass index; CI, confidence interval; ICC, intraclass/interclass correlation coefficient; KLG, Kellgren-Lawrence grade; KOOS, knee injury and osteoarthritis outcome score; MRI, magnetic resonance imaging; OA, osteoarthritis; QOL, quality of life; sports, sport and recreation; WORMS, whole organ magnetic resonance imaging score

Acknowledgements

We are very grateful to all who participated in the Iwaki Health Promotion Project, and the staff of our department who conducted the interviews and collected the data. This study was supported in part by the Ministry of Education, Culture, Sports, Science and Technology of Japan (no.: 18200044), Japanese Society for the Promotion of Science (number 21500676), Karoji Memorial Fund for Medical Research (number 5310139302), and JOA-Subsidized Science Research Project grant from the Japanese Orthopedic Association.

Authors' contributions

DC chiefly drafted the manuscript and designed the study, and performed acquisition, analysis, and interpretation of data. ET revised the manuscript critically for important intellectual content. SM acquired data and helped to draft the manuscript. ES revised the manuscript, and analyzed and interpreted data. IT chiefly organized our cohort study and helped to draft the manuscript. SN conceived the study and gave final approval of the manuscript to be submitted. YI helped to revise the manuscript and gave final approval of the manuscript to be submitted. All authors read and approved the final manuscript.

Competing interests

The authors declare that they have no competing interests.

References

1. Yoshimura N, Muraki S, Oka H, Mabuchi A, En-Yo Y, Yoshida M, et al. Prevalence of knee osteoarthritis, lumbar spondylosis, and osteoporosis in Japanese men and women: the research on osteoarthritis/osteoporosis against disability study. J Bone Miner Metab. 2009;27:620–8.
2. Hoogeboom TJ, den Broeder AA, de Bie RA, van den Ende CH. Longitudinal impact of joint pain comorbidity on quality of life and activity levels in knee osteoarthritis: data from the Osteoarthritis Initiative. Rheumatology (Oxford). 2013;52:543–6.
3. Muraki S, Akune T, Oka H, Ishimoto Y, Nagata K, Yoshida M, et al. Incidence and risk factors for radiographic knee osteoarthritis and knee pain in Japanese men and women: a longitudinal population-based cohort study. Arthritis Rheum. 2012;64:1447–56.
4. Scanzello CR, Goldring SR. The role of synovitis in osteoarthritis pathogenesis. Bone. 2012;51:249–57.
5. Roemer FW, Kassim Javaid M, Guermazi A, Thomas M, Kiran A, Keen R, et al. Anatomical distribution of synovitis in knee osteoarthritis and its association with joint effusion assessed on non-enhanced and contrast-enhanced MRI. Osteoarthritis Cartilage. 2010;18:1269–74.
6. Hunter DJ, Zhang W, Conaghan PG, Hirko K, Menashe L, Li L, et al. Systematic review of the concurrent and predictive validity of MRI biomarkers in OA. Osteoarthritis Cartilage. 2011;19:557–88.
7. Turan Y, Bal S, Gurgan A, Topac H, Koseoglu M. Serum hyaluronan levels in patients with knee osteoarthritis. Clin Rheumatol. 2007;26:1293–8.
8. Inoue R, Ishibashi Y, Tsuda E, Yamamoto Y, Matsuzaka M, Takahashi I, et al. Knee osteoarthritis, knee joint pain and aging in relation to increasing serum hyaluronan level in the Japanese population. Osteoarthritis Cartilage. 2011;19:51–7. http://dx.doi.org/10.1016/j.joca.2010.10.021.
9. Ishijima M, Watari T, Naito K, Kaneko H, Futami I, Yoshimura-Ishida K, et al. Relationships between biomarkers of cartilage, bone, synovial metabolism and knee pain provide insights into the origins of pain in early knee osteoarthritis. Arthritis Res Ther. 2011;13:R22.
10. D'Agostino MA, Conaghan P, Le Bars M, Baron G, Grassi W, Martin-Mola E, et al. EULAR report on the use of ultrasonography in painful knee osteoarthritis. Part 1: prevalence of inflammation in osteoarthritis. Ann Rheum Dis. 2005;64:1703–9.

11. Conaghan P, D'Agostino MA, Ravaud P, Baron G, Le Bars M, Grassi W, et al. EULAR report on the use of ultrasonography in painful knee osteoarthritis. Part 2: exploring decision rules for clinical utility. Ann Rheum Dis. 2005;64:1710–4.
12. Peterfy CG, Guermazi A, Zaim S, Tirman PF, Miaux Y, White D, et al. Whole-Organ Magnetic Resonance Imaging Score (WORMS) of the knee in osteoarthritis. Osteoarthritis Cartilage. 2004;12:177–90.
13. Kellgren JH, Lawrence JS. Radiological assessment of osteo-arthrosis. Ann Rheum Dis. 1957;16:494–502.
14. Roos EM, Roos HP, Lohmander LS, Ekdahl C, Beynnon BD. Knee Injury and Osteoarthritis Outcome Score (KOOS)–development of a self-administered outcome measure. J Orthop Sports Phys Ther. 1998;28:88–96.
15. Nakamura N, Takeuchi R, Sawaguchi T, Ishikawa H, Saito T, Goldhahn S. Cross-cultural adaptation and validation of the Japanese Knee Injury and Osteoarthritis Outcome Score (KOOS). J Orthop Sci. 2011;16:516–23.
16. Zhang Y, Nevitt M, Niu J, Lewis C, Torner J, Guermazi A, et al. Fluctuation of knee pain and changes in bone marrow lesions, effusions, and synovitis on magnetic resonance imaging. Arthritis Rheum. 2011;63:691–9.
17. Javaid MK, Kiran A, Guermazi A, Kwoh CK, Zaim S, Carbone L, et al. Individual magnetic resonance imaging and radiographic features of knee osteoarthritis in subjects with unilateral knee pain: the health, aging, and body composition study. Arthritis Rheum. 2012;64:3246–55. doi:10.1002/art.34594.
18. Sowers M, Karvonen-Gutierrez CA, Jacobson JA, Jiang Y, Yosef M. Associations of anatomical measures from MRI with radiographically defined knee osteoarthritis score, pain, and physical functioning. J Bone Joint Surg Am. 2011;93:241–51.
19. Lo GH, McAlindon TE, Niu J, Zhang Y, Beals C, Dabrowski C, et al. Bone marrow lesions and joint effusion are strongly and independently associated with weight-bearing pain in knee osteoarthritis: data from the osteoarthritis initiative. Osteoarthritis Cartilage. 2009;17:1562–9.
20. Naredo E, Cabero F, Palop MJ, Collado P, Cruz A, Crespo M. Ultrasonographic findings in knee osteoarthritis: A comparative study with clinical and radiographic assessment. Osteoarthritis Cartilage. 2005;13:568–74.
21. Bevers K, Bijlsma JW, Vriezekolk JE, van den Ende CH, den Broeder AA. Ultrasonographic features in symptomatic osteoarthritis of the knee and relation with pain. Rheumatology (Oxford). 2014;53:1625–9.
22. Hall M, Doherty S, Courtney P, Latief K, Zhang W, Doherty M. Synovial pathology detected on ultrasound correlates with the severity of radiographic knee osteoarthritis more than with symptoms. Osteoarthritis Cartilage. 2014;22:1627–33.
23. Zweers MC, de Boer TN, van Roon J, Bijlsma JW, Lafeber FP, Mastbergen SC. Celecoxib: considerations regarding its potential disease-modifying properties in osteoarthritis. Arthritis Res Ther. 2011;13:239.
24. Roemer FW, Guermazi A, Felson DT, Niu J, Nevitt MC, Crema MD, et al. Presence of MRI-detected joint effusion and synovitis increases the risk of cartilage loss in knees without osteoarthritis at 30-month follow-up: the MOST study. Ann Rheum Dis. 2011;70:1804–9. doi:10.1136/ard.2011.150243.
25. Atukorala I, Kwoh CK, Guermazi A, Roemer FW, Boudreau RM, Hannon MJ, et al. Synovitis in knee osteoarthritis: a precursor of disease? Ann Rheum Dis. 2014;75:390–5. doi:10.1136/annrheumdis-2014-205894.
26. Wang X, Blizzard L, Halliday A, Han W, Jin X, Cicuttini F, et al. Association between MRI-detected knee joint regional effusion-synovitis and structural changes in older adults: a cohort study. Ann Rheum Dis. 2014;75:519–25.
27. Kumm J, Tamm A, Lintrop M, Tamm A. Association between ultrasonographic findings and bone/cartilage biomarkers in patients with early-stage knee osteoarthritis. Calcif Tissue Int. 2009;85:514–22.

17

Is local platelet-rich plasma injection clinically superior to hyaluronic acid for treatment of knee osteoarthritis?

Yalong Di[1†], Changxu Han[2†], Liang Zhao[2] and Yizhong Ren[2*]

Abstract

Background: In this study, we evaluated whether platelet-rich plasma (PRP) is superior to hyaluronic acid (HA) in the treatment of knee osteoarthritis.

Methods: The Cochrane Central Register of Controlled Trials, PubMed, and Embase databases were searched for English-language, human in vivo studies on the treatment of symptomatic knee osteoarthritis with intra-articular PRP compared with HA. The following keywords were used for the search: "platelet-rich plasma," "PRP," "platelet-rich fibrin," "PRF," "platelet," "plasma," "arthritis," "osteoarthritis," "gonarthrosis," and "degeneration."

Results: Seven articles reporting 908 patients and 908 knees were analyzed, including 44% men and 56% women with a mean age of 59.8 years. All studies met the minimal clinically important difference criteria and showed statistically significant improvements in clinical outcomes, including pain, physical function, and stiffness, with PRP treatment. All except two studies showed significant differences between PRP and HA regarding clinical outcomes of pain and function.

Conclusions: PRP intra-articular injection of the knee may be an effective alternative treatment for knee OA, especially in patients with mild knee OA. Although some studies suggested that the effect of PRP was no better than HA, we found that it was no worse. A large, multicenter, randomized trial is needed to further assess the efficacy of PRP treatment for patients with knee OA.

Keywords: Knee, Osteoarthritis, Platelet-rich plasma, Hyaluronic acid

Background

Osteoarthritis (OA) is a multifactorial chronic bone and joint disease characterized by articular cartilage degeneration that adversely impacts patient mobility and quality of life [1]. OA has been estimated to affect 27 million people in the United States [2]. In addition, the cartilage is avascular in this condition, and the cells have low mitotic activity. Healing potential is limited once the cartilage is injured, eventually leading to irreversible damage. These effects have a major impact on the functioning and independence of patients [2], especially the elderly. The prevalence of knee OA is 50% among patients aged above 65 years [3], and its main symptoms are knee pain, swelling, and limited mobility; furthermore, it is accompanied by a high prevalence of wide, late, and extensive functional disability.

The goal of treatment for knee OA is to relieve pain, improve function and quality of life, and reduce disability. Intra-articular injection of hyaluronic acid

* Correspondence: 270397188@qq.com
[†]Di Yalong and Han Changxu contributed equally to this work.
[2]Department of Sports Medicine, Second Affiliated Hospital of Inner Mongolia Medical University, Huhehaote 010030, China
Full list of author information is available at the end of the article

(HA) [4], corticosteroids, and platelet-rich plasma (PRP); oral nonsteroidal anti-inflammatory drugs; and physical therapy are important nonsurgical treatment options for knee OA. PRP is an autologous blood product produced by centrifugation of whole blood [5] that yields a concentration of platelets above the baseline value [6, 7].

PRP lacks proper standardization and definition. Differences between some of the key characteristics, including platelet concentration, anticoagulant and coagulation activation agent type, presence of inflammatory white blood cells, and activation level, can significantly affect the biological effect.

Local injection of autologous PRP in animal models has been shown to significantly improve the biomechanical behavior of cartilage and chondrocyte proliferation and to repair cartilage injury [8–10]. Although the relevant literature has moderate applicability and strength of evidence, the current guidelines of the American Association of Orthopedic Surgeons do not recommend or oppose the use of PRP in the treatment of knee OA. However, comparison studies conducted on the use of intra-articular injection of PRP compared with HA for mild or moderate knee OA showed a higher clinical outcome score with PRP than with the latter [11–14]. Therefore, the aim of this systematic review was to analyze randomized controlled trials (RCTs) of PRP and HA to determine whether PRP is superior to HA in the treatment of knee OA.

Methods

Research design

We conducted a systematic review in 2016 to investigate the effectiveness of PRP and HA for the treatment of knee OA.

Study search

This systematic review was registered with PROSPERO on October 4, 2016 (registration ID CRD42016048394). The Preferred Reporting Items for Systematic Reviews guidelines were followed. The Cochrane Central Register of Controlled Trials (CENTRAL) (The Cochrane Library, 2016), PubMed, and Embase (January 2005 to August 2016) databases were searched for English-language, human in vivo studies on the treatment of symptomatic knee OA with intra-articular PRP in comparison with HA treatment. The following keywords were used for the search: "platelet-rich plasma," "PRP," "platelet-rich fibrin," "PRF," "platelet," "plasma," "arthritis," "osteoarthritis," "gonarthrosis," and "degeneration." In addition, presentations and abstracts from annual meetings of the American Academy of Orthopaedic Surgeons, the European League against Rheumatism, the American Academy of Physical Medicine and Rehabilitation, the American College of Rheumatology, and the Osteoarthritis Research Society International (OARSI) were manually searched. The search was performed independently by two reviewers. The search results were reviewed to determine which articles were ultimately included in the study according to inclusion criteria.

Inclusion and exclusion criteria

Inclusion criteria for this study were as follows: (1) RCTs in which knee OA was identified; (2) studies that compared the use of autologous PRP with HA; (3) studies involving PRP and HA intra-articular injection; and (4) English-language, original, randomized comparative trials. The exclusion criteria were as follows: studies with unknown data and methodology and those conducted on patients with knee OA who had additional diseases, such as those with pain or swelling associated with knee joint disease, ligament or meniscus injury, arthritis, blood diseases, serious cardiovascular disease, or infection or those receiving immunosuppressive or anticoagulation therapy.

Outcome measures

The main outcome of the efficacy and response to treatment for recovery used in this systematic review were the Western Ontario and McMaster Universities Osteoarthritis Index (WOMAC) [15], International Knee Documentation Committee (IKDC) [16], Knee Injury and Osteoarthritis Outcome Score (KOOS) [17], EuroQol visual analogue scale (EQ VAS) [18], and Tegner score [19].

Data extraction

On the basis of inclusion and exclusion criteria of the study, two reviewers independently examined the titles and abstracts of studies. The selected studies were included in the systematic review. In case of a difference of opinion between the two reviewers, a third party acted as a referee, and the dispute was resolved by discussion. The following data were extracted from all eligible studies:

1. General study information: title, authors, publication year, and registration number
2. Study characteristics: study design, study setting, and inclusion/exclusion criteria
3. Details of the interventions: dose, frequency of administration, and duration of treatment
4. Primary and secondary outcome measures, including the results for the intervention and the comparison groups from baseline to follow-up, with the effect sizes [20]

The difference between the means, Cohen's *d*, was calculated as follows: M1 – M2/s, where M is the mean value of either group and s is the standard deviation of either group. The other values calculated were the minimum clinically important difference [21] (with an effect size of 0.5) and *P* value.

Effect size (ES) is a name given to a family of indices that measure the magnitude of a treatment effect. Unlike significance tests, these indices are independent of sample size. ES measures are the common currency of meta-analyses that summarize the findings in a specific area of research.

Quality assessment

Two independent reviewers assessed the quality of the included studies using the Cochrane Collaboration risk-of-bias tool as follows:

1. *Strong evidence*: Provided by at least two studies with a low risk of bias and by generally consistent findings in all studies (≥ 75% of the studies reporting consistent findings)
2. *Moderate evidence*: Provided by one study with a low risk of bias and/or at least two studies with a high risk of bias and by generally consistent findings in all studies (≥ 75% of the studies reporting consistent findings)
3. *Limited evidence*: Provided by only one study with a high risk of bias
4. *Conflicting evidence*: Inconsistent findings in multiple studies (≥ 75% of the studies reporting consistent findings)
5. *No evidence*: No studies found

Results

Search results

Of the 242 nonduplicate citations identified from the literature, 17 clinical trials were screened for eligibility (Fig. 1). Of these, 10 articles were excluded for the following reasons: introduction of PRP by arthroscopic surgery (not by injection) (one study), Chinese language (not English) (one study), assessment of PRP in comparison with placebo (not HA) (one study), conference proceeding that did not provide any data (one study), and non-RCTs (six studies).

Description of studies

The characteristics of the included studies, excluded studies, and ongoing studies are provided in the online supplementary materials.

Data analysis

All studies except those by Cerza et al. [22] and Filardo et al. [11] provided the registration numbers. In total, seven articles (908 patients, 908 knees) were analyzed (Table 1), and the study population included 44% men and 56% women with a mean age of 59.8 years. The number of injections and the interval and volume of PRP injection are shown in Table 1. The safety data, which summarize the adverse events for each study, are shown in Table 2.

One study used the Ahlbäck classification system of knee OA and showed that 50.0% of patients had grade I, 36.8% had grade II, and 13.2% had grade III. Six studies used the Kellgren-Lawrence classification of knee OA and showed that 8.7% had grade I, 40.7% had grade II, 37.9% had grade III, and 12.7% had grade IV. Filardo et al. [11] reported only the

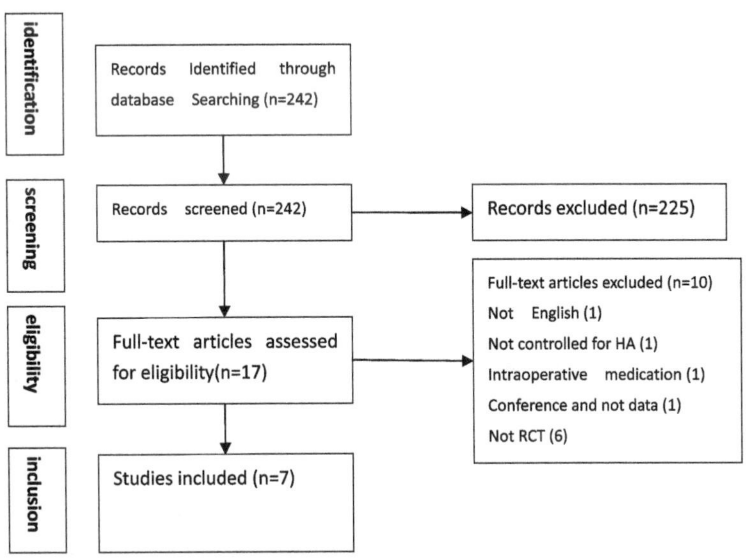

Fig. 1 Search strategy results. *HA* Hyaluronic acid, *RCT* Randomized controlled trial

Table 1 Demographics and methods of included clinical trials

	Cerza et al., 2012 [22]	Filardo et al., 2012 [11]	Sanchez et al., 2012 [24]	Vaquerizo et al., 2013 [25]	Filardo et al., 2015 [23]	Raeissadat et al., 2015 [13]	Montañez-Heredia, et al. 2016 [14]
Registered	Not recorded	Not recorded	Real Decreto 223/2004	Real Decreto 223/2004	ClinicalTrials.gov, NCT01670578	IRCT2014012113442N5	ClinicalTrials.gov, NCT02448407
Subject enrollment date	September 2009–September 2010	Not recorded	January 2008–November 2009	Not recorded	2009–2013	Not recorded	January to March 2014
Country	Italy	Italy	Spain	Spain	Italy	Iran	Spain
Conflict of interest	None	None	None	Not mentioned	Not mentioned	None	None
No. of subjects (knees)	120 (120)	109 (109)	176 (176)	96 (96)	183 (183)	160 (160)	55 (55)
Sex: male, female	53, 67	68, 41	85, 91	38, 58	112, 71	23, 116	21, 32
Mean age, yr	66.4	56.5	59.8	63.6	55.34	58.79	63.9
BMI, kg/m^2	Not recorded	26.5	28.0	30.9	25.7	27.68	29.7
Bilateral vs. unilateral knee injections	Unilateral	Unilateral	Unilateral	Unilateral	Unilateral	Unilateral	Unilateral
Ultrasound-guided injections or not	Not mentioned	Not mentioned	Not mentioned	Not mentioned	Not mentioned	Not mentioned	No
Study group 1	60 Patients	54 Patients	87 Patients	48 Patients	96 Patients	87 Patients	28 Patients
Study group 2	60 Patients	55 Patients	89 Patients	48 Patients	96 Patients	73 Patients	27 Patients
Baseline characteristic differences between groups	No differences	No differences	No differences	No differences	No differences except for age	No differences except for age, sex, WOMAC (pain, function)	No differences
Radiographic classification	Kellgren-Lawrence	Kellgren-Lawrence	Ahlbäck	Kellgren-Lawrence	Kellgren-Lawrence	Kellgren-Lawrence	Kellgren-Lawrence
	Grade I: 25	Average of grade	Grade I: 87	Grade II: 32	Average of grade	Grade I: 6	Grade I: 7
	Grade II: 22	2.2 for PRP group and 2.1 for HA group	Grade II: 64	Grade III: 47	2.0 for PRP group and 2.0 for HA group	Grade II: 91	Grade II: 19
	Grade III: 13		Grade III: 23	Grade IV: 17		Grade III: 75	Grade III: 27
						Grade IV: 28	

Table 1 Demographics and methods of included clinical trials *(Continued)*

	Cerza et al., 2012 [22]	Filardo et al., 2012 [11]	Sanchez et al., 2012 [24]	Vaquerizo et al., 2013 [25]	Filardo et al., 2015 [23]	Raeissadat et al., 2015 [13]	Montañez-Heredia, et al. 2016 [14]
Length of follow-up	24 Weeks	12 Months	6 Months	48 Weeks	12 Months	52 Weeks	6 Months
Outcome scores used	WOMAC	IKDC, Tegner, KOOS, EQ VAS	WOMAC, VAS	WOMAC, Lequesne, OMERACT-OARSI	IKDC, KOOS, EQ VAS, Tegner score	WOMAC, SF-36	VAS, KOOS, EuroQol
Prior surgeries	No	63 Subjects	None in last year	Not recorded	101 Subjects	Not recorded	No
Prior injections	No	Not recorded	None in prior 6 months	None in prior 6 months	Conservative	None in prior 2 weeks	No
PRP no. of injections	4	3	3	3	3	2	3
PRP volume per Injection	5.5 ml	8 ml	12 ml	8 ml	5 ml	4–6 ml	5 ml
Injection interval, wk	1	1	1	2	1	4	2
Injection approach	Superolateral	Not recorded	Superolateral	Superolateral	Not recorded	Anteromedial or lateral midpatellar	Not recorded
Primary and secondary outcomes	WOMAC score before infiltration and at 4, 12, and 24 weeks after first injection	IKDC, EQ VAS, Tegner, and KOOS scores, range of motion and knee circumference changes were evaluated at 2, 6, and 12 months	WOMAC scores at 1, 2, and 6 months	WOMAC and Lequesne scores at 24 and 48 weeks	IKDC, KOOS, EQ VAS, and Tegner scores at baseline and then at 2, 6, and 12 months after last injection	WOMAC and SF-36 scores at 52 weeks	VAS, KOOS, EuroQol following the third infiltration and after 3 and 6 months following final infiltration

Abbreviations: EQ VAS EuroQol visual analogue scale, *IKDC* International Knee Documentation Committee, *KOOS* Knee Injury and Osteoarthritis Outcome Score, *OMERACT-OARSI* Outcome Measures in Rheumatology Osteoarthritis Research Society International, *PRP* Platelet-rich plasma, *SF-36* 36-Item Short Form Health Survey, *VAS* Visual analogue scale, *WOMAC* Western Ontario and McMaster Universities Osteoarthritis Index

Table 2 Safety data

Study	Adverse events
Cerza et al. [22]	No adverse reactions. None were observed in our series.
Filardo et al., 2012 [11]	Only minor adverse events were detected in some patients, such as mild pain and effusion after the injections, in particular in the PRP group, where a significantly higher post-injective pain reaction was observed ($P = 0.039$). However, this reaction was self-limiting within a few days and did not compromise the overall outcome.
Sanchez et al.. [24]	Adverse events were generally mild and evenly distributed between the groups ($P < 0.811$). Most of these adverse events (96% in the PRGF-Endoret® group and 92% in the HA group) were not related to the type of treatment.
Vaquerizo et al. [25]	Sixteen adverse events, 8 in the PRGF-Endoret® group and 8 in the HA group, were reported during the study. Adverse events were generally mild and evenly distributed between the groups ($P = 0.610$). Seven of 8 adverse events in the HA group and all the events in the PRGF-Endoret® group were related to pain associated with the infiltration.
Filardo et al., 2015 [23]	Two patients reported severe pain and swelling after HA injections, while no major adverse events were noted in the PRP group. However, PRP presented overall significantly more postinjection swelling and pain.
Raeissadat et al......... [13]	The present authors had previously performed studies to evaluate the clinical application of PRP, and recorded safety and positive findings. It was a prospective study published in 2013 on 60 patients treated with two injections of PRP (1 every 4 weeks).
Montañez-Heredia et al. [14]	Adverse events relating to infiltration were infrequent, mild and appeared immediately, and their distribution between both groups did not show significant differences. There was pain related to infiltration in nine of 27 PRP injections and in four of 26 for HA, but only one patient (in PRP group) had transitory swelling that resolved itself. No relationship between these events and the growth factor or blood cell composition of PRP was found.

HA Hyaluronic acid, *PRGF-Endoret®* Plasma rich in growth factors, *PRP* Platelet-rich plasma

average Kellgren-Lawrence grades for HA and PRP groups (2.1 and 2.2, respectively), and therefore their study was not included in the grade-percentage stratification mentioned above. Six articles reported a body mass index < 32 kg/m^2 (26.5, 28.0, 30.9, 25.7, 27.68, and 29.7 kg/m^2), and one article did not report the body mass index (Filardo et al. [11]). The average age ranged from 55 to 67 years.

Of the of seven articles, four studies used the WOMAC for outcome scores, two used the IKDC, three used the KOOS, one used the 36-item Short Form Health Survey, one used Tegner scoring, four used the VAS, and one used the Lequesne index.

Regardless of the outcome measures, all studies consistently demonstrated the efficacy of PRP in improving function and quality of life and reducing pain among patients with knee OA. Five studies showed that PRP is superior to HA in the treatment of knee OA, and two studies (by the same authors) showed no difference between the two treatments (Table 3).

In one study, the two groups that reached the minimum clinically important difference also showed a statistically significant difference in WOMAC scores, with a greater effect in the PRP group [22]. Two studies reported that both groups had clinical improvement at follow-up evaluation, but the comparison between the two groups did not show a statistically significant difference in all scores evaluated [11, 23]. In the study by Sanchez et al. [24], the rate of response to PRGF-Endoret® (BTI Biotechnology Institute, Blue Bell, PA, USA) was 14.1% higher than that of HA (95% CI, 0.5–27.6; $P = 0.044$). Regarding the secondary outcome measures, the rate of response to PRGF-Endoret® was higher than that to HA in all cases, although the difference did not reach statistical significance [24].

One study showed that at 24 and 48 weeks, the rate of response to PRGF-Endoret® was significantly higher than that to HA for all parameters, including pain, stiffness, and physical function, on the WOMAC, Lequesne index, and OMERACT-OARSI scales [25]. At the 12-month follow-up, Raeissadat et al. [13] reported that the WOMAC pain score significantly improved in both the PRP and HA groups. Although all achieved the minimum clinically important difference, but the results were significantly better in the PRP group (ES, 1.1) than in the HA (ES, 0.5) group ($P < 0.001$) [13]. Montañez-Heredia et al. [14] reported that at 3 and 6 months after treatment completion, the results in the PRP group was superior to those in the HA group in terms of VAS and KOOS scores [14]. Some studies showed that PRP was not beneficial to all participants and was associated with degree of knee OA [11, 14, 22, 24].

Risk of bias

The risk of bias in the two RCTs that contributed to the cessation meta-analysis was low across all domains [11, 24]. In the 2012 study by Filardo et al. [11], there were three uncertain risk biases. Categorization of the included studies by the nature of their design showed that all studies were at high risk of selection bias. Three of these studies did not blind participants or personnel; considering the nature of the studies, follow-up measures, and contact with researchers, these studies were found to have a risk

Table 3 WOMAC, KOOS, Tegner, Lequesne, IKDC, and SF-36 scores

Study	Pretreatment	Early (0–6 wk)	Middle (6–12 wk)	Late (12–26 wk)	Extended (26–52 wk)
Cerza et al. [22]	ACP: WOMAC 76.9 ± 9.5	ACP: WOMAC 49.6 ± 17.7 ES: 2.8	ACP: WOMAC 39.1 ± 17.8	ACP: WOMAC 36.5 ± 17.9	DNC
		HA: WOMAC 55.2 ± 12.3	ES: 4.0	ES: 4.3	
	HA: WOMAC 75.4 ± 10.7	ES: 1.9 ($P < 0.001$) between groups	HA: WOMAC 57 ± 11.7	HA: WOMAC 65.1 ± 10.6	
			ES: 1.7 ($P < 0.001$) between groups	ES: 1.0 ($P < 0.001$) between groups	
Filardo et al. [11]	PRP: IKDC score 50.2 ± 15.7	DNC	PRP: IKDC score 62.8 ± 17.6 ES: 0.8	PRP: IKDC score 64.3 ± 16.4 ES: 0.9	PRP: IKDC score 64.9 ± 16.8 ES: 0.9
	KOOS symptoms 64.0 ± 17.9		KOOS symptoms 71.9 ± 17.0 ES: 0.4	KOOS symptoms 73.0 ± 18.3 ES: 0.5	KOOS symptoms 71.3 ± 17.9 ES: 0.4
	Pain 65.4 ± 17.7		Pain 71.9 ± 17.0 ES: 0.4	Pain 74.2 ± 19.6 ES: 0.5	Pain 74.0 ± 19.4 ES: 0.5
	ADL 69.9 ± 20.0		ADL 81.2 ± 17.9 ES: 0.6	ADL 79.1 ± 19.0 ES: 0.5	ADL 77.9 ± 20.6 ES: 0.4
	Sport 37.6 ± 24.7		Sport 48.8 ± 25.9 ES: 0.5	Sport 48.7 ± 29.5 ES: 0.5	Sport 47.4 ± 28.2 ES: 0.4
	QOL 34.9 ± 18.8		QOL 48.8 ± 25.9 ES: 0.7	QOL 48.0 ± 23.1 ES: 0.7	QOL 50.5 ± 22.6 ES: 0.8
	Tegner score 2.9 ± 1.4				Tegner score 3.8 ± 1.3 ES: 0.6
	HA: IKDC score 47.4 ± 15.7		HA: IKDC score 61.4 ± 16.2	HA: IKDC score 61.0 ± 18.2	HA: IKDC score 61.7 ± 19.0
			ES: 0.9	ES: 0.9	ES: 0.9
	KOOS		KOOS	KOOS	KOOS
	Symptoms 67.8 ± 15.7		Symptoms 71.6 ± 16.3 ES: 0.2	Symptoms 74.3 ± 16.0 ES: 0.4	Symptoms 74.2 ± 17.5 ES: 0.4
	Pain 63.1 ± 17.4		Pain 71.1 ± 18.6 ES: 0.5	Pain 73.2 ± 18.1 ES: 0.6	Pain 74.0 ± 19.4 ES: 0.6
	ADL 67.8 ± 21.0		ADL 78.2 ± 17.4 ES: 0.5	ADL 77.3 ± 18.6 ES: 0.5	ADL 77.3 ± 19.8 ES: 0.5
	Sport 34.2 ± 23.9		Sport 45.0 ± 24.1 ES: 0.5	Sport 44.7 ± 27.8 ES: 0.5	Sport 46.6 + −27.9 ES: 0.5
	QOL 33.6 ± 18.0		QOL 45.5 ± 23.9 ES: 0.7	QOL 48.5 ± 24.7 ES: 0.8	QOL 49.2 ± 26.0 ES: 0.9
	Tegner score 2.6 ± 1.2				Tegner score 3.4 ± 1.6 ES: 0.7
					P values not recorded
Sanchez et al. [24]	PRGF: WOMAC	DNC	DNC	PRGF: WOMAC 74.0 ± 42.7 ES: 1.1	DNC
	121.8 ± 44.4			38.2% of patients had 50% decrease in WOMAC pain score 57.3% of patients had 20% decrease in WOMAC pain score	
	Lequesne 9.5 ± 3.0			Lequesne 5.2 ± 3.4 ES: 1.4	
	HA: WOMAC			HA: WOMAC 78.3 ± 48.1	

Table 3 WOMAC, KOOS, Tegner, Lequesne, IKDC, and SF-36 scores *(Continued)*

Study	Pretreatment	Early (0–6 wk)	Middle (6–12 wk)	Late (12–26 wk)	Extended (26–52 wk)
	115.6 ± 45.1			ES: 0.8	
				24.1% of patients had 50% decrease in WOMAC pain score, 52.9% of patients had 20% decrease in WOMAC pain score	DNC
	Lequesne 9.1 ± 3.2			Lequesne 5.4 ± 3.3 ES: 1.2	
				Differences between PRGF and HA for 50% decrease in WOMAC pain score ($P = 0.044$), for 20% decrease ($P = 0.555$), for total WOMAC score ($P = 0.561$), and for Lequesne score ($P = 0.714$)	
Vaquerizo et al. [25]	PRGF: WOMAC 45.9 ± 12.7 Lequesne 12.8 ± 3.8 HA: WOMAC 50.8 ± 18.4 Lequesne 13.1 ± 38	DNC	DNC	For patients with 30% decrease in: WOMAC summed score: rate of response of PRGF was 66, 43, and 23 percentage points higher than that of HA for pain, physical function and stiffness, respectively ($P < 0.001$, $P < 0.001$, $P = 0.02$, respectively). Lequesne score: PRGF group is 56 percentage points higher than HA group ($P < 0.001$) For patients with 50% decrease in: WOMAC summed score: rate of response of PRGF was 43, 29, and 19 percentage points higher than that of HA for pain, physical function and stiffness, respectively ($P < 0.001$, $P = 0.001$, $P = 0.035$, respectively). Lequesne score: PRGF group is 25 percentage points higher than HA group ($P = 0.002$)	For patients with 30% decrease in: WOMAC summed score: rate of response of PRGF was 46, 37, and 40 percentage points higher than that of HA for pain, physical function and stiffness, respectively ($P < .001$, $P < .001$, $P < 0.001$, respectively). Lequesne score: PRGF group 46 percentage points higher than HA group ($P < 0.001$) For patients with 50% decrease in: WOMAC summed score: rate of response of PRGF was 29, 31, and 28 percentage points higher than that of HA for pain, physical function and stiffness, respectively ($P < 0.001$, $P < 0.001$, $P = 0.001$, respectively). Lequesne score: 19 and 2 percentage points in the PRGF and HA groups, respectively
Filardo et al. [23]	PRP: IKDC score 52.4 ± 14.1	DNC	PRP: IKDC score 63.2 ± 16.6 ES: 0.8	PRP: IKDC score 65.0 ± 16.1 ES: 0.9	PRP: IKDC score 66.2 ± 16.7 ES: 1.0
	KOOS Symptoms 65.5 ± 16.6		KOOS Symptoms 72.9 ± 17.0 ES: 0.4	KOOS Symptoms 74.7 ± 16.9 ES: 0.6	KOOS Symptoms 73.9 ± 17.2 ES: 0.5
	Pain 66.1 ± 17.9		Pain 73.8 ± 19.9 ES: 0.4	Pain 74.7 ± 19.3 ES: 0.5	Pain 74.9 ± 19.3 ES: 0.5
	ADL 70.6 ± 19.4		ADL 79.0 ± 19.8 ES: 0.4	ADL 79.1 ± 19.6 ES: 0.4	ADL 78.4 ± 20.7 ES: 0.4
	Sport 37.9 ± 25.0		Sport 48.0 ± 26.1 ES: 0.4	Sport 49.6 ± 28.6 ES: 0.5	Sport 49.3 ± 28.6 ES: 0.5
	QOL 36.0 ± 19.4		QOL 48.4 ± 23.1 ES: 0.6	QOL 49.2 ± 23.4 ES: 0.7	QOL 50.8 ± 24.0 ES: 0.8
	EQ VAS score 73.2 ± 12.0		EQ VAS score 76.3 ± 12.7	EQ VAS score 76.2 ± 12.9	EQ VAS score 77.6 ± 11.1
			ES: 0.3	ES: 0.3	ES: 0.4
	Tegner score 2.9 ± 1.3		Tegner score3.6 ± 1.4 ES: 0.5	Tegner score 3.7 ± 1.5 ES: 0.6	Tegner score 3.7 ± 1.3 ES: 0.6
	ROM 129.6 ± 12.2		ROM 130.6 ± 11.8	ROM 130.3 ± 10.7	ROM 130.2 ± 11.1

Table 3 WOMAC, KOOS, Tegner, Lequesne, IKDC, and SF-36 scores *(Continued)*

Study	Pretreatment	Early (0–6 wk)	Middle (6–12 wk)	Late (12–26 wk)	Extended (26–52 wk)
	TPC 410.0 ± 34.3		TPC 411.4 ± 35.2	TPC 407.2 ± 35.6 ES: 0.1	TPC 402.3 ± 33.4 ES: 0.1
	HA: IKDC score 49.7 ± 13.0		HA: IKDC score 63.5 ± 15.2 ES: 0	HA: IKDC score 63.5 ± 17.1 ES: 0	HA: IKDC score 64.2 ± 18.0 ES: 0
	KOOS Symptoms65.8 ± 16.3		KOOS Symptoms 70.9 ± 16.6 ES: 0.3	KOOS Symptoms 72.7 ± 17.4 ES: 0.4	KOOS Symptoms73.9 ± 18.4 ES: 0.5
	Pain 64.1 ± 16.5		Pain 72.6 ± 17.9 ES: 0.5	Pain74.8 ± 17.6 ES: 0.7	Pain 75.4 ± 19.0 ES: 0.7
	ADL 68.2 ± 20.2		ADL 78.0 ± 17.9 ES: 0.5	ADL78.4 ± 18.6 ES: 0.5	ADL 78.4 ± 19.3 ES: 0.5
	Sport 35.7 ± 24.6		Sport 44.0 ± 25.5 ES: 0.3	Sport 45.1 ± 27.0 ES: 0.4	Sport 46.3 ± 28.1 ES: 0.4
	QOL 35.7 ± 18.2		QOL 47.7 ± 22.1 ES: 0.7	QOL 49.9 ± 23.1 ES: 0.8	QOL 50.9 ± 24.4 ES: 0.8
	EQ VAS score 71.6 ± 13.4		EQ VAS score 73.9 ± 13.7 ES: 0.2	EQ VAS score74.1 ± 15.1 ES: 0.2	EQ VAS score 73.4 ± 15.2 ES: 0.1
	Tegner score 2.8 ± 1.3		Tegner score3.3 ± 1.5 ES: 0.4	Tegner score 3.5 ± 1.5 ES: 0.5	Tegner score 3.4 ± 1.5 ES: 0.5
	ROM 128.2 ± 12.2		ROM 129.0 ± 10.9	ROM 128.0 ± 11.4	ROM 127.4 ± 12.0
	TPC 415.0 ± 34.7		TPC 413.3 ± 34.1	TPC 408.7 ± 32.5	No statistical significance between groups
	No statistical significance between groups		No statistical significance between groups	No statistical significance between groups	
Raeissadat et al. [13]	PRP: WOMAC 39.5 ± 17.06	DNC	DNC	DNC	PRP: WOMAC 18.44 ± 14.35 (*P* < 0.001) ES: 1.2
	Pain 8.46 ± 4.17				Pain 4.03 ± 3.36 (*P* < 0.001) ES: 1.1
	Physical function 2.2 ± 1.76				Physical function 1.19 ± 1.4 (*P* < 0.001) ES: 0.6
	Stiffness 28.91 ± 12.63				Stiffness 13.19 ± 10.39 (*P* < 0.001) ES: 1.2
	SF-36 (PCS) 178.14 ± 81.0				SF-36 (PCS) 255.96 ± 77.59 (*P* < 0.001) ES: 1.0
	SF-36 (MCS) 229.22 ± 95.62				SF-36 (MCS) 269.92 ± 91.48 (*P* < 0.001) ES: 0.4
	HA: WOMAC 28.69 ± 16.69 pain 6.91 ± 3.82 physical function 1.88 ± 1.72 stiffness 19.88 ± 12.32 SF-36 (PCS) 180.4 ± 68.52 SF-36 (MCS) 226.43 ± 97.39				HA: WOMAC 27.46 ± 16.36 (*P* = 0.78) pain 5.08 ± 3.71 (*P* = 0.029) ES: 0.5 physical function 2.14 ± 1.66 (*P* = 0.16) stiffness 19.51 ± 11.9 (*P* = 0.919) SF-36 (PCS) 189.39 ± 103.73 (*P* = 0.37) SF-36 (MCS) 216.91 ± 100.9 (*P* = 0.74) ES: 0.1
Montañez-Heredia et al. [14]	DNC	PRP: EQ Worsening 7.4%	DNC	PRP: EQ Worsening 3.7%	PRP: EQ Worsening 7.4%

Table 3 WOMAC, KOOS, Tegner, Lequesne, IKDC, and SF-36 scores *(Continued)*

Study	Pretreatment	Early (0–6 wk)	Middle (6–12 wk)	Late (12–26 wk)	Extended (26–52 wk)
		Similar 74.1%		Similar 48.1%	Similar 48.1%
		Improvement 18.5%		Improvement 48.1%	Improvement 44.4%
		50% decrease VAS: 55.5%		50% decrease VAS: 55.5%	50% decrease VAS: 44.4%
		HA: EQ Worsening 0%		HA: EQ Worsening 11.5%	HA: EQ Worsening 15.4%
		Similar 65.4%		Similar 53.8%	Similar 50.0%
		Improvement 34.6%		Improvement 34.6%	Improvement 34.6%
		50% decrease VAS: 57.7%		50% decrease VAS: 30.7%	50% decrease VAS: 42.3%
				KOOS: For patients with arthritis grade II, ADL at 3-month follow-up improved significantly on the KOOS scale in the PRP group as compared with the HA group ($P = 0.040$)	KOOS: At 6 months follow-up, pain decreased for arthritis grade II patients injected with PRP ($P = 0.012$) with improvements in function in daily living ($P = 0.013$) and function in sport and recreation ($P = 0.021$)

Abbreviations: ACP Autologous conditioned plasma, *DNC* study did not collect data during this time period, *ADL* Activities of daily living, *EQ VAS* EuroQol visual analogue scale, *ES* Effect size, *HA* Hyaluronic acid, *IKDC* International Knee Documentation Committee, *KOOS* Knee Injury and Osteoarthritis Outcome Score, *MCS* Mental Component Summary, *OMERACT-OARSI* Outcome Measures in Rheumatology Osteoarthritis Research Society International, *PCS* Physical Component Summary *PRP* Platelet-rich plasma, *QOL* Quality of life, *ROM* Range of motion, *SF-36* 36-Item Short Form Health Survey, *TPC* Transpatellar circumference, *VAS* Visual analogue scale, *WOMAC* Western Ontario and McMaster Universities Osteoarthritis Index

of selection or performance bias or both. In the other studies, the lack of intervention or contact with researchers was assumed to reflect an unlikely significant performance or detection bias.

With regard to random sequence generation (selection bias), 85.71% of RCTs had low bias and 14.29% had high bias. With regard to allocation concealment (selection bias), 57.14% of RCTs had low bias, 28.57% had uncertain bias, and 14.29% had high bias. For blinding of participants and personnel (performance bias), 57.14% of RCTs had low bias and 42.86% had high bias. For blinding of outcome assessment (detection bias), 57.14% of RCTs had low bias and 42.86% had uncertain bias. For incomplete outcome data (attrition bias), 42.86% of RCTs had low bias, 28.57% had uncertain bias, and 28.57% had high bias. With regard to selective reporting (reporting bias), 71.43% of RCTs had low bias, 14.29% had uncertain bias, and 14.29% had high bias. Finally, for other biases, 28.57% of RCTs had low bias, 57.14% had uncertain bias, and 14.29% had high bias. Figure 2 illustrates the bias for each included study.

Discussion

The main aim of the present study was to investigate a novel biological approach to the treatment of knee OA. In recent years, there has been an increase in the prevalence of the use of autologous blood products that might supply cellular and humoral mediators (blood growth factors) for tissue healing in a variety of applications [26]. PRP is a blood product that provides a simple, low-cost, minimally invasive alternative to obtain a concentration of many of these growth factors [27].

This systematic review shows that intra-articular injection of PRP has a modest effect in the treatment of knee OA and is superior to HA [13, 14, 22, 24, 25]. All studies except two by the same authors [11, 23] found PRP to be especially effective in patients with mild knee OA. The main findings of this systematic review are that multiple sequential intra-articular PRP knee injections (range, two to four injections) improved functional outcome scores (WOMAC) at a minimum of 24 weeks [13, 22, 24, 25]. However, no benefit of PRP was observed over the control treatment in terms of other pain measures such as IKDC, KOOS, and VAS.

With regard to the injection protocol in all studies, the present review evaluated the efficacy of once-weekly intra-articular PRP injection administered at least three times at 2–3 months after the first injection, because this regimen and time frame of PRP provide the greatest efficacy. Of the included studies, four used frozen PRP and three used fresh PRP, and four used leukocyte-poor PRP and three used leukocyte-rich PRP (Table 4). Such differences could have resulted from the preparation techniques (frequency/speed/length of centrifugation or the use of ancillary activating/anticoagulant agents), administration techniques (volume/frequency/delivery in terms of means of administration), postadministration rehabilitation protocols, participants' baseline characteristics (age, sex, activity level, or OA grade), and the methodological rigor of

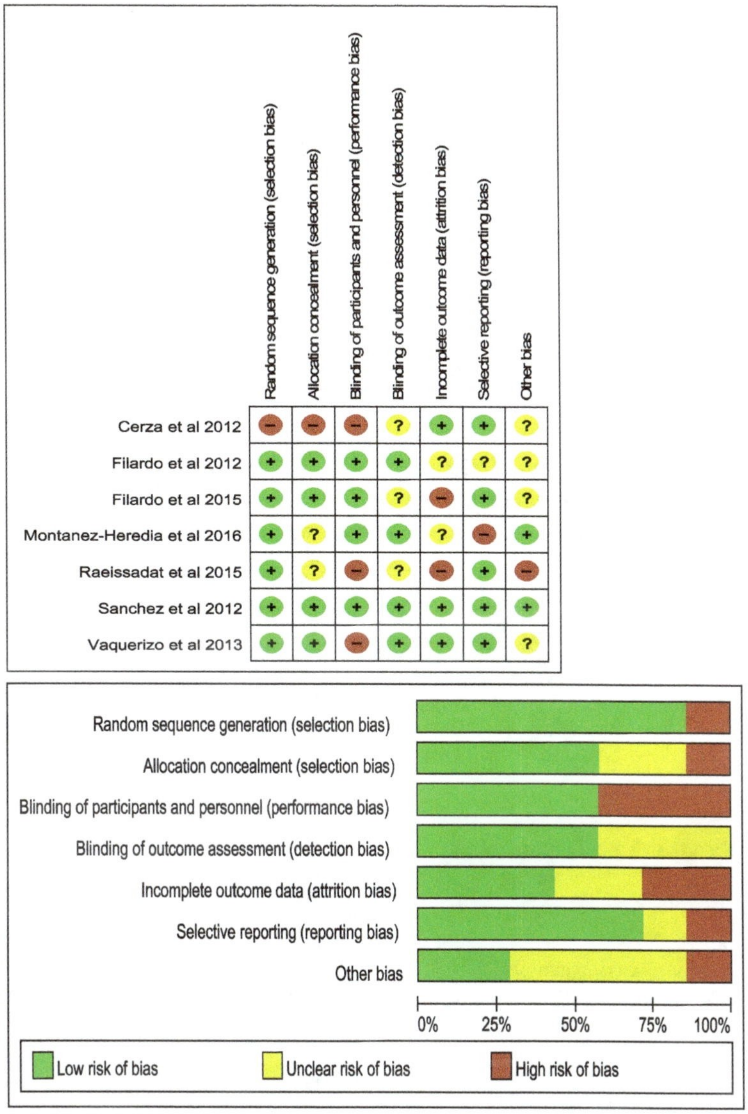

Fig. 2 Risk-of-bias summary: review authors' judgments about each risk-of-bias item for each included study

Table 4 PRP type

Study	Leukocyte-poor/rich PRP	Fresh/frozen PRP
Cerza et al. [22]	Leukocyte-poor PRP	Frozen PRP
Filardo et al. [23]	Leukocyte-rich PRP	Fresh PRP
Sanchez et al. [24]	Leukocyte-poor PRP	Fresh PRP
Vaquerizo et al. [25]	Leukocyte-poor PRP	Frozen PRP
Filardo et al. [23]	Leukocyte-rich PRP	Frozen PRP
Raeissadat et al. [13]	Leukocyte-rich PRP	Fresh PRP
Montañez-Heredia et al. [14]	Leukocyte-poor PRP	Frozen PRP

PRP Platelet-rich plasma

the study. Safety is an important aspect of evaluating PRP as a conservative treatment. In this review, we found no serious adverse local or systemic reactions during and after injection in both the short and long term.

Limitations

This study has a few limitations that need to be addressed. First, only English-language RCTs with high-grade evidence were included, which increases the risk of selection bias. Second, the pooled sample size for this review was limited, with the control arm of PRP including 460 patients and the arm control of HA including 448 patients. This small sample size can limit the power to detect changes that might reach the threshold for a minimal clinically important difference in outcome measures. The third limitation of this study is the lack of a placebo group, meaning that there is no clear evidence that PRP is indeed effective in traumatic or degenerative cartilage lesions. The majority (75%) of the overall treatment effect in OA RCTs is attributable to contextual effects rather than to the specific effect of treatments [21]. However, this review only included studies of high quality that used established outcome measures.

Conclusions

PRP intra-articular injection of the knee may be an effective alternative treatment for knee OA, especially in patients with mild knee OA. However, some studies suggested that PRP is not more effective than HA. A large, multicenter, randomized trial study is needed to further assess the efficacy of PRP treatment for patients with knee OA.

Abbreviations

EQ VAS: EuroQol visual analogue scale; ES: Effect size; HA: Hyaluronic acid; IKDC: International Knee Documentation Committee; KOOS: Knee Injury and Osteoarthritis Outcome Score; OA: Osteoarthritis; OARSI: Osteoarthritis Research Society International; PRGF-Endoret®: Plasma rich in growth factors technology; PRP: Platelet-rich plasma; RCT: Randomized controlled trial; WOMAC: Western Ontario and McMaster Universities Osteoarthritis Index

Acknowledgements

We thank the native English-speaking scientists of Elixigen Company (Huntington Beach, CA, USA) for editing the manuscript.

Funding

This research was not supported by any specific grant from funding agencies in the public, commercial, or not-for-profit sectors.

Authors' contributions

RYZ conceived of and designed the study, performed the analysis, interpreted the results, and wrote the manuscript. DYL and HCX performed the literature search and data extraction and wrote the manuscript. DYL, HCX, and ZL revised the manuscript and acquired data. All authors read and approved the final manuscript.

Competing interests

The authors declare that they have no competing interests.

Author details

[1]Department of Medical Imaging, Hebei General Hospital, Shijiazhuang 050051, China. [2]Department of Sports Medicine, Second Affiliated Hospital of Inner Mongolia Medical University, Huhehaote 010030, China.

References

1. Richmond J, Hunter D, Irrgang J, et al. American Academy of Orthopaedic Surgeons clinical practice guideline on the treatment of osteoarthritis (OA) of the knee. J Bone Joint Surg Am. 2010;92(4):990–3.
2. Van Manen MD, Nace J, Mont MA. Management of primary knee osteoarthritis and indications for total knee arthroplasty for general practitioners. J Am Osteopath Assoc. 2012;112(11):709–15.
3. Arden N, Nevitt MC. Osteoarthritis: epidemiology. Best Pract Res Clin Rheumatol. 2006;20(1):3–25.
4. Jevsevar D. Treatment of Osteoarthritis of the Knee: Evidence-based Guideline, 2nd Edition. J Am Acad Orthop Surg. 2013;21(9):571–6.
5. Marx R. Platelet-rich plasma (PRP): what is PRP and what is not PRP? Implant Dent. 2001;10(4):225–8.
6. Nguyen US, Zhang Y, Zhu Y, Niu J, Zhang B, Felson DT. Increasing prevalence of knee pain and symptomatic knee osteoarthritis: survey and cohort data. Ann Intern Med. 2011;155(11):725–32.
7. van Buul GM, Koevoet WL, Kops N, et al. Platelet-rich plasma releasate inhibits inflammatory processes in osteoarthritic chondrocytes. Am J Sports Med. 2011;39(11):2362–70.
8. Perdisa F, Filardo G, Di Matteo B, Marcacci M, Kon E. Platelet rich plasma: a valid augmentation for cartilage scaffolds? A systematic review. Histol Histopathol. 2014;29(7):805–14.
9. Mifune Y, Matsumoto T, Takayama K, et al. The effect of platelet-rich plasma on the regenerative therapy of muscle derived stem cells for articular cartilage repair. Osteoarthritis Cartilage. 2013;21(1):175–85.
10. Kwon DR, Park GY, Lee SU. The effects of intra-articular platelet-rich plasma injection according to the severity of collagenase-induced knee osteoarthritis in a rabbit model. Ann Rehabil Med. 2012;36(4):458–65.
11. Filardo G, Kon E, Martino A, et al. Platelet-rich plasma vs hyaluronic acid to treat knee degenerative pathology: study design and preliminary results of a randomized controlled trial. BMC Musculoskelet Disord. 2012;13(1):229.
12. Patel S, Dhillon MS, Aggarwal S, Marwaha N, Jain A. Treatment with platelet-rich plasma is more effective than placebo for knee osteoarthritis: a prospective, double-blind, randomized trial. Am J Sports Med. 2013;41(2):356–64.
13. Raeissadat SA, Rayegani SM, Hassanabadi H, et al. Knee osteoarthritis injection choices: platelet-rich plasma (PRP) versus hyaluronic acid (a one-year randomized clinical trial). Clin Med Insights Arthritis Musculoskelet Disord. 2015;8:1–8.
14. Montañez-Heredia E, Irízar S, Huertas PJ, et al. Intra-articular injections of platelet-rich plasma versus hyaluronic acid in the treatment of osteoarthritic knee pain: a randomized clinical trial in the context of the Spanish National Health Care System. Int J Mol Sci. 2016;17(7):1064.
15. Bellamy N, Buchanan W, Goldsmith C, Campbell J, Stitt L. Validation study of WOMAC: a health status instrument for measuring clinically important patient relevant outcomes to antirheumatic drug therapy in patients with osteoarthritis of the hip or knee. J Rheumatol. 1988;15(12): 1833–40.
16. Hefti E, Müller W, Jakob RP, Stäubli HU. Evaluation of knee ligament injuries with the IKDC form. Knee Surg Sports Traumatol Arthrosc. 1993;1(3–4):226.
17. Roos EM, Lohmander LS. The Knee injury and Osteoarthritis Outcome Score (KOOS): from joint injury to osteoarthritis. Health Qual Life Outcomes. 2003;1(1):64.
18. Group E. EuroQol—a new facility for the measurement of health-related quality of life. Health Policy. 1999;16(3):199–208.
19. Tegner Y, Lysholm J. Rating systems in the evaluation of knee ligament injuries. Clin Orthop Relat Res. 1985;198(198):43–9.
20. Cohen J. Statistical power analysis for the behavioral sciences. 2nd ed. Hillsdale: Lawrence Erlbaum Associates; 1988.
21. Zou K, Wong J, Abdullah N, et al. Examination of overall treatment effect and the proportion attributable to contextual effect in osteoarthritis: meta-analysis of randomised controlled trials. Ann Rheum Dis. 2016;75(11):1964–70.
22. Cerza F, Carnì S, Carcangiu A, et al. Comparison between hyaluronic acid and platelet-rich plasma, intra-articular infiltration in the treatment of gonarthrosis. Am J Sports Med. 2012;40(12):2822–7.
23. Filardo G, Matteo B, Martino A, et al. Platelet-rich plasma intra-articular knee injections show no superiority versus viscosupplementation: a randomized controlled trial. Am J Sports Med. 2015;43(7):e79945.
24. Sanchez M, Fiz N, Azofra J, et al. A randomized clinical trial evaluating plasma rich in growth factors (PRGF-Endoret) versus hyaluronic acid in the short-term treatment of symptomatic knee osteoarthritis. Arthroscopy. 2012; 28(8):1070–8.
25. Vaquerizo V, Plasencia MA, Arribas I, et al. Comparison of intra-articular injections of plasma rich in growth factors (PRGF-Endoret) versus Durolane hyaluronic acid in the treatment of patients with symptomatic osteoarthritis: a randomized controlled trial. Arthroscopy. 2013;29(10):1635–43.
26. Bendinelli P, Matteucci E, Dogliotti G, et al. Molecular basis of anti-inflammatory action of platelet-rich plasma on human chondrocytes: mechanisms of NF-κB inhibition via HGF. J Cell Physiol. 2010;225(3):757–66.
27. Schmidt MB, Chen EH, Lynch SE. A review of the effects of insulin-like growth factor and platelet derived growth factor on in vivo cartilage healing and repair. Osteoarthritis Cartilage. 2006;14(5):403–12.

18

Sex differences in the association of skin advanced glycation endproducts with knee osteoarthritis progression

Charles B. Eaton[1,2,3*], Maria Sayeed[4], Syeda Ameernaz[3], Mary B. Roberts[3], John D. Maynard[5], Jeffrey B. Driban[6] and Timothy E. McAlindon[6]

Abstract

Background: The accumulation of advanced glycation endproducts in articular cartilage has been suggested as an etiologic factor in the development and progression of knee osteoarthritis (KOA).

Methods: We conducted a prospective cohort study of skin advanced glycation endproducts (sAGEs) measured non-invasively by skin intrinsic fluorescence and the relationship between sAGE KOA progression in 160 men and 287 women in a sub-cohort of the Osteoarthritis Initiative at a single site. KOA progression was measured by yearly changes in Osteoarthritis Research Society International (OARSI)-defined joint space narrowing (JSN) and by yearly changes in joint space width (JSW) from baseline to 48 months. Sex-stratified repeated measures, mixed models to account for correlation between the knees within persons and adjusted for age, body mass index (BMI), Kellgren-Lawrence (KL) grade, beam angle and rim-to-rim distance were utilized.

Results: Increasing tertiles of sAGE measured at 36 months were associated with greater JSN over 4 years in men but not in women. The percentage of knees with JSN at 48 months, by tertiles of sAGE, were 7.0%, 16.0% and 17.7% in men (p for linear trend = 0.03) and 11.4%, 14.4% and 8.4% in women (p for linear trend = 0.33). Using change in JSW as the outcome, a similar trend was found in men but it was not statistically significant in fully adjusted models and no association was found in women.

Conclusion: This study provides preliminary evidence that sAGEs independent of age and BMI, are associated with knee JSN in men but not in women.

Keywords: Advanced glycation endproducts, Knee osteoarthritis, Progression, Sex differences

Background

Osteoarthritis (OA) is characterized by the progressive destruction of articular cartilage and is strongly and positively associated with chronological age, but the mechanism by which aging contributes to this increased susceptibility is largely unknown. Recently the hypothesis has been promulgated that accumulation of advanced glycation endproducts (AGEs) that are associated with cumulative glycemic exposure, oxidative stress and aging might explain some or most of this association [1]. Alterations in the extracellular matrix and loss of resident cells to repair this matrix damage induced by oxidative stress and AGEs have been suggested as explanations for the progressive articular damage associated with aging. AGEs are the endproducts of spontaneous reactions of reducing sugars with proteins, or non-enzymatic glycation found in tissues throughout the human body. These sugar-protein products are stabilized in humans through a group of complicated biochemical reactions (Maillard reactions) that produce a range of pigmented, fluorescent and glucose-derived protein cross-links that are collectively known as AGEs. Most AGEs have not been characterized in human systems; therefore a few markers of the non-enzymatic glycation process have been used to study their effects on human biology. AGEs form at accelerated rates in many tissues in patients with diabetes mellitus

* Correspondence: CEaton@CareNE.org
[1]Alpert Medical School of Brown University, Providence, USA
[2]School of Public Health of Brown University, Providence, USA
Full list of author information is available at the end of the article

and therefore have been largely studied to better understand this disease and its complications [2–4]. AGEs have been associated with the several other age-related chronic diseases including Alzheimer's dementia, and cardiovascular disease [5–8]. Pentosidine, a fluorescent AGE formed by lysine and arginine residues, is a highly sensitive marker of AGE and is often used to characterize the whole family of AGEs in human tissues. Pentosidine has been shown to accumulate in the collagen matrix of skin, lens, and articular cartilage [1].

Of particular importance in OA, low turnover tissues such as articular cartilage appear to be particularly sensitive to the accumulation of AGEs regardless of glucose metabolic status [1, 7]. Several lines of evidence have been reported that suggest that the accumulation of AGEs in articular cartilage might be an important mechanism in the association between aging and OA. First, articular chondrocytes express the receptors of advanced glycation endproducts in humans [9]. Second, in dog models of experimentally induced OA, elevated levels of AGEs lead to more severe OA based upon histologic grading, increased collagen damage and enhanced release of proteoglycans [10]. Third, human articular cartilage incubated in AGEs demonstrates a dose-dependent increase in AGEs that is associated with increased stiffness of the collagen network and decreases in the tensile strength of the collagen network suggesting that accumulation of AGE crosslinks might be an important putative mechanism in the development or progression of OA [11]. Senoult et al. [12] found increased levels of pentosidine, an advanced glycation endproduct in the serum and synovial fluid of patients with knee OA compared to controls. Both the serum and synovial fluid pentosidine levels correlated with synovial fluid cartilage oligomeric matrix protein (COMP) but not with radiographic staging of the knee OA. Vos et al. found in cross-sectional analysis that skin pentosidine was associated with increased severity and progression of knee and hip OA [13, 14].

This evidence adds additional support to the concept that AGEs may act as novel biomarkers of the incidence and progression of knee OA. However, not all studies are supportive of this hypothesis. Hunter et al. did not find correlation between urinary pentosidine and cartilage loss in the Boston Osteoarthritis of the Knee Study [15]. In addition, Vos et al. identified an inverse relationship of cartilage pentosidine levels and microscopic, histological and biochemical cartilage damage in samples obtained in total knee replacement [16].

Advanced glycation endproduct serum assays are not widely available due to a complex mixture of trace compounds in tissue proteins and the sophisticated and expensive techniques, such as gas chromatography and mass spectrometry, which are needed to reliably and precisely measure these products. However, when pentosidine is exposed to light in the near-UV and blue spectrum, it emits characteristic wavelengths of light called autofluorescence. Levels of the pentosidine found in skin biopsy specimens are highly correlated with collagen-linked fluorescence of the skin. Recently several groups have developed non-invasive means to measure skin fluorescence and thus indirectly measure skin AGE levels [17–19]. These skin fluorescence levels have been shown to be correlated with collagen-linked fluorescence of the skin and AGE levels in skin biopsy specimens in both human and animal models [20, 21].

We were therefore interested in exploring the association of skin fluorescence with the progression of knee OA by measuring changes in joint space narrowing (JSN) and changes in joint space width (JSW) over a 4-year period.

Methods

Cohort description

This is an approved ancillary study to the Osteoarthritis Initiative (OAI) performed at a single clinical center, the Brown University, Pawtucket, Rhode Island site ($n = 1000$ participants, 2000 knees). Detailed information about the OAI protocol is available (http://oai.epi-ucsf.org) [22]. Briefly, the OAI is a multi-center, longitudinal, prospective observational study of knee OA. The overall aim of the OAI is to develop a public domain research resource to facilitate the scientific evaluation of biomarkers for osteoarthritis as potential surrogate endpoints for disease onset and progression. In 2004–2006, the OAI collected baseline data from four study sites (i.e. Baltimore MD, Columbus OH, Pittsburgh PA and Pawtucket RI, USA) totaling 4796 patients with established OA or at risk of developing knee OA.

Skin intrinsic fluorescent measurements were performed at 36 months at a single clinical center in Pawtucket RI in 728 of the 1000 participants. Knees were excluded from this analysis if they had (1) severe radiographic OA, as evidenced by a baseline Kellgren/Lawrence (K/L) grade of 4 (n = 38) or (2) primarily lateral JSN at any point from baseline to 48 months (n = 94). Additionally, specific follow-up knee data were excluded if there was missing or unsatisfactory knee positioning on the follow-up radiograph (n = 250). Unsatisfactory knee positioning was indicated if the difference in rim distance (from the tibial plateau to the tibial rim closest to the femoral condyle) between that follow-up visit and the baseline visit was >2 mm. This is done to minimize possible effects of knee position on measurement error in the measurement of joint space width (JSW). The analytic cohort comprised 447 participants (733 knees) with a K/L grade of 0–3, and who had skin AGE (sAGE) data available at 36 months (see flow diagram, Fig. 1).

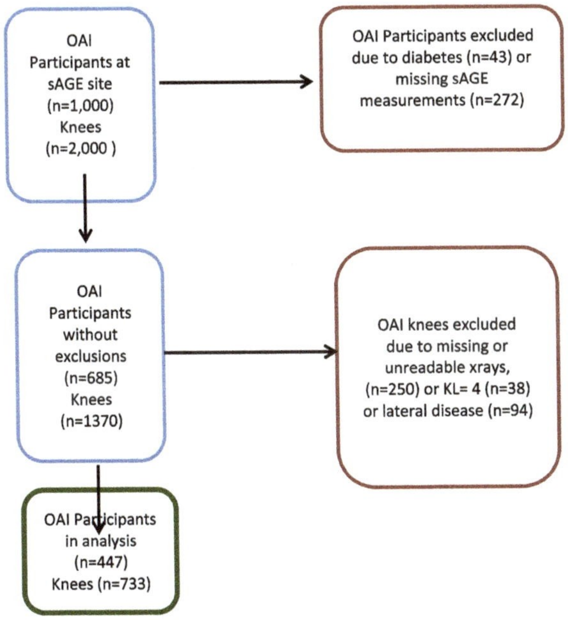

Fig. 1 Flow diagram for determination of Ostearthritis Initiative (OAI) participants used in analysis. *sAGE* skin advanced glycation endproduct, *KL* Kellgren/Lawrence grade

Repeated radiographic measurements at 12, 24, 36 and 48 months were included in this analysis. Due to potential alterations in sAGEs, 43 patients with diabetes mellitus were removed from the analytic dataset.

Radiographic assessment of knees

In the OAI, current assessment of radiographs involved both semi-quantitative assessment of JSN and quantitative assessment of JSW. Using the semi-quantitative approach, JSN was scaled at grade intervals of 0.2 (i.e. 1.2, 1.4, etc.) and any change by grade 0.2 in the medial compartment was considered progression [23].

A quantitative approach was used to provide a precise measure of JSW in millimeters between the adjacent bones of the knee [24, 25]. Multiple JSWs were measured at fixed locations along the joint in the medial compartment, denoted as JSW(x), at intervals of 0.025 for $x = 0.15–0.30$. The reproducibility of this technique and the responsiveness to change have been documented elsewhere [26–28] including one study using OAI data, which demonstrated responsiveness that compared favorably to magnetic resonance imaging (MRI) [26]. We used medial JSW at $x = 0.25$ with the best responsiveness of change to quantify the progression of OA [28]. We defined the repeated measures of the changes in JSW from baseline to 12, 24, 36 and 48 months as one of the outcome variables. To account for changes in beam angle and alignment at each visit, which introduces measurement error in serial JSW measurement and JSN assessments, we also adjusted for changes of the beam angles and rim distances (from the tibial plateau to the tibial rim closest to the femoral condyle between follow-up visits and baseline). For these analyses, we used the publically available quantitative JSW measurements (version 06/17/2013, online at http://oai.epi-ucsf.org) and the semi-quantitative JSN readings (kXR_SQ_BU, version 06/17/2013, online at http://oai.epi-ucsf.org.

Skin intrinsic fluorescence measurement

Levels of AGEs were determined using spectroscopic measurement of sAGEs at the 36-month visit [19, 21]. We measured sAGE using the SCOUT DS (VeraLight Inc., Albuquerque, NM). sAGE measures skin intrinsic fluorescence using a specifically designed fiber-optic probe that sends near-UV and blue excitation light to the forearm skin of the subject and the resulting skin fluorescence and diffuse reflectance is detected by a charge-coupled device array. In addition, a white-light-emitting diode (LED) illuminated the skin to measure the subject's skin tone and correct the measured fluorescence for skin tone to yield skin intrinsic fluorescence.

The sequentially illuminated, excitation LEDs in the instrument have peak wavelengths of 375, 405, 420, 435, and 460 nm. The optical radiation emitted from the skin is dispersed in a modified research-grade spectrometer. A mathematical algorithm is applied to spectrum results to adjust for hemoglobin, skin pigmentation and light scattering. Thus, the subject-specific distortion of the emitted fluorescence is normalized by the measured skin tone to yield the intrinsic fluorescence. For our analysis, we used the excitation wavelength of 375 nm and emission wavelengths of 435–660 nm, which are correlated with crosslinks of collagen, flavin adenine dinucleotide (FAD) and nicotinamide adenine dinucleotide hydride (NADH) and thus, represent sAGEs and oxidative stress most likely associated with accumulation in articular cartilage. The output is scaled 0–100, with higher levels associated with higher levels of AGEs.

Covariates

Sociodemographic factors measured at baseline included race/ethnicity, age, sex, smoking status, education years, and income. Race/ethnicity (African American, white or other race) was self-reported. Age, sex and smoking status (never, past or current) were self-reported. Body mass index (BMI) was measured by physical exam and was calculated from measured height and weight (weight (kg)/height (m)^2) was classified into normal weight (BMI 18.5–24.9), overweight (BMI 25.0–29.9), or obese (BMI ≥30). Waist circumference was measured at the umbilicus twice and the average taken. sAGE levels were examined by smoking status and found to be equivalent in current and past smokers. The smoking status variable was restructured for further analysis into never smoked versus current and past smoking.

Statistical analysis

The focus of the analysis was to assess the association between sAGEs and change in JSN and JSW over the study period. As sAGEs were not normally distributed we rank-ordered the data and categorized sAGEs into sex-specific tertiles. The outcomes were repeated measures of the change in JSN and JSW from baseline to 12, 24, 36 and 48 months. We tested for interaction by sex using the F test and found it was significant ($p = 0.007$ for JSN and $p = 0.008$ for JSW). Therefore, separate models of repeated measures for men and women were used to test the independent association between sAGEs and the change in JSN and JSW over time. Because of the hierarchical structure of the data (participant, knee, measures over time), linear mixed models were used to account for within-subject correlation and for the correlation of repeated measures at the knee for JSW and logistic mixed models for JSN. We additionally adjusted for beam angle and rim-to-rim distance to account for changes in JSW and JSN due to changes in position.

We evaluated crude models and models adjusted for age, BMI, and baseline K/L grade to evaluate the effect of increasing tertiles of sAGEs on JSN and JSW over the 4-year period from baseline to year 4. While smoking status and hypertension were associated with sAGE levels, they were not associated with progression of knee OA in men, and when added to our models in women they did not change the results of the analysis, and therefore these variables were not incorporated into our multiple variable models. All data analyses were conducted using SAS, version 9.2 (Cary, NC, USA).

Results

sAGE scores ranged from 18.7 to 69.5 in men and 17.8 to 59.7 in women. We evaluated 160 men (255 knees) and 287 women (478 knees). Sex-specific ranges for each tertile of sAGEs and the cross-sectional associations between sAGEs and baseline characteristics are given in Table 1. Only older age and hypertension were associated with increasing levels of sAGEs in both sexes. Past and current smoking was associated with increasing levels of sAGEs in men only. Of note in women, the lowest tertile of sAGEs was associated with the greatest abdominal circumference and the percentage of women with obesity, contrary to the direction that was expected.

Due to multiple exclusions and measurement of sAGEs at a single site, we were concerned about potential selection bias and issues of generalizability. We therefore compared our sample to those excluded and to the overall OAI sample (Additional file 1: Table S1). The analytic sample differed from those excluded at the site where sAGEs were measured in terms being a slightly younger age compared to the excluded sample, and we noted fewer changes in JSW over the 4 years of measurement in the analytic sample when compared to the excluded sample at the site of measurement of sAGEs. The participants at the site where sAGEs were measured differed from the eligible participants in the overall OAI sample in that a higher percentage were women, there were fewer African Americans, more past or present smokers, greater abdominal circumference, lower diastolic blood pressure, less hypertension, lower K/L grades and less change in JSW.

The percentage of men and women with worsening JSN are given by tertile of sAGEs in Table 2, comparing a crude model and fully adjusted models of age, BMI, K/L grade, rim distance and beam angle. In all models there was a monotonically increased relationship between worsening JSN and sAGEs in men but not in women, with 9%, 16.9% and 20.9% progression in men in the base models and 13.7%, 19.6% and 13.4% in women in the base models. Adjusting for age, BMI, and K/L grade individually in men had little effect on the estimates and with full adjustment the test for trend remained statistically significant ($p = 0.03$). For women the null results (p for trend = 0.93) persisted with adjustment for potential confounding (p for trend = 0.33).

Measured change in JSW at a fixed point in the medial tibia as a measure of progression of OA by tertile of sAGEs are given in Table 3, comparing crude, and fully adjusted models of age, BMI, and K/L grade. In the crude model in men there was a significant monotonically increased relationship between JSW by tertile of sAGEs (p for trend = 0.02). However in the full model (p for linear trend = 0.15) the relationship was no longer statistically significant. Similar to the JSN analysis, there was no relationship between tertiles of sAGEs and loss of JSW in women over serial yearly measurements.

We performed several sensitivity analyses, adding patients with diabetes mellitus to our study population, and only evaluating the white participants due to concerns that the skin autofluorescence would be affected by skin pigmentation. Including patients with diabetes mellitus did not materially affect our results, with a significant p value for trend for association between tertiles of sAGEs and JSN in men (p trend = 0.02) and no relationship in women ($p = 0.27$). Similarly, in comparing tertiles of sAGEs and changes in JSW there was a non-significant trend ($p = 0.14$) in men and no relationship in women ($p = 0.84$). Evaluating white participants only reduced the sample size, and while a similar result was found in terms of trends in men compared to women, they were no longer statistically significant ($p = 0.08$ and 0.39, respectively, for JSN and $p = 0.26$ and 0.94, respectively, for changes in JSW.

Table 1 Tertile of sAGEs and baseline characteristics by sex

	Men				Women				*P* value for sex
	Tertile 1 18.7–28.0	Tertile 2 28.1–33.7	Tertile 3 33.9–69.5	*P* value	Tertile 1 17.8–24.8	Tertile 2 24.9 – 28.9	Tertile 3 29.0–59.7	*P* value	
Subjects, *n*	56	50	54		104	86	97		
Knees, *n*	88	81	86		171	146	161		
BMI, mean (sd)	29.0 (3.4)	29.6 (4.1)	29.5 (3.8)	0.65	30.1 (5.4)	29.0 (5.4)	29.0 (5.5)	0.26	0.98
Age, years, mean (sd)	55.6 (7.7)	61.7 (8.5)	66.2 (8.8)	<0.01	58.8 (9.3)	63.1 (8.4)	64.6 (8.0)	<0.01	0.28
Ethnicity-Hispanic, *n* (%)	1 (1.8)	2 (4.0)	1 (1.9)	0.71	0 (0.0)	2 (2.3)	1 (1.0)	0.29	0.26
Race, *n* (%)									
White	54 (96.4)	49 (98.0)	48 (88.9)	0.21	100 (96.2)	85 (98.8)	91 (93.8)	0.01	0.45
Black	0 (0.0)	0 (0.0)	3 (5.6)		0 (0.0)	0 (0.0)	3 (3.1)		
Other	2 (3.6)	1 (2.0)	3 (5.5)		4 (3.8)	1 (1.2)	3 (3.1)		
Past or current smoking, *n* (%)	21 (37.5)	27 (54.0)	35 (64.8)	0.02	50 (48.1)	43 (50.0)	56 (57.7)	0.36	0.99
Abdominal circumference, mean (sd)	102.26 (9.83)	104.97 (11.28)	105.18 (10.99)	0.28	108.56 (13.53)	106.13 (14.02)	105.79 (12.78)	0.28	0.02
WC > sex cut, *n* (%)	30 (53.6)	33 (66.0)	37 (68.5)	0.22	100 (96.2)	79 (91.9)	91 (93.8)	0.45	<0. 01
Systolic BP, mean (sd)	122 (14.1)	125 (15.9)	128 (13.1)	0.13	122 (14.7)	123 (14.2)	124 (17.8)	0.70	0.12
Diastolic BP, mean (sd)	76 (9.1)	74 (10.4)	73 (9.5)	0.20	71 (8.1)	70 (8.7)	70 (10.6)	0.41	<0.01
HTN, *n* (%)	25 (44.6)	31 (62.0)	43 (79.6)	<0.01	48 (46.2)	53 (61.6)	58 (59.8)	0.06	0.18
Dyslipidemia, *n* (%)	14 (25.0)	16 (32.0)	21 (38.9)	0.29	25 (24.0)	24 (27.9)	32 (33.0)	0.37	0.42
BMI category, *n* (%)									
Normal	3 (8.9)	7 (14.0)	6 (11.1)	0.63	23 (22.1)	23 (26.7)	25 (25.8)	0.65	<0.01
Overweight	32 (57.1)	21 (42.0)	26 (48.2)		28 (26.9)	27 (31.4)	32 (33.0)		
Obese	19 (33.9)	22 (44.0)	22 (40.7)		53 (61.0)	36 (41.9)	40 (41.2)		
Knee K/L grade									
0–1	49 (55.7)	35 (43.2)	40 (46.5)	0.35	73 (42.7)	51 (34.9)	67 (41.6)	0.41	0.02
2–3	39 (44.3)	46 (56.8)	46 (53.5)		98 (57.3)	95 (65.1)	94 (58.4)		
Baseline joint space width, mean (se)	6.069 (0.164)	6.247 (0.170)	6.403 (0.166)	0.36	5.159 (0.114)	5.298 (0.116)	5.329 (0.108)	0.52	<0.01
Baseline joint space narrowing (*n*, %)									
OARSI 0	50 (56.8)	34 (42.0)	35 (40.7)	0.06	99 (57.9)	71 (48.6)	76 (47.2)	0.24	0.90
OARSI 1	23 (26.1)	27 (33.3)	28 (32.6)		38 (22.2)	44 (30.1)	48 (29.8)		
OARSI 2	15 (17.1)	20 (24.7)	23 (26.7)		34 (19.9)	31 (21.2)	37 (23.0)		

BMI **body mass index,** ***BP*** **blood pressure,** ***OARSI*** **Osteoarthritis Research Society International,** ***HTN*** **Hypertension,** ***WC*** **Waist Circumference**

Table 2 Change in joint space narrowing over 4 years by tertile of skin advanced glycation end products (sAGEs)

sAGEs	Crude model	Trend *p* value	Fully adjusted model	Trend *p* trend
Men				
Tertile 1: 18.7–28.0	9.02%	0.010	6.99%	0.028
Tertile 2: 28.1–33.7	16.88%		15.98%	
Tertile 3: 33.9–69.5	20.92%		17.72%	
Women				
Tertile 1: 17.8–24.8	13.67%	0.932	11.39%	0.328
Tertile 2: 24.9–28.9	19.6%		14.39%	
Tertile 3: 29.0–59.7	13.39%		8.44%	

Discussion

In this study of progression of knee OA, using semi-quantitative measurements (of JSN) we found that higher levels of skin AGEs were associated with progression of medial-tibial knee OA in men but not in women, and identified a trend using serial measurements of loss of JSW. These results provide preliminary evidence supporting the hypothesis that AGEs may play an important role in the progression of knee OA, particularly in men.

In the CHECK cohort, Vos et al. [13, 14] demonstrated an association between skin pentosidine and more severe knee OA at baseline, but only a modest association with progression of a combined score of hip and knee OA. Using skin biopsies and measurements of skin pentosidine levels, they did show a weak association ($r = 0.167$, $p = 0.02$) between skin pentosidine levels and K/L score for progression in the hip and knee. This relationship persisted when adjusted for age and BMI. They did not present any sex-specific findings or evaluate a sex-based interaction effect. Using measurements of urinary pentosidine, Hunter et al. did not find any association with cartilage loss in the knee [15]. However, the ability of urinary pentosidine in the setting of normal renal function to reflect the effect of AGEs on cartilage is unknown.

In our study, we identified progression of OA with increased skin AGE levels in men and not in women, suggesting sex differences in the effect of skin AGEs on the progression of OA. This finding could be spurious or could suggest that there are unique sex-specific mechanistic pathways that may lie behind such differences. Sex differences in the prevalence, incidence and severity of radiographic and clinical OA are well-described [29, 30], but specific examination of sex differences in MRI biomarkers or in biomarkers of joint metabolism are few, and results vary considerably [31, 32].

Men compared women have less prevalent and incident knee OA and less severe OA after the age of 55 years [29, 30]. MRI suggests that women have a smaller volume of lower knee cartilage compared to men [31]. Women have higher levels of bone resorption biomarkers [32] whereas men have higher levels of serum hyaluronan (HA), an indicator of synovial inflammation [33]. Karvonen-Guteirrez, Sowers and Heeringa [34] reported relationships between cardiometabolic risk factors and knee OA that were unique to each gender and to obesity status. In non-obese men, BMI and homeostasis model assessment-insulin resistance (HOMA-IR) and leptin, were the risk factors related to knee OA. In obese men,

Table 3 Change in joint space width over 4 years by tertile of skin advanced glycation end products (sAGEs)

sAGEs	Crude model	Trend *p* value	Fully adjusted model	Trend *p* value
Men				
Tertile 1: 18.7–28.0	0.208 (0.058)	0.023	0.247 (0.060)	0.154
Tertile 2: 28.1–33.7	0.288 (0.059)		0.292 (0.058)	
Tertile 3: 33.9–69.5	0.384 (0.057)		0.374 (0.059)	
Women				
Tertile 1: 17.8–24.8	0.216 (0.034)	0.523	0.209 (0.035)	0.838
Tertile 2: 24.9–28.9	0.246 (0.036)		0.219 (0.036)	
Tertile 3: 29.0–59.7	0.184 (0.035)		0.194 (0.035)	

Mean change in joint space width (SE) in mm

BMI was not related to knee OA, but HOMA-IR was strongly related to it. In non-obese and obese women, BMI continued to be a strong predictor of knee OA; however, HOMA-IR was inversely related to knee OA in obese women. In non-obese and obese men, leptin was found to be inversely related to the presence of radiographic OA, whereas leptin was positively associated with radiographic knee OA in obese women. These findings suggest that the effects of metabolic factors on knee OA are different in men and women, similar to our findings related to sAGEs. Indeed, insulin resistance, elevated insulin-like growth factor (IGF)-1, and AGEs are all related to body fat distribution and adipocyte biology, which might partially explain the gender difference found in our study [35–39].

Strengths and limitations

The strengths of this study include the novel use of skin intrinsic fluorescence as a surrogate measure of sAGEs and the use of both JSN and JSW as measures of cartilage loss and thus, progression of knee OA. The limitations include the single measurement of skin intrinsic fluorescence at 36 months, while progression was determined yearly from time zero to 48 months, and thus, a clear temporal sequence potentially reflecting a cause and effect relationship is not present in this study. It is thought that skin fluorescence captures the cumulative exposure of AGEs in collagen and is relatively stable over time compared to serum or urinary pentosidine [17–20]. However, dietary AGEs, trace metals, cigarette smoking and other enzymatic co-factors may affect sAGEs and thus, the stability of a single measurement of sAGEs needs further study. It should, however, be noted that single measures of skin fluorescence are associated with increased risk of diabetes mellitus, cardiovascular disease, renal disease and mortality [2–6].

In addition, given the large number of exclusions and the study being performed at a single site, concerns about selection bias and generalizability are of concern. The lack of difference between included and excluded individuals and between knees for most covariates within the site of measurement of sAGEs is reassuring as it suggests that selection bias is unlikely to explain our results. The lesser changes in JSW in our analytic cohort compared to those excluded at the site of measurement of sAGEs would make it harder to find a significant association, so we may be underestimating the effect of sAGEs on changes in JSW.

We identified a stronger association using semi-quantitative measurement of JSN as a measure of progression compared to the quantitative measurement of changes in JSW, due to greater sensitivity to change using JSN. This may be related to the fact that JSN measurements use serial evaluation of knee radiographs by experienced musculoskeletal radiologists ordered by time, whereas JSW is measured independent of time using a computerized grid system. When comparing changes in JSW, subtle progression of OA that may be missed due to alignment issues obscuring these changes over the same time period may be picked up by experienced musculoskeletal radiologists.

The differences in sex, race and baseline K/L grade in our sample when compared to the overall OAI sample limits the generalizability of our findings and highlights the need for replication of our findings in additional cohorts. Indeed, while the sex differences appear strong they may be spurious due to the relatively small sample size. Elevated sAGEs are associated with pre-diabetes mellitus and diabetes mellitus [2–5]. To account for confounding related to the association between diabetes mellitus with OA and with sAGEs, we excluded participants with known diabetes mellitus; however, this reduced our sample size. We therefore performed additional sensitivity analyses including the 43 patients known to have diabetes mellitus, and the results were nearly identical.

Conclusion

While biomechanical factors are clearly involved in the development and progression of knee osteoarthritis, systemic pathways including innate immunity, inflammation and advanced glycation endproducts are increasingly being recognized as playing a potentially important role in the natural history of osteoarthritis. This study adds credence to this view of the pathophysiology of knee osteoarthritis and suggests that future studies should be performed to examine the advanced glycation endproduct hypothesis.

Abbreviations

AGEs: Advanced glycation endproducts; BMI: Body mass index; FAD: Flavin adenine dinucleotide; JSN: Joint space narrowing; JSW: Joint space width; K/L: Kellgren/Lawrence; KOA: Knee osteoarthritis; LED: Light-emitting diode; MRI: magnetic resonance imaging; NADH: Nicotinamide adenine dinucleotide hydride; OA: Osteoarthritis; OAI: Osteoarthritis Initiative; OARSI: Osteoarthritis Research Society International; sAGE: Skin advanced glycation endproducts

Acknowledgements

VeraLight Corporation provided the Scout DS instrument for data acquisition at no cost.

Funding

Funding for this analysis was provided by contract HHSN2682010000XXC - Reference Number: BAA-NHLBI-AR-10-06 - National Institute of Arthritis and Musculoskeletal and Skin Diseases.

Authors' contributions

CBE designed the study, performed data acquisition, developed the analysis plan, led the interpretation of the results, provided critical revisions to the manuscript and provided the funding for the project. MS wrote the initial manuscript and helped with interpretation of the results. SA helped with the interpretation of the results and provided critical revisions to the manuscript. MBR contributed to the analytic plan, performed the statistical analysis and reviewed/edited the manuscript. JM assisted in data acquisition, reviewed the manuscript and provided critical revisions. JBD contributed to the analysis plan and interpretation of the results, reviewed/edited the manuscript and provided critical revisions. TEMc contributed to the analysis plan and to interpretation of the results, reviewed/edited the manuscript and provided critical revisions to the manuscript. All authors read and approved the final manuscript.

Authors' information

All authors read and approved this manuscript.

Competing interests

John Maynard is former VP of VeraLight and provided the Scout DS skin autofluorsecent machine for data acquisition and data analytic support on the wavelengths to be utilized for skin intrinsic fluorescence, to represent advanced glycation endproducts associated with crosslinking collagen in the skin most similar to articular cartilage. He was not involved in data interpretation or any of the statistical analysis that was un-blinded to outcomes. Charles B. Eaton, MD, Maria Sayeed, MD, Syeda Ameernaz, MD, Mary B. Roberts, MS, Jeffrey B. Driban, PhD, ATC, CSCS and Timothy A. McAlindon, MD have no competing interests.

Author details

[1]Alpert Medical School of Brown University, Providence, USA. [2]School of Public Health of Brown University, Providence, USA. [3]Center of Primary Care and Prevention, Memorial Hospital of Rhode Island, 111 Brewster Street, Pawtucket, RI 02860, USA. [4]Department of Medicine, Memorial Hospital of Rhode Island, 111 Brewster Street, Pawtucket, RI, USA. [5]Vera Light Inc., 800 Bradbury Dr SE # 217, Albuquerque, NM, USA. [6]Division of Rheumatology, Tufts Medical Center, 800 Washington Street, Box 406, Boston, MA, USA.

References

1. Verzijl N, Bank R, TeKoppele J, DeGroot J. AGEing and osteoarthritis: a different perspective. Curr Opin Rheumatol. 2003;15:616–22.
2. Monnier VM, Bautista O, Kenny D, Sell DR, Fogarty J, Dahms W, et al. Skin collagen glycation, glycoxidation, and cross linking are lower in subjects with long-term intensive versus conventional therapy of type 1 diabetes: relevance of glycated collagen products versus HbA1c as markers of diabetic complications. Diabetes. 1999;48:870–80.
3. Genuth S, Sun W, Cleary P, Sell DR, Dahms W, Malone J, et al. Glycation and carboxymethyllsine levels in skin collagen predict the risk of future 10-year progression of diabetic retinopathy and nephropathy in the diabetes control and complications trial and epidemiology of diabetes interventions and complications participants with type 1 diabetes. Diabetes. 2005;54:3103–11.
4. Meerwaldt R, Links TP, Graaff R, Hoogenberg K, Lefrandt JD, Baynes JW, et al. Increased accumulation of skin advanced glycation end products precedes and correlates with clinical manifestation of diabetic neuropathy. Diabetologia. 2005;48:1637–44.
5. Meerwaldt R, Lutgers H, Links T, Graaff R, Baynes J, Gans R, et al. Skin auto fluorescence is a strong predictor of cardiac mortality in diabetes. Diabetes Care. 2007;30:107–12.
6. Asif M, Egan J, Vasan S, Jyothirmayi GN, Masurekar MR, Lopez S, et al. An advanced glycation end product cross-link breaker can reverse age-related increases in myocardial stiffness. Proc Natl Acad Sci U S A. 2000;97:2809–13.
7. Sell DR, Monnier VM. Structure elucidation of a senescence cross-link from human extracellular matrix: implication of pentoses in the aging process. J Biol Chem. 1989;264:21597–602.
8. Nagai R, Hayashi CM, Xia L, Takeya M, Horiuchi S. Identification in human atherosclerotic lesions of GA-pyridine, a novel structure derived from glycoladehyde-modifies proteins. J Biol Chem. 2002;277:48905–12.
9. Loeser R, Yammani R, Carlson C, Chen H, Cole A, Im H, et al. Articular chondrocytes express the receptor for advanced glycation end products, potential role in osteoarthritis. Arthritis Rheum. 2005;52:2376–85.
10. DeGroot J, Verzijl N, Wenting-van M, Jacobs K, Van El B, Van Roermund P, et al. Accumulation of advanced glycation end products as a molecular mechanism for aging as a risk factor in osteoarthritis. Arthritis Rheum. 2004;50:1207–15.
11. Verzijl N, DeGroot J, Zaken C, Braun-Benjamin O, Maroudas A, Bank R, et al. Crosslinking by advanced glycation end products increases the stiffness of the collagen network in human articular cartilage, a possible mechanism through which age is a risk factor for osteoarthritis. Arthritis Rheum. 2002;46:114–23.
12. Senolt L, Braun M, Olejárová M, Forejtová S, Gatterová J, Pavelka K. Increased pentosidine, an advanced glycation end product, in serum and synovial fluid from patients with knee osteoarthritis and its relation with cartilage oligomeric matrix protein. Ann Rheum Dis. 2005;64:886–90.
13. Vos PA, DeGroot J, Huisman AM, Oostveen JC, Marijnissen AC, Bijlsma JW, et al. Skin and urine pentosidine weakly correlate with joint damage in a cohort of patients with early signs of osteoarthritis (CHECK). Osteoarthritis Cartilage. 2010;18:1329–36.
14. Vos PA, Welsing PM, deGroot J, Huisman AM, Oostveen JC, Reijman M, et al. Skin pentosidine in very early hip/knee osteoarthritis (CHECK) is not a strong independent predictor of radiographic progression over 5 years follow-up. Osteoarthr Cartil. 2013;21:823–30.
15. Hunter DJ, LaValley M, Li J, Zhang Y, Bauer D, Nevitt M, et al. Urinary pentosidine does not predict cartilage loss among subjects with symptomatic knee OA: the BOKS study. Osteoarthr Cartil. 2007;15:93–7.
16. Vos PA, Mastbergen SC, Huisman AM, Boer TN, Degroot J, Polak AA, et al. In end stage osteoarthritis, cartilage tissue pentosidine levels are inversely related to parameters of cartilage damage. Osteoarthr Cartil. 2012;20:233–40.
17. Cleary PA, Braffett BH, Orchard T, Lyons TJ, Maynard J, Cowie C, et al. Clinical and technical factors associated with skin intrinsic fluorescence in subjects with type 1 diabetes from the DCCT/EDIC study. Diabetes Technol Ther. 2013;15:466–74.
18. Meerwaldt R, Graaff R, Oomen PH, Links TP, Jager JJ, Alderson NL, et al. Simple non-invasive assessment of advanced glycation endproduct accumulation. Diabetologia. 2004;47:1324–30.
19. Beisswenger PJ, Howell S, Mackenzie T, Corstjens H, Muizzuddin N, Matsui MS. Two fluorescent wavelengths, 440(ex)/520(em) nm and 370(ex)/440(em) nm, reflect advanced glycation and oxidation end products in human skin without diabetes. Diabetes Technol Ther. 2012;14:285–92.
20. Hull EL, Ediger MN, Unione AHT, Deemer EK, Stroman ML, Baynes JW. Noninvasive, optical detection of diabetes: model studies with porcine skin. Opt Express. 2004;12:4496–510.
21. Maynard J, Rohrscheib M, Way J, Nguyen C, Ediger M. Noninvasive type 2 diabetes screening, superior sensitivity to fasting plasma glucose and A1C. Diabetes Care. 2007;30:1120–4.
22. Duryea J, Zaim S, Genant HK. New radiographic-based surrogate outcome measures for osteoarthritis of the knee. Osteoarthr Cartil. 2003;11:102–10.
23. The Osteoarthritis Initiative protocol for the cohort study. http://oai.epi-ucsf.org/datarelease/docs/StudyDesignProtocol.pdf.
24. Felson DT, Gale DR, Elon Gale M, Niu J, Hunter DJ, Goggins J, et al. Osteophytes and progression of knee osteoarthritis. Rheumatology (Oxford). 2005;44:100–4.
25. Sharp JT, Angwin J, Boers M, Duryea J, von Ingersleben G, Hall JR, et al. Computer based methods for measurement of joint space width: update of an ongoing OMERACT project. J Rheumatol. 2007;34:874–83. PMID: 17407243.
26. Duryea J, Neumann G, Niu J, Totterman S, Tamez J, Dabrowski C, et al. Comparison of radiographic joint space width with magnetic resonance imaging cartilage morphometry: analysis of longitudinal data from the Osteoarthritis Initiative. Arthritis Care Res (Hoboken). 2010;62:932–7.
27. Duryea J, Li J, Peterfy CG, Gordon C, Genant HK. Trainable rule-based algorithm for the measurement of joint space width in digital radiographic images of the knee. Med Phys. 2000;27:580–91.
28. Neumann G, Hunter D, Nevitt M, Chibnik LB, Kwoh K, Chen H, et al. Location specific radiographic joint space width for osteoarthritis progression. Osteoarthritis Cartilage. 2009;17:761–5.

29. Srikanth VK, Fryer JL, Zhai G, Winzenberg TM, Hosmer D, Jones G. A meta analysis of sex differences prevalence, incidence and severity of osteoarthritis. Osteoarthr Cartil. 2005;13:769–81.
30. Oliveria SA, Felson DT, Reed JI, Cirillo PA, Walker AM. Incidence of symptomatic hand, hip, and knee osteoarthritis among patients in a health maintenance organization. Arthritis Rheum. 1995;38:1134–41.
31. Maleki-Fischbach M, Jordan JM. New developments in osteoarthritis. Sex differences in magnetic resonance imaging-based biomarkers and in those of joint metabolism. Arthritis Res Ther. 2010;12:212–20.
32. Karsdal MA, Byrjalsen I, Bay-Jensen AC, Henriksen K, Riis BJ, Christiansen C. Biochemical markers identify influences on bone and cartilage degradation in osteoarthritis- the effect of sex, Kellgren-Lawrence (KL) score, body mass index (BMI), oral salmon calcitonin (Sct) treatment and diurnal variation. BMC Musculoskelet Disord. 2010;11:125. doi:10.1186/1471-2474-11-125.
33. Elliot AL, Kraus VB, Luta G, Stabler T, Renner JB, Woodward J, Dragomir AD, Helmick CG, Hockberg MC, Jordan JM. Serum hyaluronan levels and radiographic knee and hip osteoarthritis in African Americans and Caucasians in the Johnston County Osteoarthritis Project. Arthritis Rheum. 2005;52:105–11.
34. Karvonen-Gutierrez CA, Sowers MR, Heeringa SG. Sex dimorphism in the association of cardiometabolic characteristics and osteophytes-defined radiographic knee osteoarthritis among obese and non-obese adults: NHANES III. Osteoarthritis Cartilage. 2012;20:614.
35. Pagura SM, Thomas SG, Woodhouse LJ, Ezzat S, Marks P. Circulating and synovial levels of IGF-I, cytokines, physical function and anthropometry differ in women awaiting total knee arthroplasty when compared to men. J Orthop Res. 2005;23:397–405.
36. Issa RI, Griffin TM. Pathobiology of obesity and osteoarthritis: integrating biomechanics and inflammation. Pathobiol Aging Age Relat Dis. 2012;2. doi:10.3402/pba.v2i0.17470.
37. Berenbaum F, Eymard F, Houard X. Osteoarthritis, inflammation and obesity. Curr Opin Rheumatol. 2013;25:114–8.
38. de Boer TN, van Spil WE, Huisman AM, Polak AA, Bijlsma JWJ, Lafeber FPJG, et al. Serum adipokines in osteoarthritis; comparison with controls and relationship with local parameters of synovial inflammation and cartilage damage. Osteoarthritis Cartilage. 2012;20:846–52.
39. Conde J, Scotece M, Gomez R, Lopez V, Gomez-Reino JJ, Gualillo O. Adipokines and osteoarthritis: novel molecules involved in the pathogenesis and progression of disease. Arthritis. 2011;2011:203901. doi:10.1155/2011/203901. Epub 2011 Aug 18.

Synovial fluid adipokines are associated with clinical severity in knee osteoarthritis: a cross-sectional study in female patients with joint effusion

Joan Calvet[1,2*], Cristóbal Orellana[1], Jordi Gratacós[1,2], Antoni Berenguer-Llergo[3], Assumpta Caixàs[4], Juan José Chillarón[2,5], Juan Pedro-Botet[2,5], María García-Manrique[1], Noemí Navarro[1] and Marta Larrosa[1]

Abstract

Background: Adipokines are related to knee osteoarthritis, but their exact role is not well known. The aim of this study was to evaluate the association between adipokines in synovial fluid and clinical severity in patients with knee osteoarthritis with joint effusion.

Methods: Cross-sectional study with systematic inclusion of female patients with symptomatic primary knee osteoarthritis with ultrasound-confirmed joint effusion. Age, physical exercise, knee osteoarthritis symptoms duration, classical cardiovascular risk factors and different anthropometric measurements were collected. Metabolic syndrome was defined in accordance to National Cholesterol Education Program-Adult Treatment Panel III. Radiographic severity was evaluated according to Kellgren-Lawrence scale and Lequesne index was used to assess clinical severity. Seven adipokines (leptin, adiponectin, resistin, visfatin, osteopontin, omentin and chemerin) and three inflammatory markers (tumor necrosis factor α, interleukin 6 and high sensitivity C-reactive protein) were measured by enzyme-linked immunosorbent assay in synovial fluid.

Results: Kellgren-Lawrence grade, physical exercise, all anthropometric measurements (especially waist circumference), tumor necrosis factor α, and high levels of leptin, resistin, and ostepontin were related to knee osteoarthritis severity. After adjustment for clinical confounders (age, symptom duration, and radiology), anthropometric measurements, inflammatory markers, and all evaluated adipokines, there were independent associations with clinical severity for resistin (directly associated) and visfatin (inversely associated). No other adipokines or inflammatory markers were independently associated with Lequesne index. The association of radiological parameters, physical exercise, and waist circumference with Lequesne index remained after adjustment.

Conclusions: Resistin was directly associated, and visfatin was inversely associated, with clinical severity in female patients with knee osteoarthritis with joint effusion. These associations were more important after adjustment for confounders, especially when all adipokines were evaluated.

Keywords: Knee osteoarthritis, Adipokines, Inflammation, Synovial fluid, Clinical severity

* Correspondence: joan.calvet.fontova@gmail.com
[1]Rheumatology Department, Parc Tauli Sabadell University Hospital, Institute for Research and Innovation Parc Tauli (I3PT), Universitat Autónoma de Barcelona (UAB), 08208 Sabadell, Spain
[2]Departament de Medicina, Universitat Autónoma de Barcelona (UAB), 08003 Barcelona, Spain
Full list of author information is available at the end of the article

Background

Osteoarthritis (OA) is the most prevalent articular disease, and the most common cause of disability in developed and developing countries [1], with knee involvement being the most prevalent and disabling condition [2]. The prevalence of knee osteoarthritis (KOA) increases with age, and, given the aging of population, an even greater impact is expected in the future [3]. The etiology of OA is multifactorial, classically related to mechanical factors, trauma, or overload [2]. Genetic and, more recently, anthropometric, metabolic, and local inflammatory factors have been implicated in the pathophysiology of OA [4]. Different epidemiologic studies have shown a high prevalence of cardiovascular risk factors, such as hypertension, dyslipidemia, diabetes, obesity, and metabolic syndrome (MetS), in patients with KOA [5, 6]. MetS and its individual components are related to severity as measured by pain, disability, and radiography [7]. More recently, some authors have suggested that OA and MetS share a similar biochemical and inflammatory profile, which could explain associations between them and their influence in the severity or progression of the disease [8]. Obesity is, together with age, the most important risk factor related to KOA [9, 10]. In this respect, adipokines such as leptin, adiponectin, resistin, visfatin, and osteopontin, both in plasma and in synovial fluid, have been associated with the frequency and severity of KOA, usually measured by radiographic damage. However, studies of adipokines in synovial fluid were performed in patients with advanced disease undergoing prosthetic surgery and were not focused on severity or on the inflammatory profile of KOA [11–17].

Markers of inflammation in synovial fluid, such as interleukin (IL)-6, tumor necrosis factor α (TNF-α), or high-sensitivity C-reactive protein (hs-CRP), have been associated with severity in KOA in recent studies [18, 19]. In fact, a significant percentage of patients with KOA present with joint effusion, which could be considered as a marker of local inflammation. Patients with KOA with persisting joint effusion could be a particular subset of KOA with special characteristics compared with patients without effusion. These patients make up a group of patients of particular interest in investigations of metabolic inflammation in KOA.

The exact role of adipokines in KOA is not well known, but they may play a significant role indirectly via their link to obesity and directly on OA pathways in many patients. Researchers in different studies have evaluated the relationship between adipokines individually or controlled by some metabolic and other cytokines and clinical severity, but they did not assess the possible interactions when a significant number of adipokines were evaluated or their relationship to local inflammation. The main aim of this study was to evaluate the association of synovial adipokines with clinical severity in patients with KOA and persistent joint effusion. For this purpose, the effect on clinical severity and the biological interactions of adipokines previously studied in KOA were investigated.

Methods

Patients and study design

We conducted a cross-sectional study with systematic inclusion of female patients with symptomatic primary KOA according to American College of Rheumatology criteria [20] who visited our hospital for a monographic OA consultation. The women were aged 50–85 years and had evidence of significant joint effusion based on physical examination and confirmed by ultrasound (≥4 mm on midline suprapatellar line). Symptomatic OA was defined as pain intensity rated as ≥4 on a 10-cm visual analogue scale despite the use of prescribed analgesic drugs for at least 3 months. Only patients reporting persisting knee effusion or with documented effusion in several consultations were entered into the study. Patients with secondary OA were excluded, such as those with a history of trauma, meniscal injury, inflammatory rheumatic or septic conditions, previous knee surgery, any condition that could interfere with pain perception, systemic glucocorticoid intake in the last 6 months, or intra-articular glucocorticoid or hyaluronic acid injection in the last 3 or 6 months, respectively. The recruitment period was October 2013 to June 2015. We included only female patients to homogenize the sample, as there are differences between men and women related to pain perception, anthropometric measures, and fat content and distribution that might influence the adipokine profile [21–23]. This study was approved by the local ethics committee at the Parc Tauli Sabadell University Hospital. All patients included were verbally informed about the study and signed informed consent forms.

Assessments

Information on the following variables was collected: age, physical exercise (never, occasional [less than 150 minutes per week], or regular), tobacco exposure, and KOA symptom duration. Each participant's medical history, specifically regarding the presence of cardiovascular risk factors, was recorded. A diagnosis of hypertension, dyslipidemia, or diabetes was established if already diagnosed or if the participant was receiving treatment for any of these conditions. Anthropometric measurements included weight (kg), height (cm), body mass index (BMI) (kg/m^2), waist circumference (WC) (cm), hip circumference (cm), waist-to-hip ratio (WHR), and percentage of body fat measured using a bioimpedance analyzer (BC-418 MA; Tanita, Arlington Heights, IL, USA) according to a standard protocol. Obesity was defined as a BMI ≥30 kg/m^2. In accordance with the modified criteria of the National Cholesterol Education Program Adult Treatment Panel III, MetS was defined as having three or more of the following conditions: fasting plasma glucose ≥100 mg/dl or treatment with glucose-lowering drugs, arterial blood pressure ≥130/85 mmHg or antihypertensive medication, fasting plasma triglycerides ≥150 mg/dl (1.7 mmol/L) or drug treatment for hypertriglyceridemia, high-density lipoprotein (HDL) cholesterol <50 mg/dl (1.28 mmol/L) or drug therapy to raise HDL cholesterol concentration, and WC ≥88 cm [24]. Radiographic severity was evaluated by anteroposterior knee x-ray examination with the patient in standing position performed in the last 18 months and graded according to the Kellgren-Lawrence (KL) scale (grades 1–4). Time between radiologic evaluation and visit was considered for adjustment in the statistical analysis. Two rheumatologists (JC, CO) evaluated x-rays independently. The Lequesne algofunctional index, a simple and validated questionnaire for pain and disability in KOA with scores ranging from 0 (best) to 24 (worst), was used to assess clinical severity.

Joint aspiration was performed during the visit and at the same time of the day for proper evaluation of synovial adipokines. Synovial fluid was analyzed to ensure noninflammatory fluid (joint cell count <2500 cells) and absence of microcrystals. Synovial samples were stored at −80 °C. Seven adipokines and three inflammatory markers were measured by enzyme-linked immunosorbent assay (ELISA) in accordance with the manufacturers' recommendations for synovial fluid dilutions: leptin (Biocompare, South San Francisco, CA, USA), adiponectin (eBioscience, San Diego, CA, USA), resistin (RayBiotech, Norcross, GA, USA), osteopontin (eBioscience), visfatin (Phoenix Pharmaceuticals, Burlingame, CA, USA), omentin (CUSABIO, Wuhan, China), chemerin (Elabscience, Bethesda, MD, USA), hs-CRP (DRG Diagnostics, Marburg, Germany), and IL-6 and TNF-α (Milliplex HCYTOMAG-60 K-03; Merck Millipore, Billerica, MA, USA) (see Additional file 1 for detailed description). For technical reasons related to ELISA technology (configuration of the plates used), none of these markers could be assessed at the same time for all patients. In order to control for technical variability, the rounds of measurement were considered as an adjustment factor in the statistical analyses.

Statistical methods

Clinical data and laboratory parameters and their association with Lequesne index score were summarized using nonparametric methods. Medians, interquartile ranges, and Spearman's correlations (r) were used for continuous measures, while frequencies and Mann-Whitney or Kruskal-Wallis tests were applied to categorical variables. For estimation of adjusted effects, linear models were fitted with suitable transformation of explanatory variables when necessary in order to fit the model assumptions. The covariates included in the multivariate analyses were age at recruitment, KL grade, time from visit to date of radiologic assessment, and KOA symptom duration. Using this model as a starting point, a stepwise algorithm was used sequentially with the rest of the potential confounders in two stages: first, only anthropometric and metabolic parameters were evaluated; second, inflammatory markers were considered in the resulting model, then each adipokine was added one at a time to the resulting model to assess its association with KOA severity (Table 3, "Adjusted effects" column). Finally, all adipokines were added to the model to assess their association with the Lequesne index after controlling for the anthropometric, metabolic, and inflammatory markers found to be informative in the previous steps, as well as for the rest of the adipokines ("Multivariate model" column in Table 3). For interpretation purposes, the partial correlation coefficient (PCC) was used as a measure of association for continuous variables. Associations for adipokines and inflammatory markers were adjusted by measurement round in all cases. Owing to high collinearity observed between adiponectin and omentin (PCC 0.792), only one of them at a time was included in a linear model. When selection of confounders was needed, a stepwise algorithm was carried out using Akaike's information criterion for model selection. Associations were assessed in the linear models using the corresponding F and Wald tests. Tests were performed at the 5 % significance level. All statistical analyses were conducted using R software (see Additional file 2 for detailed description).

Results

One hundred fifteen women were included (Table 1). The percentages of obesity and dyslipidemia were 57.4 % and 47.8 %, respectively. The prevalence of MetS was 40.9 %. The median BMI, WC, and WHR were in the obesity range (30.5 kg/m^2, 100.5 cm, and 0.91, respectively). The median Lequesne index score was 14. The predominant KL grades were 2 and 3 (41.7 % each), and only 3.5 % of our sample were classified in KL grade 4. Because of batch measurement adjustments, we could not consider reference values or cutoff points for inflammatory markers or adipokines, but adjusted values are shown in Table 1.

Table 2 displays associations between Lequesne index; demographic, radiographic, and cardiovascular risk factors; and anthropometric measurements. Intensity of physical exercise showed a significant inverse association with clinical severity, and more severe KL grade was significantly associated with Lequesne index. All anthropometric

Table 1 Demographic variables, cardiovascular risk factors, radiographic and clinical severity, anthropometric measurements, inflammatory markers, and adipokines levels in synovial fluid

Variables	Category		Median (IQR) or n (%)
Age, years			68.8 (11.1)
KOA symptoms duration, months			50.0 (73.0)
Tobacco exposure	Yes		8 (7.0 %)
Physical exercise	Never		53 (46.1 %)
	Occasional		28 (24.3 %)
	Regular		34 (29.6 %)
Cardiovascular risk factors	DM		12 (10.4 %)
	DL		55 (47.8 %)
	Obesity		65 (56.5 %)
	HT		63 (54.8 %)
	Crit MetS	0	10 (8.7 %)
		1	28 (24.3 %)
		2	31 (27.0 %)
		3	32 (27.8 %)
		4	14 (12.2 %)
	MetS		47 (40.9 %)
Anthropometric measurements	Body fat, %		41.8 (6.5)
	BMI, kg/m^2		30.5 (6.4)
	Weight, kg		72.2 (13.5)
	WC, cm		100.5 (14.5)
	HC, cm		107.0 (14.0)
	WHR		0.91 (0.09)
Radiographic severity	KL grade	1	15 (13.1 %)
		2	48 (41.7 %)
		3	48 (41.7 %)
		4	4 (3.5 %)
Clinical severity	Lequesne index		14.0 (5.0)
Inflammatory markers in SF[a]	IL-6, pg/ml		106.0 (302.6)
	TNF-α, pg/ml		10.2 (8.0)
	hs-CRP, mg/ml		0.91 (0.76)
Adipokines in SF[a]	Leptin, pg/ml		42079.4 (29566.0)
	Adiponectin, ng/ml		1734.8 (1352.5)
	Resistin, pg/ml		2225.7 (2205.8)
	Visfatin, ng/ml		1.5 (1.2)
	Osteopontin, ng/ml		57.7 (83.2)
	Omentin, pg/ml		3396.0 (3550.4)
	Chemerin, ng/ml		102.7 (82.5)

Abbreviations: DM Diabetes mellitus, *DL* Dyslipidemia, *HT* Hypertension, *Crit MetS* Number of individual criteria for metabolic syndrome, *MetS* Metabolic syndrome, *KL* Kellgren-Lawrence scale, *BMI* Body mass index, *WC* Waist circumference, *HP* Hip circumference, *WHR* Waist-to-hip ratio. *IL-6* Interleukin 6, *SF* Synovial fluid, *TNF-α* Tumor necrosis factor-α, *hs-CRP* High-sensitivity C-reactive protein
Medians and interquartile ranges (IQR) were used to describe continuous variables; categorical data were summarized using absolute frequencies (n) and percentages (%)
[a]Levels of inflammatory markers and adipokines in synovial fluid were adjusted by measure round

parameters achieved significance, with WC being the one showing the strongest association ($r = 0.404$, $p < 0.0001$). It is worth noting that all these anthropometric measures were highly intercorrelated (r values 0.630–0.883). Weak, nonsignificant trends for association were found for MetS, obesity, and hypertension with Lequesne index ($p = 0.072$, $p = 0.071$, and $p = 0.059$, respectively). Among all the inflammatory markers under study, only TNF-α showed a significant association with Lequesne index after controlling by measurement batch (PCC 0.273, $p = 0.0057$). No association with severity was found for age, KOA symptom duration, MetS factors, dyslipidemia, or diabetes mellitus.

Among all the anthropometric measures evaluated in a multivariate model, WC was the most strongly associated with clinical severity, accounting for an estimated increase of 0.9 points in the Lequesne index for every 5-cm increase in WC before simultaneous evaluation of inflammatory markers and adipokines (PCC 0.338, $p = 0.0003$). Although the percentage of body fat was also selected as a confounder according to model selection criteria, it was not significantly associated to severity in the multivariate model.

Table 3 shows the association between the Lequesne index and each adipokine for three different settings: in a univariate fashion (estimates were adjusted only by measurement batch), adjusting by selected confounders (a different model was fitted for each compound), and controlling by selected confounders as well as the rest of the adipokines (a unique model was fitted to perform all estimations). This sequential analysis allowed us to evaluate the relationship between each adipokine and OA severity while assessing the effect of confounders in these associations. Variables selected for adjustment of the adipokines' effects included age, KL grade, time from recruitment to date of radiologic assessment, KOA symptom duration, WC, percentage of body fat, physical exercise, TNF-α, and batch of ELISA measurements.

Regarding adipokines, leptin showed a significant strong association according to the univariate-like analysis (PCC 0.413, $p < 0.0001$) (Fig. 1a). However, significance was highly attenuated after adjustment by confounding variables, especially after inclusion of WC, as revealed by a detailed examination of the model (see Additional file 3: Table S2).

Similarly, in univariate analysis, resistin showed a highly significant correlation with Lequesne index (PCC 0.324, $p = 0.0005$) that was markedly reduced after adjustment by confounders. Nevertheless, resistin became the strongest positively associated adipokine when all of them were jointly evaluated (PCC 0.265, $p = 0.0184$) (Fig. 1b; see Additional file 3: Table S3).

A nonsignificant association between visfatin and Lequesne index in the univariate analysis or after adjustment by selected confounders was found. Nevertheless,

Table 2 Associations between Lequesne index and demographic, radiographic, and cardiovascular risk factors; anthropometric measurements; and inflammatory markers

	Category	Median or correlation (95 % CI)	*p* Value
Age		0.118 (−0.078, 0.313)	0.2090
KOA symptom duration (months)		−0.008 (−0.178, 0.176)	0.9345
Tobacco exposure	No	14.0 (13.0–15.0)	0.0608
	Yes	12.5 (7.0–15.0)	
Physical exercise	Never	15.0 (13.0–16.0)	0.0401
	Occasional	14.0 (12.0–16.0)	
	Regular	13.0 (10.0–14.0)	
Radiographic severity (KL grade)	1	13.0 (9.0–15.0)	0.1721
	2	13.0 (12.0–15.0)	
	3–4[a]	14.0 (13.0–16.0)	
DM	Yes	13.5 (11.0–18.0)	0.7480
	No	14.0 (13.0–15.0)	
DL	Yes	14.0 (12.0, 16.0)	0.8551
	No	14.0 (13.0–15.0)	
Obesity	Yes	14.0 (13.0–16.0)	0.0705
	No	13.0 (12.0–15.0)	
HT	Yes	14.0 (13.0–16.0)	0.0589
	No	13.0 (12.0–14.0)	
MetS	Yes	15.0 (13.0–16.0)	0.0722
	No	13.0 (12.0–14.0)	
Crit MetS	0	12.5 (9.0–16.0)	0.1490
	1	14.0 (13.0–15.0)	
	2	13.0 (11.0–14.0)	
	3	15.5 (14.0–17.0)	
	4	12.5 (10.0–18.0)	
Percent body fat		0.243 (0.062–0.422)	0.0088
BMI		0.277 (0.097–0.435)	0.0027
Weight		0.249 (0.082–0.407)	0.0072
WC		0.404 (0.237–0.567)	<0.0001
HC		0.252 (0.078–0.412)	0.0065
WHR		0.221 (0.026–0.392)	0.0177
IL-6		0.146 (−0.045, 0.327)	0.1259
TNF-α		0.273 (0.078–0.448)	0.0057
hs-CRP		0.139 (−0.051, 0.320)	0.1429

Definition of abbreviations: KL Kellgren-Lawrence scale, *DM* Diabetes mellitus, *DL* Dyslipidemia, *HT* Hypertension, *Crit MetS* Number of individual criteria for metabolic syndrome, *MetS* Metabolic syndrome, *BMI* Body mass index, *WC* Waist circumference, *HP* Hip circumference, *WHR* Waist-to-hip ratio, *IL-6* Interleukin 6, *TNF-α* Tumor necrosis factor-α, *hs-CRP* High-sensitivity C-reactive protein

Correlations for continuous variables, medians for groups and their corresponding 95 % confidence (95 % CI) are shown. The partial correlation coefficient after adjustment by measure round was used to assess associations for IL-6, TNF-α, and hs-CRP. Spearman's correlation coefficient is shown for the rest of the continuous measures

[a]Because only four patients were classified as KL grade 4, KL grades 3 and 4 were combined in one category

an inverse association became evident after inclusion of all adipokines in the model (PCC −0.298, $p = 0.0075$) (Fig. 1c). A detailed study of the model showed that this effect reached statistical significance after controlling for resistin levels (Fig. 2) (see Additional file 3: Table S4).

Osteopontin achieved a significant correlation with Lequesne index in the univariate and adjusted models (PCC 0.350, $p = 0.0002$, and PCC 0.245, $p = 0.0187$, respectively) (Fig. 1d). However, only a trend for association remained when it was evaluated in the complete model (PCC 0.197, $p = 0.0824$) (see Additional file 3: Table S5).

No relationship between adiponectin or omentin and Lequesne index was observed in the univariate or adjusted analyses, but a nonsignificant trend arose for both when the rest of the adipokines were included in the model (PCC 0.212, $p = 0.0612$, and PCC 0.216, $p = 0.0562$, respectively). Finally, chemerin showed no association with KOA clinical severity in any of the settings studied.

Regarding inflammatory markers, TNF-α showed a weak but statistically significant association with Lequesne index, which remained after adjustment by confounders (PCC 0.249, $p = 0.0162$). Nonetheless, there was no independent association between Lequesne index and TNF-α when controlled by the effect of adipokines. Specifically, a detailed study of the complete model revealed that TNF-α did not show an independent association for osteopontin and resistin (see Additional file 3: Table S1).

Last, the covariates that retained a significant association with Lequesne index after the inclusion of TNF-α and the adipokines in the complete model were physical exercise, with an estimated decrease of nearly 3 Lequesne index points among patients doing regular exercise versus sporadic or no exercise ($p = 0.0016$); WC, which showed an increase of 0.5 Lequesne index points for every 5-cm increment (PCC 0.230, $p = 0.0419$); and radiographic severity, with an average increase of 1 point in the Lequesne index for every change in KL grade ($p = 0.0265$) (see Additional file 3: Tables S6, S7, and S10).

Discussion

In this study, we evaluated the relationship between clinical severity of KOA as measured by the Lequesne index and different adipokines and inflammatory markers in synovial fluid, anthropometric measurements, cardiovascular risk factors, and MetS in a cohort of women with KOA and persistent joint effusion. Our results show that, among all the adipokines measured, high levels of resistin, leptin, and osteopontin were related to greater clinical severity of KOA. Of these, resistin showed an effect independent from all adjusted variables; the association with leptin was attenuated by WC and was eliminated by TNF-α, while the effect of osteopontin did not remain once the rest of the adipokines were evaluated

Table 3 Association between adipokines and Lequesne index in three different settings

	Univariate effects		Adjusted effects		Multivariate model	
	PCC (95 % CI)	*p* Value	PCC (95 % CI)	*p* Value	PCC (95 % CI)	*p* Value
Leptin	0.413 (0.238–0.561)	<0.0001	0.182 (−0.033, 0.382)	0.0891	0.192 (−0.036, 0.402)	0.0897
Adiponectin	0.035 (−0.155, 0.222)	0.7170	0.134 (−0.078, 0.334)	0.2027	0.212 (−0.016, 0.419)	0.0612
Resistin	0.324 (0.143–0.483)	0.0005	0.179 (−0.031, 0.375)	0.0875	0.265 (0.040–0.464)	0.0184
Visfatin	0.066 (−0.125, 0.252)	0.4915	−0.179 (−0.374, 0.032)	0.0886	−0.298 (−0.492, −0.077)	0.0075
Osteopontin	0.350 (0.172–0.505)	0.0002	0.245 (0.037–0.432)	0.0187	0.197 (−0.032, 0.406)	0.0824
Omentin	0.013 (−0.179, 0.204)	0.8925	0.173 (−0.040, 0.371)	0.1028	0.216[a] (−0.012, 0.422)	0.0562[a]
Chemerin	0.071 (−0.124, 0.260)	0.4674	0.037 (−0.179, 0.249)	0.7327	0.012 (−0.215, 0.239)	0.9133

For univariate effects, adipokine associations were assessed separately, adjusting their effects by measurement batch only. For adjusted effects, estimation of adipokine effects was additionally adjusted by potential confounders: age, knee osteoarthritis symptom duration, Kellgren-Lawrence grade (divided into three categories: 1, 2, and 3 + 4 combined), time from recruitment to radiology, waist circumference, percentage of body fat, physical exercise, and tumor necrosis factor α. In the multivariate model, effects were simultaneously estimated using a single model that included previous confounders and all adipokines except omentin (due to high collinearity observed with adiponectin: partial correlation coefficient [PCC] 0.792)

[a]Multivariate association for omentin was assessed in an analogous model in which adiponectin was excluded. The PCC after adjustment by measure round was used to assess associations between Lequesne index and adipokines

simultaneously. In addition, high levels of visfatin were found to be associated with lesser clinical severity for patients with similar levels of resistin. Regarding the rest of the clinical parameters, only WC among all anthropometric measurements was independently associated with Lequesne index score. Radiographic damage was also independently associated with clinical severity, while intensity of physical exercise was inversely related to Lequesne index score.

In our opinion, this cohort of patients is very homogeneous and has four distinctive features compared with previous studies. First, all patients in our sample had synovial effusion, which is usually considered an inflammatory feature, and this differentiates our study from others [25–27]. Second, our patients were very symptomatic in contrast to other series in which symptomatic status was not evaluated and only radiographic or diagnostic criteria were assessed [28–30]. Third, most patients were not in the final stage of the disease, with more than 50 % in KL grade 1 or 2, in contrast to other series where most patients had advanced disease or were undergoing prosthetic surgery. Fourth, all patients were women. As previous researchers have reported, there are differences regarding pain evaluation or anthropometric measures related to gender [31].

Resistin was the adipokine most clearly associated with the Lequesne index in our study. A previous study showed an association between Western Ontario and McMaster Universities Osteoarthritis Index (WOMAC) total score and synovial fluid resistin, but, in contrast to our study, it was conducted with patients undergoing arthroscopic lavage and was not focused on patients with joint effusion, and the relationship with Lequesne index was not evaluated [15]. Other authors have reported an association between resistin and IL-6 with severity scores of KOA [32], but patients were in a final stage of the disease, and the synovial fluid was collected during surgery. In contrast, other authors who have evaluated the role of synovial fluid IL-6 and TNF-α in patients with KOA stages similar to those of our sample found no relationship between IL-6 and WOMAC subscales of pain or disability [33]. Thus, the role of resistin in KOA clinical severity was not explained by the possible association with IL-6, which might be more important in more advanced disease [34].

Our analyses seem to unveil a probable protective effect of visfatin in KOA regarding clinical severity. Visfatin has been related to cartilage degradation [17], and synovial fluid levels of visfatin have been associated with hip pain, but not with knee pain [35]. In contrast to our study, in these studies all patients were classified in KL grade 3 or 4 and undergoing joint arthroplasty. In vitro studies had evaluated the relationship between visfatin and different pain mechanisms in OA, such as nerve growth factor stimuli and nicotinamide phosphoribosyltransferase enzyme activity [36, 37]. Nevertheless, to our knowledge, its association with OA severity has not been clinically evaluated. Interestingly, the association with visfatin becomes evident only when controlled by TNF-α and the rest of the adipokines in the analysis, especially resistin. We do not know the mechanism behind this effect, but this result suggests the existence of interrelationships among these compounds regarding their role in KOA clinical severity. Overall, these findings may provide new and promising hypotheses for exploration in future research into how inflammation is activated or blocked by visfatin. In this respect, it might be interesting to assess the association of synovial fluid visfatin levels with anti-inflammatory factors, such as IL-10 [38].

Previous studies have related synovial fluid osteopontin with KOA severity [16, 39], although the patients differed from those in our series because of synovial fluid

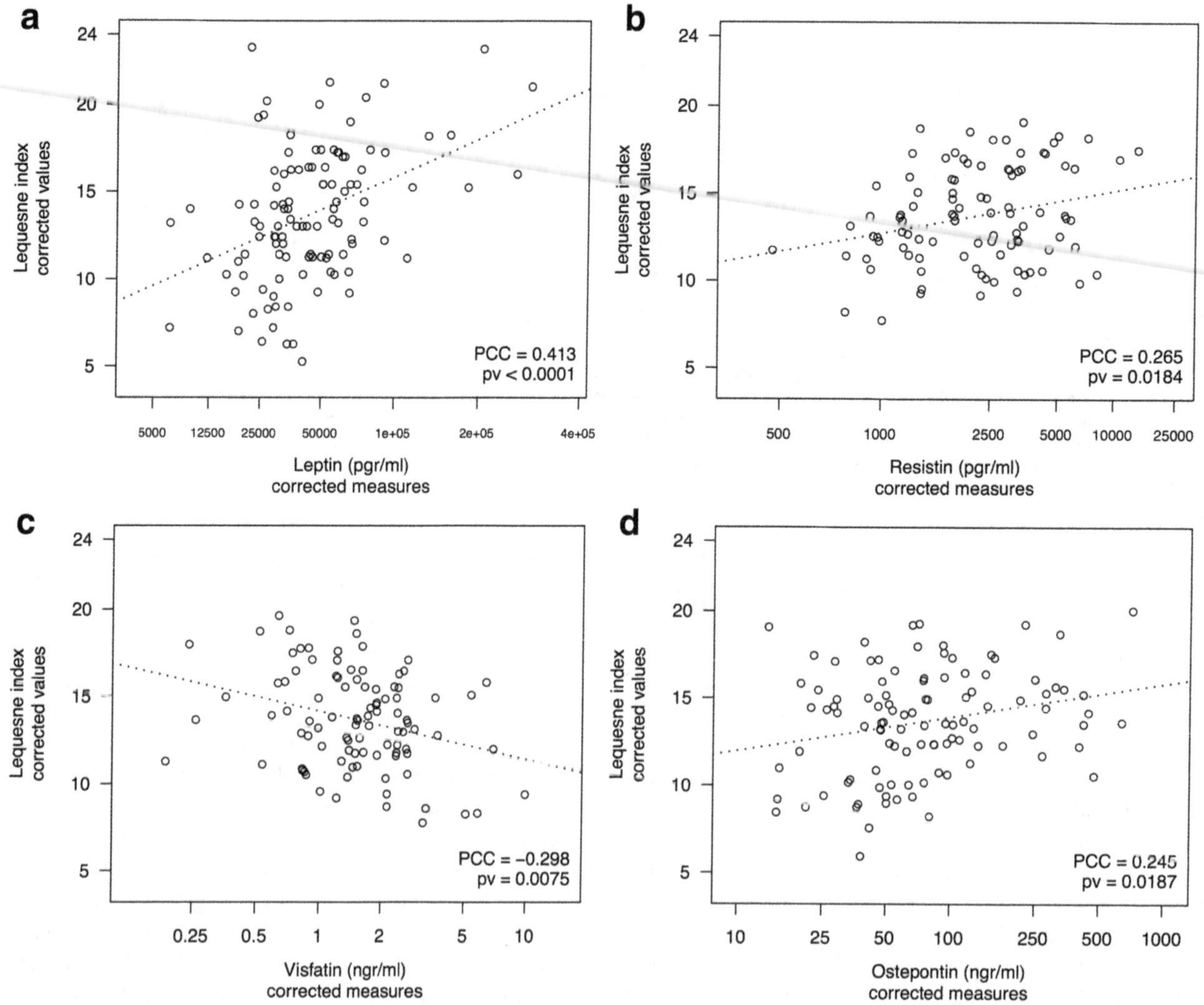

Fig. 1 Scatterplots showing significant associations between adipokines and knee osteoarthritis severity: effect of leptin on Lequesne index score in the univariate setting (adjusted by round of measurement only (**a**), association for resistin (**b**), and visfatin (**c**) independently of clinical, anthropometric, metabolic, and inflammatory factors as well as the rest of the adipokines; association between Lequesne index and osteopontin after adjustment by clinical, anthropometric, metabolic, and inflammatory factors, but not the rest of the adipokines (**d**)). In all cases, values were corrected for confounders using the corresponding linear model. Adipokine values were drawn in the scale of the corresponding Taylor transformation. Labels along *x*-axes are shown in the original scale of the adipokines. *PCC* Partial correlation coefficient, *pv* Association *p* value according to *F*-test derived from the linear model

presence and KOA stage. In our study, osteopontin showed a clear association with clinical KOA severity that decreased when adjusted by other adipokines, again suggesting the existence of biological or clinical interrelationships between adipokines. An interaction between osteopontin and resistin has been shown in vascular disease [40], and it is possible that synovial osteopontin could also be controlled by other adipokines in KOA or that they could share mechanisms of action.

A relationship between leptin and clinical severity in knee OA has already been reported [35, 41], but, to our knowledge, this is the first study where synovial leptin has been studied simultaneously with a significant number of adipokines. After proper control by WC, the association with leptin was highly attenuated and lost statistical significance when controlled by TNF-α. Interaction between leptin and BMI in knee OA has been described previously using serum samples and related to radiologic KOA, but clinical severity was not evaluated, and this study was not controlled by the presence of inflammatory features such as joint effusion [42]. Leptin and anthropometric measurements may share pathways influencing clinical severity in KOA, but our results could indicate that WC may have a more important association than leptin in patients with joint effusion.

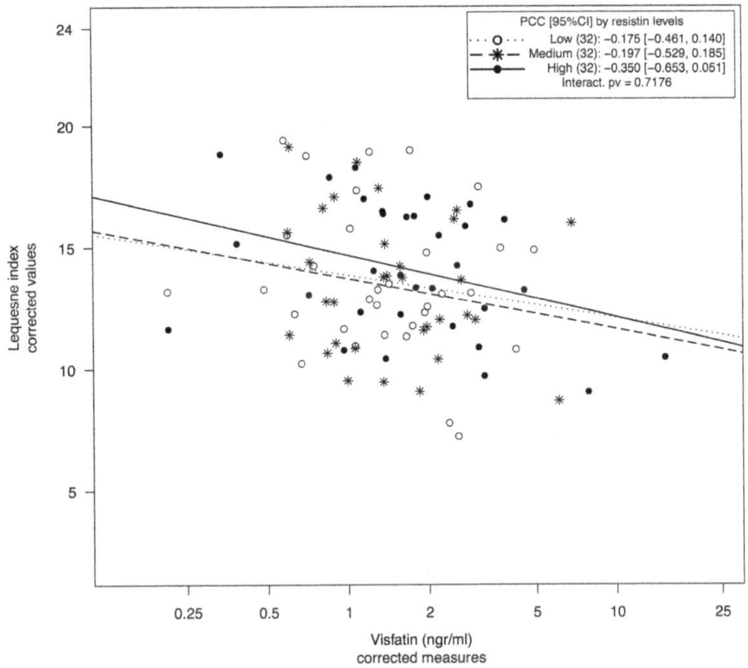

Fig. 2 Scatterplot of visfatin vs Lequesne index after stratification by resistin levels. Values were corrected for confounders, except for resistin, using the complete model (multivariate model in Table 3). Levels of resistin were defined using tertiles after correction of their values by measurement round using the complete model. *PCC* Partial correlation coefficient, *95 % CI* PCC interval at 95 % confidence, *Interact. pv p* Value for the interaction between visfatin and resistin according to an *F*-test derived from the linear model

Regarding resistin, visfatin, leptin, and osteopontin, it is important to highlight that when a model excluding anthropometric measures or inflammatory factors was applied (see Additional file 3: Tables S8 and S9), the association of clinical severity with resistin and visfatin persisted, suggesting that their effects were not completely explained by obesity or TNF-α. The association between Lequesne index and leptin was highly increased in the two models when the effect of leptin was not controlled by anthropometric or inflammatory variables, indicating that the pathway of leptin in clinical severity could be shared by TNF-α and obesity. The relationship of clinical severity and osteopontin was higher when not controlled by anthropometric measures, but it was attenuated when not controlled by TNF-α, indicating a possible common pathway between obesity and osteopontin [43].

A nonsignificant trend toward an association between adiponectin and omentin with Lequesne index was observed when other adipokines were considered. Adiponectin has been found to be associated with inflammatory synovial parameters, but not with clinical severity [12, 44]. Researchers in one previous study found that synovial fluid omentin was associated with less pain and disability as measured by WOMAC but that it was not controlled by other adipokines [45]. One important deduction from our results is that, in order to evaluate the effect of adipokines properly, as many of them as possible should be assessed together and controlled by anthropometric variables and inflammatory markers.

The association of Lequesne index with TNF-α remained significant after controlling for clinical, anthropometric, and metabolic factors. Nevertheless, this association did not appear to be independent from the effect of adipokines, especially ostepontin and resistin. In a previous study with a group of patients comparable to ours, investigators found a relationship between TNF-α, pain, and disability as measured using WOMAC subscales, but it was not controlled by other adipokines [33]. Further work might be required to unveil the role of TNF-α in clinical KOA severity and its relationship to adipokines [29].

Among all anthropometric measurements, WC was the most strongly associated with clinical severity. Different anthropometric measurements have been related to KOA prevalence in prior studies, and their relationship to Lequesne index has been described previously [30, 46, 47]. WC could represent a better measurement of visceral and abdominal fat, which is known to be related to low-grade systemic inflammation [9, 10], and could have more relevance in our group of patients with local inflammation.

Several studies have connected physical exercise with less pain and disability in KOA. It has been suggested that this effect could be related to better muscle strength

[48]. In our study, physical exercise was associated with a better Lequesne index score.

Cross-sectional studies are not the best way to evaluate radiographic implication in pain, but disability may be evaluated. In our study, the relationship between radiologic and clinical severity was assessed in a group of female patients with KOA with effusion. We used the Lequesne index, in which disability has a relative weight greater than that of pain, and we found that radiographic severity was associated with Lequesne index, in accordance with previous studies [49], although they were not conducted with patients with KOA with synovial effusion.

Cardiovascular risk factors and MetS have been associated with the presence of OA [6, 7], and in some cases with higher pain levels, especially in patients with diabetes. Association between MetS and KOA was not evaluated in this study, but MetS and its individual components were very prevalent in our patients. No individual cardiovascular risk factor was related to Lequesne index, although hypertension and obesity showed a trend toward association. Neither MetS nor the addition of its individual components was significantly associated with clinical severity in our group of female patients with KOA on the basis of synovial fluid measurements. It is important to highlight that the association between MetS and OA may change depending on the diagnostic criteria used, so it would be important to standardize criteria for future studies [46, 50].

The main limitation of our study arises from its cross-sectional nature and therefore its inability to establish causality. Accordingly, conclusions can be drawn only in terms of associations. A selection bias toward greater disease severity could exist, as all patients were referred from primary care or other specialists to our rheumatology unit and were systematically included. These results warrant replication in other groups of patients with KOA, such as men or patients with lesser WC, BMI, or pain. In this study, information on OA at other sites, which could interfere with the evaluation of clinical severity, was not adequately collected to be analyzed. There may be technical concerns regarding measures in synovial fluid that are inherent to ELISA technology; nonnegligible effects associated with time of measurement were identified. For this reason, we corrected these measures by round in the statistical models to make values of adipokines and inflammatory markers totally comparable across samples. Although this correction resulted in reliable estimations of association for these measures, it was not possible to establish either their real range of variability or meaningful cutoffs that could be extrapolated to other datasets.

A remarkable strength of this work is that a highly homogeneous sample of patients with KOA was studied, which increased the statistical power to detect associations of a moderate magnitude. Another strength is the availability of patient information relevant to outcome, which makes this study singular among others, as it allowed for a simultaneous analysis of a high number of clinical, anthropometric, metabolic, and inflammatory factors and their relationship to up to seven different adipokines.

Conclusions

To the best of our knowledge, this is the first study of the relationship between seven adipokines in synovial fluid and clinical severity of KOA controlled by three inflammatory markers in synovial fluid, anthropometric measurements, and metabolic factors. Resistin and visfatin were independently associated with the Lequesne index. Leptin and osteopontin were associated with clinical severity of KOA until all adipokines were evaluated together, pointing to potential biologic interrelationships among them. Therefore, simultaneous study of different adipokines should be recommended in future research. Further evaluation of different adipokines both in synovial fluid and in serum in future studies and in different populations, such as male patients, patients without synovial effusion, or patients with lower levels of pain are warranted.

Abbreviations

BMI: Body mass index; DL: Dyslipidemia; DM: Diabetes mellitus; HC: Hip circumference; HDL: High-density lipoprotein; hs-CRP: High-sensitivity C-reactive protein; HT: Hypertension; IL: Interleukin; KL: Kellgren-Lawrence; KOA: Knee osteoarthritis; MetS: Metabolic syndrome; OA: Osteoarthritis; PCC: Partial correlation coefficient; pv: *p* value; *r*: Spearman's correlation coefficient; SF: Synovial fluid; TNF-α: Tumor necrosis factor α; WC: Waist circumference; WHR: Waist-to-hip ratio; WOMAC: Western Ontario and McMaster Universities Osteoarthritis Index

Acknowledgements

The authors acknowledge Néstor Albiñana, coordinator of Unitat Científico-Tècnica in Parc Taulí Sabadell University Hospital; the Institute for Research and Innovation Parc Tauli (I3PT) Research Institute, Universitat Autónoma de Barcelona (UAB), for kit acquisition, supervision of the ELISA technique, synovial fluid management, and referral of patients for monographic consultation; Cristina Aymerich, a nurse in the Hospital de Dia of Rheumatology at Parc Taulí Sabadell University Hospital; and Carlos Galisteo, Enrique Casado, Eduard Graell, Mireia Moreno, and Antonio Gómez, who are members of the Rheumatology Department of Parc Taulí Sabadell University Hospital. Without these contributions, the study would not have been possible.

Funding

This study was partially funded by the 2013 and 2014 Osteoarthritis Grant of the Catalan Rheumatology Society and by the Bioiberica collaboration.

Authors' contributions
JC and CO participated in the conception and design of the study, acquisition of data, analysis and interpretation of the results, drafting of the manuscript and revising it critically for important intellectual content, and final approval of the version to be submitted for publication. JG participated in the conception and design of the study, interpretation of the results, critical revision of the manuscript for important intellectual content, and final approval of the version to be submitted for publication. ABL participated in the design of the study, analysis and interpretation of the results, critical revision of the manuscript for important intellectual content, and final approval of the version to be submitted for publication. AC participated in the conception of the study, acquisition of data, critical revision of the manuscript for important intellectual content, and final approval of the version to be submitted for publication. JJC participated in the conception and design of the study, analysis of the results, critical revision of the manuscript for important intellectual content, and final approval of the version to be submitted for publication. JBP participated in the conception and design of the study, critical revision of the manuscript for important intellectual content, and final approval of the version to be submitted for publication. MGM participated in acquisition of data, interpretation of the results, critical revision of the manuscript for important intellectual content, and final approval of the version to be submitted for publication. NN participated in acquisition of data, drafting of the manuscript, and final approval of the version to be submitted for publication. ML participated in the conception and design of the study, interpretation of the results, critical revision of the manuscript for important intellectual content, and final approval of the version to be submitted for publication.

Authors' information
Not applicable.

Competing interests
The authors declare that they have no competing interests.

Author details
[1]Rheumatology Department, Parc Tauli Sabadell University Hospital, Institute for Research and Innovation Parc Tauli (I3PT), Universitat Autónoma de Barcelona (UAB), 08208 Sabadell, Spain. [2]Departament de Medicina, Universitat Autónoma de Barcelona (UAB), 08003 Barcelona, Spain. [3]Biostatistics and Bioinformatics Unit, Institute for Research in Biomedicine Barcelona (IRB Barcelona), 08028 Barcelona, Spain. [4]Endocrinology and Nutrition Department, Parc Tauli Sabadell University Hospital, Institute for Research and Innovation Parc Tauli (I3PT), Universitat Autónoma de Barcelona (UAB), 08208 Sabadell, Spain. [5]Endocrinology and Nutrition Department, Hospital del Mar, 08003 Barcelona, Spain.

References
1. Sharma L, Kapoor D, Issa S. Epidemiology of osteoarthritis: an update. Curr Opin Rheumatol. 2006;18(2):147–56.
2. Bijlsma JW, Berenbaum F, Lafeber FP. Osteoarthritis: an update with relevance for clinical practice. Lancet. 2011;377(9783):2115–26.
3. Felson DT, Lawrence RC, Dieppe PA, Hirsch R, Helmick CG, Jordan JM, Kington RS, Lane NE, Nevitt MC, Zhang Y, et al. Osteoarthritis: new insights. Part 1: the disease and its risk factors. Ann Intern Med. 2000;133(8):635–46.
4. Zhuo Q, Yang W, Chen J, Wang Y. Metabolic syndrome meets osteoarthritis. Nat Rev Rheumatol. 2012;8(12):729–37.
5. Singh G, Miller JD, Lee FH, Pettitt D, Russell MW. Prevalence of cardiovascular disease risk factors among US adults with self-reported osteoarthritis: data from the Third National Health and Nutrition Examination Survey. Am J Manag Care. 2002;8(15 Suppl):S383–91.
6. Calvet J, Orellana C, Larrosa M, Navarro N, Chillarón JJ, Pedro-Botet J, Galisteo C, García-Manrique M, Gratacós J. High prevalence of cardiovascular co-morbidities in patients with symptomatic knee or hand osteoarthritis. Scand J Rheumatol. 2016;45(1):41–4.
7. Yoshimura N, Muraki S, Oka H, Tanaka S, Kawaguchi H, Nakamura K, Akune T. Accumulation of metabolic risk factors such as overweight, hypertension, dyslipidaemia, and impaired glucose tolerance raises the risk of occurrence and progression of knee osteoarthritis: a 3-year follow-up of the ROAD study. Osteoarthritis Cartilage. 2012;20(11):1217–26.
8. Katz JD, Agrawal S, Velasquez M. Getting to the heart of the matter: osteoarthritis takes its place as part of the metabolic syndrome. Curr Opin Rheumatol. 2010;22(5):512–9.
9. Berenbaum F, Eymard F, Houard X. Osteoarthritis, inflammation and obesity. Curr Opin Rheumatol. 2013;25(1):114–8.
10. Courties A, Gualillo O, Berenbaum F, Sellam J. Metabolic stress-induced joint inflammation and osteoarthritis. Osteoarthritis Cartilage. 2015;23(11):1955–65.
11. Abella V, Scotece M, Conde J, López V, Lazzaro V, Pino J, et al. Adipokines, metabolic syndrome and rheumatic diseases. J Immunol Res. 2014;2014:343746.
12. Staikos C, Ververidis A, Drosos G, Manolopoulos VG, Verettas DA, Tavridou A. The association of adipokine levels in plasma and synovial fluid with the severity of knee osteoarthritis. Rheumatology (Oxford). 2013;52(6):1077–83.
13. Lübbeke A, Finckh A, Puskas GJ, Suva D, Lädermann A, Bas S, Fritschy D, Gabay C, Hoffmeyer P. Do synovial leptin levels correlate with pain in end stage arthritis? Int Orthop. 2013;37(10):2071–9.
14. Zheng S, Xu J, Xu S, Zhang M, Huang S, He F, Yang X, Xiao H, Zhang H, Ding C. Association between circulating adipokines, radiographic changes, and knee cartilage volume in patients with knee osteoarthritis. Scand J Rheumatol. 2016;45(3):224–9.
15. Song YZ, Guan J, Wang HJ, Ma W, Li F, Xu F, Ding LB, Xie L, Liu B, Liu K, et al. Possible involvement of serum and synovial fluid resistin in knee osteoarthritis: cartilage damage, clinical, and radiological links. J Clin Lab Anal. 2015;15. doi:10.1002/jcla.21876.
16. Hasegawa M, Segawa T, Maeda M, Yoshida T, Sudo A. Thrombin-cleaved osteopontin levels in synovial fluid correlate with disease severity of knee osteoarthritis. J Rheumatol. 2011;38(1):129–34.
17. Duan Y, Hao D, Li M, Wu Z, Li D, Yang X, Qiu G. Increased synovial fluid visfatin is positively linked to cartilage degradation biomarkers in osteoarthritis. Rheumatol Int. 2012;32(4):985–90.
18. Larsson S, Englund M, Struglics A, Lohmander LS. Interleukin-6 and tumor necrosis factor α in synovial fluid are associated with progression of radiographic knee osteoarthritis in subjects with previous meniscectomy. Osteoarthritis Cartilage. 2015;23(11):1906–14.
19. Jiang L, Bao J, Zhou X, Xiong Y, Wu L. Increased serum levels and chondrocyte expression of nesfatin-1 in patients with osteoarthritis and its relation with BMI, hsCRP, and IL-18. Mediators Inflamm. 2013;2013:631251.
20. Altman R, Asch E, Bloch D, Bole G, Borenstein D, Brandt K, Christy W, Cooke TD, Greenwald R, Hochberg M. Development of criteria for the classification and reporting of osteoarthritis: classification of osteoarthritis of the knee. Arthritis Rheum. 1986;29(8):1039–49.
21. Glass N, Segal NA, Sluka KA, Torner JC, Nevitt MC, Felson DT, Bradley LA, Neogi T, Lewis CE, Frey-Law LA. Examining sex differences in knee pain: the multicenter osteoarthritis study. Osteoarthritis Cartilage. 2014;22(8):1100–6.
22. Fang WH, Huang GS, Chang HF, Chen CY, Kang CY, Wang CC, Lin C, Yang JH, Su W, Kao S, et al. Gender differences between WOMAC index scores, health-related quality of life and physical performance in an elderly Taiwanese population with knee osteoarthritis. BMJ Open. 2015;5(9):e008542.
23. Gross JB, Guillaume C, Gégout-Pottie P, Mainard D, Presle N. Synovial fluid levels of adipokines in osteoarthritis: association with local factors of inflammation and cartilage maintenance. Biomed Mater Eng. 2014;24(1 Suppl):17–25.
24. Grundy SM, Cleeman JI, Daniels SR, Donato KA, Eckel RH, Franklin BA, Gordon DJ, Krauss RM, Savage PJ, Smith SC, et al. Diagnosis and management of the metabolic syndrome: an American Heart Association/ National Heart, Lung, and Blood Institute scientific statement. Circulation. 2005;112(17):2735–52.
25. Suh DH, Han KD, Hong JY, Park JH, Bae JH, Moon YW, Kim JG. Body composition is more closely related to the development of knee osteoarthritis in women than men: a cross-sectional study using the Fifth Korea National Health and Nutrition Examination Survey (KNHANES V-1, 2). Osteoarthritis Cartilage. 2016;24(4):605–11.
26. Wesseling J, Bastick AN, ten Wolde S, Kloppenburg M, Lafeber FP, Bierma-Zeinstra SM, Bijlsma JW. Identifying trajectories of pain severity in

early symptomatic knee osteoarthritis: a 5-year followup of the Cohort Hip and Cohort Knee (CHECK) study. J Rheumatol. 2015;42(8):1470–7.
27. Van Spil WE, Nair SC, Kinds MB, Emans PJ, Hilberdink WK, Welsing PM, Lafeber FP. Systemic biochemical markers of joint metabolism and inflammation in relation to radiographic parameters and pain of the knee: data from CHECK, a cohort of early osteoarthritis subjects. Osteoarthritis Cartilage. 2015;23(1):48–56.
28. Oak SR, Ghodadra A, Winalski CS, Miniaci A, Jones MH. Radiographic joint space width is correlated with 4-year clinical outcomes in patients with knee osteoarthritis: data from the osteoarthritis initiative. Osteoarthritis Cartilage. 2013;21(9):1185–90.
29. de Lange-Brokaar BJ, Ioan-Facsinay A, Yusuf E, Visser AW, Kroon HM, van Osch GJ, Zuurmond AM, Stojanovic-Susulic V, Bloem JL, Nelissen RG, et al. Association of pain in knee osteoarthritis with distinct patterns of synovitis. Arthritis Rheumatol. 2015;67(3):733–40.
30. Lohmander LS, Gerhardsson de Verdier M, Rollof J, Nilsson PM, Engström G. Incidence of severe knee and hip osteoarthritis in relation to different measures of body mass: a population-based prospective cohort study. Ann Rheum Dis. 2009;68(4):490–6.
31. Presle N, Pottie P, Dumond H, Guillaume C, Lapicque F, Pallu S, Mainard D, Netter P, Terlain B. Differential distribution of adipokines between serum and synovial fluid in patients with osteoarthritis: contribution of joint tissues to their articular production. Osteoarthritis Cartilage. 2006;14(7):690–5.
32. Koskinen A, Vuolteenaho K, Moilanen T, Moilanen E. Resistin as a factor in osteoarthritis: synovial fluid resistin concentrations correlate positively with interleukin 6 and matrix metalloproteinases MMP-1 and MMP-3. Scand J Rheumatol. 2014;43(3):249–53.
33. Orita S, Koshi T, Mitsuka T, Miyagi M, Inoue G, Arai G, Ishikawa T, Hanaoka E, Yamashita K, Yamashita M, et al. Associations between proinflammatory cytokines in the synovial fluid and radiographic grading and pain-related scores in 47 consecutive patients with osteoarthritis of the knee. BMC Musculoskelet Disord. 2011;12:144.
34. Siqueira MB, Frangiamore S, Klika AK, Gajewski N, Barsoum WK, Higuera CA. Comparison of Synovial Fluid Cytokine Levels between Traumatic Knee Injury and End-Stage Osteoarthritis. J Knee Surg. 2016;34. doi:10.1055/s-0036-1583269.
35. Bas S, Finckh A, Puskas GJ, Suva D, Hoffmeyer P, Gabay C, Lübbeke A. Adipokines correlate with pain in lower limb osteoarthritis: different associations in hip and knee. Int Orthop. 2014;38(12):2577–83.
36. Pecchi E, Priam S, Gosset M, Pigenet A, Sudre L, Laiguillon MC, Berenbaum F, Houard X. Induction of nerve growth factor expression and release by mechanical and inflammatory stimuli in chondrocytes: possible involvement in osteoarthritis pain. Arthritis Res Ther. 2014;16(1):R16.
37. Laiguillon MC, Houard X, Bougault C, Gosset M, Nourissat G, Sautet A, Jacques C, Berenbaum F, Sellam J. Expression and function of visfatin (Nampt), an adipokine-enzyme involved in inflammatory pathways of osteoarthritis. Arthritis Res Ther. 2014;16(1):R38.
38. Helmark IC, Mikkelsen UR, Børglum J, Rothe A, Petersen MC, Andersen O, Langberg H, Kjaer M. Exercise increases interleukin-10 levels both intraarticularly and peri-synovially in patients with knee osteoarthritis: a randomized controlled trial. Arthritis Res Ther. 2010;12(4):R126.
39. Gao SG, Li KH, Zeng KB, Tu M, Xu M, Lei GH. Elevated osteopontin level of synovial fluid and articular cartilage is associated with disease severity in knee osteoarthritis patients. Osteoarthritis Cartilage. 2010;18(1):82–7.
40. Park SY, Kim KH, Seo KW, Bae JU, Kim YH, Lee SJ, Lee WS, Kim CD. Resistin derived from diabetic perivascular adipose tissue up-regulates vascular expression of osteopontin via the AP-1 signalling pathway. J Pathol. 2014;232(1):87–97.
41. Vuolteenaho K, Koskinen A, Moilanen T, Moilanen E. Leptin levels are increased and its negative regulators, SOCS-3 and sOb-R are decreased in obese patients with osteoarthritis: a link between obesity and osteoarthritis. Ann Rheum Dis. 2012;71(11):1912–3.
42. Fowler-Brown A, Kim DH, Shi L, Marcantonio E, Wee CC, Shmerling RH, Leveille S. The mediating effect of leptin on the relationship between body weight and knee osteoarthritis in older adults. Arthritis Rheumatol. 2015;67(1):169–75.
43. Kiefer FW, Zeyda M, Todoric J, Huber J, Geyeregger R, Weichhart T, Aszmann O, Ludvik B, Silberhumer GR, Prager G, et al. Osteopontin expression in human and murine obesity: extensive local up-regulation in adipose tissue but minimal systemic alterations. Endocrinology. 2008;149(3):1350–7.
44. de Boer TN, van Spil WE, Huisman AM, Polak AA, Bijlsma JW, Lafeber FP, Mastbergen SC. Serum adipokines in osteoarthritis; comparison with controls and relationship with local parameters of synovial inflammation and cartilage damage. Osteoarthritis Cartilage. 2012;20(8):846–53.
45. Li ZG, Zhao DW, Xia CJ, Wang TN, Liu YP, Zhang Y, Wang BJ. Decreased synovial fluid omentin-1 concentrations reflect symptomatic severity in patients with knee osteoarthritis. Scand J Clin Lab Invest. 2012;72(8):623–8.
46. Abourazzak FE, Talbi S, Lazrak F, Azzouzi H, Aradoini N, Keita S, Errasfa M, Harzy T. Does metabolic syndrome or its individual components affect pain and function in knee osteoarthritis women? Curr Rheumatol Rev. 2015;11(1):8–14.
47. Batsis JA, Zbehlik AJ, Barre LK, Mackenzie TA, Bartels SJ. The impact of waist circumference on function and physical activity in older adults: longitudinal observational data from the osteoarthritis initiative. Nutr J. 2014;13:81.
48. Alkatan M, Baker JR, Machin DR, Park W, Akkari AS, Pasha EP, Tanaka H. Improved function and reduced pain after swimming and cycling training in patients with osteoarthritis. J Rheumatol. 2016;43(3):666–72.
49. Wesseling J, Bierma-Zeinstra SM, Kloppenburg M, Meijer R, Bijlsma JW. Worsening of pain and function over 5 years in individuals with 'early' OA is related to structural damage: data from the Osteoarthritis Initiative and CHECK (Cohort Hip & Cohort Knee) study. Ann Rheum Dis. 2015;74(2):347–53.
50. Han CD, Yang IH, Lee WS, Park YJ, Park KK. Correlation between metabolic syndrome and knee osteoarthritis: data from the Korean National Health and Nutrition Examination Survey (KNHANES). BMC Public Health. 2013;13:603.

Permissions

All chapters in this book were first published in AR&T, by BioMed Central; hereby published with permission under the Creative Commons Attribution License or equivalent. Every chapter published in this book has been scrutinized by our experts. Their significance has been extensively debated. The topics covered herein carry significant findings which will fuel the growth of the discipline. They may even be implemented as practical applications or may be referred to as a beginning point for another development.

The contributors of this book come from diverse backgrounds, making this book a truly international effort. This book will bring forth new frontiers with its revolutionizing research information and detailed analysis of the nascent developments around the world.

We would like to thank all the contributing authors for lending their expertise to make the book truly unique. They have played a crucial role in the development of this book. Without their invaluable contributions this book wouldn't have been possible. They have made vital efforts to compile up to date information on the varied aspects of this subject to make this book a valuable addition to the collection of many professionals and students.

This book was conceptualized with the vision of imparting up-to-date information and advanced data in this field. To ensure the same, a matchless editorial board was set up. Every individual on the board went through rigorous rounds of assessment to prove their worth. After which they invested a large part of their time researching and compiling the most relevant data for our readers.

The editorial board has been involved in producing this book since its inception. They have spent rigorous hours researching and exploring the diverse topics which have resulted in the successful publishing of this book. They have passed on their knowledge of decades through this book. To expedite this challenging task, the publisher supported the team at every step. A small team of assistant editors was also appointed to further simplify the editing procedure and attain best results for the readers.

Apart from the editorial board, the designing team has also invested a significant amount of their time in understanding the subject and creating the most relevant covers. They scrutinized every image to scout for the most suitable representation of the subject and create an appropriate cover for the book.

The publishing team has been an ardent support to the editorial, designing and production team. Their endless efforts to recruit the best for this project, has resulted in the accomplishment of this book. They are a veteran in the field of academics and their pool of knowledge is as vast as their experience in printing. Their expertise and guidance has proved useful at every step. Their uncompromising quality standards have made this book an exceptional effort. Their encouragement from time to time has been an inspiration for everyone.

The publisher and the editorial board hope that this book will prove to be a valuable piece of knowledge for researchers, students, practitioners and scholars across the globe.

List of Contributors

Chao Zeng, Tuo Yang, Yi-lun Wang, Dong-xing Xie, Hui Li and Guang-hua Lei
Department of Orthopaedics, Xiangya Hospital, Central South University, #87 Xiangya Road, Changsha, Hunan Province 410008, China

Liang-jun Li
Department of Orthopaedics, Xiangya Hospital, Central South University, #87 Xiangya Road, Changsha, Hunan Province 410008, China
Department of Orthopaedics, Changsha Central Hospital, Changsha, Hunan 410000, China

Jie Wei
Health Management Center, Xiangya Hospital, Central South University, Changsha, Hunan Province 410008, China
Department of Epidemiology and Health Statistics, Xiangya School of Public Health, Central South University, Changsha, Hunan Province 410008, China

Robert Terkeltaub
VA San Diego Medical Center, San Diego, CA 92161, USA
Department of Medicine, UCSD, San Diego, CA 92161, USA

Hyon K. Choi and Yuqing Zhang
Division of Rheumatology, Allergy and Immunology, Department of Medicine, Massachusetts General Hospital, Boston, MA 02114, USA

David J. Hunter
Rheumatology Department, Royal North Shore Hospital and Institute of Bone and Joint Research, Kolling Institute, University of Sydney, Sydney, NSW 2065, Australia

Yang Cui
International Medical Center, Xiangya Hospital, Central South University, Changsha, Hunan Province 410008, China

Shinnosuke Hada, Haruka Kaneko, Mayuko Kinoshita, Ryo Sadatsuki, Ippei Futami, Hitoshi Arita, Jun Shiozawa, Yuji Takazawa and Hiroshi Ikeda
Department of Medicine for Orthopaedics and Motor Organ, Juntendo University Graduate School of Medicine, 2-1-1, Hongo, Bunkyo-ku, Tokyo 113-8421, Japan

Muneaki Ishijima and Kazuo Kaneko
Department of Medicine for Orthopaedics and Motor Organ, Juntendo University Graduate School of Medicine, 2-1-1, Hongo, Bunkyo-ku, Tokyo 113-8421, Japan
Department of Pathophysiology for Locomotive and Neoplastic Diseases, Juntendo University Graduate School of Medicine, 2-1-1 Hongo, Bunkyo-ku, Tokyo 113-8421, Japan
Sportology Center, Juntendo University Graduate School of Medicine, Tokyo, Japan

Lizu Liu
Department of Medicine for Orthopaedics and Motor Organ, Juntendo University Graduate School of Medicine, 2-1-1, Hongo, Bunkyo-ku, Tokyo 113-8421, Japan
Sportology Center, Juntendo University Graduate School of Medicine, Tokyo, Japan

Anwajan Yusup
Department of Medicine for Orthopaedics and Motor Organ, Juntendo University Graduate School of Medicine, 2-1-1, Hongo, Bunkyo-ku, Tokyo 113-8421, Japan
Research Institute for Diseases of Old Age, Juntendo University Graduate School of Medicine, Tokyo, Japan

Yasunori Okada
Department of Pathophysiology for Locomotive and Neoplastic Diseases, Juntendo University Graduate School of Medicine, 2-1-1 Hongo, Bunkyo-ku, Tokyo 113-8421, Japan

Takako Aoki
Sportology Center, Juntendo University Graduate School of Medicine, Tokyo, Japan

Tomohiro Takamura and Shigeki Aoki
Department of Radiology, Juntendo University Graduate School of Medicine, Tokyo, Japan

Hisashi Kurosawa
Department of Orthopaedics, Juntendo Tokyo Koto Geriatric Medical Center, Tokyo, Japan

Johanne Martel-Pelletier, Jean-Pierre Raynauld, François Mineau and Jean-Pierre Pelletier
Osteoarthritis Research Unit, University of Montreal Hospital Research Centre (CRCHUM), 900 Saint-Denis, Suite R11.412, Montreal, Quebec H2X 0A9, Canada

François Abram
Medical Imaging Research & Development, ArthroLab Inc, Montreal, Quebec, Canada

Patrice Paiement and Philippe Delorme
ArthroLab Inc, Montreal, Quebec, Canada

Weam Alshenibr, Mustafa M. Tashkandi, Saqer F. Alsaqer, Yazeed Alkheriji and Manish V. Bais
Department of Molecular and Cell Biology, Boston University Henry M. Goldman School of Dental Medicine, W-216, 700 Albany Street, Boston, MA 02118, USA

Amelia Wise and Louis C. Gerstenfeld
Department of Orthopaedic Surgery, School of Medicine, Boston University, Boston, MA 02118, USA

Sadanand Fulzele
Department of Orthopaedic Surgery and Institute of Regenerative and Reparative Medicine, Georgia Regents University, Augusta, GA 30912, USA

Pushkar Mehra
Department of Oral and Maxillofacial Surgery, Boston University Henry M. Goldman School of Dental Medicine, 100 East Newton Street, Boston, MA 02118, USA

Mary B. Goldring
Hospital for Special Surgery Research Institute, Weill Cornell Medical College, New York, NY 10021, USA
Department of Cell and Developmental Biology, Weill Cornell Medical College, New York, NY 10021, USA

Benny Antony, Graeme Jones and Xingzhong Jin
Menzies Institute for Medical Research, University of Tasmania, Hobart, Tasmania 7000, Australia

Changhai Ding
Menzies Institute for Medical Research, University of Tasmania, Hobart, Tasmania 7000, Australia
Institute of Bone & Joint Translational Research, Southern Medical University, Guangzhou, Guangdong, China

Ivan Shirinsky and Valery Shirinsky
Laboratory of Clinical Immunopharmacology, Federal State Budgetary Scientific Institution, Research Institute of Fundamental and Clinical Immunology, 6 Zalesskogo Street, 630047 Novosibirsk, Russia

André Struglics, Per Swärd, Richard Frobell and L. Stefan Lohmander
Department of Clinical Sciences Lund, Orthopaedics, Lund University, Faculty of Medicine, BMC C12, SE-221 84 Lund, Sweden

Anna M. Blom
Department of Translational Medicine, Division of Medical Protein Chemistry, Lund University, Faculty of Medicine, Lund, Sweden

Marcin Okroj
Department of Translational Medicine, Division of Medical Protein Chemistry, Lund University, Faculty of Medicine, Lund, Sweden
Department of Medical Biotechnology, Intercollegiate Faculty of Biotechnology UG-MUG, Medical University of Gdańsk, Gdańsk, Poland

Tore Saxne
Department of Clinical Sciences Lund, Rheumatology, Lund University, Faculty of Medicine, Lund, Sweden

Jean-Pierre Pelletier, Jean-Pierre Raynauld and Johanne Martel-Pelletier
Osteoarthritis Research Unit, University of Montreal Hospital Research Centre (CRCHUM), 900 Saint-Denis, Suite R11.412, Montreal, QC H2X 0A9, Canada

François Abram
Medical Imaging Research & Development, ArthroLab Inc, Montreal, QC, Canada

Marc Dorais
StatSciences Inc, Notre-Dame-de-l'Île-Perrot, QC, Canada

Philippe Delorme
ArthroLab Inc, Montreal, QC, Canada

Michael P. LaValley
Department of Biostatistics, Boston University School of Public Health, 801 Massachusetts Avenue 3rd Floor, Boston, MA 02118, USA

Grace H. Lo
Medical Care Line and Research Care Line, Houston VA HSR&D Center for Innovations in Quality, Effectiveness and Safety, Michael E. DeBakey Medical Center, Houston, TX 77030, USA
Section of Immunology, Allergy and Rheumatology, Baylor College of Medicine, 1 Baylor Plaza, BCM-285, Houston, TX 77030, USA

Lori Lyn Price
Institute for Clinical Research and Health Policy Studies at Tufts Medical Center, Tufts Clinical and Translational Science Institute, Tufts University, 800 Washington Street, MA 02111, USA

Jeffrey B. Driban and Timothy E. McAlindon
Division of Rheumatology Tufts Medical Center, 800 Washington Street, Boston, MA 02111, USA

Charles B. Eaton
Department of Family Medicine, Alpert Medical School of Brown University, 111 Brewster Street, Pawtucket, RI 02860, USA

Jean-Pierre Pelletier and Johanne Martel-Pelletier
Osteoarthritis Research Unit, University of Montreal Hospital Research Centre
(CRCHUM), 900 Saint-Denis, Suite R11.412, Montreal, Quebec H2X 0A9, Canada

Jean-Pierre Raynauld
Osteoarthritis Research Unit, University of Montreal Hospital Research Centre
(CRCHUM), 900 Saint-Denis, Suite R11.412, Montreal, Quebec H2X 0A9, Canada
Institut de rhumatologie de Montréal, Montreal, Quebec, Canada

André D. Beaulieu
Centre de rhumatologie St-Louis, Sainte-Foy, Quebec, Canada

Louis Bessette
Groupe de recherche en Rhumatologie et Maladies Osseuses Inc., Sainte-Foy, Quebec, Canada

Frédéric Morin
Centre de recherche musculo-squelettique, Trois-Rivières, Quebec, Canada

Artur J. de Brum-Fernandes
Service de rhumatologie, Centre hospitalier universitaire de Sherbrooke (CHUS), Sherbrooke, Quebec, Canada

Philippe Delorme, Patrice Paiement and François Abram
ArthroLab Inc., Montreal, Quebec, Canada

Marc Dorais
StatSciences Inc., Notre-Dame de l'Île-Perrot, Quebec, Canada

Pawan Kumar Gupta, Anoop Chullikana, Mathiyazhagan Rengasamy, Prasanth Kulapurathu Vellotare, Devi Damodaran, Pachaiyappan Viswanathan, Sudha Balasubramanian and Anish Sen Majumdar
Stempeutics Research Pvt Ltd, Akshay Tech Park, No. 72 & 73, 2nd Floor, EPIP Zone, Phase I-Area, Whitefield, Bangalore 560066, India

Charan Thej
Stempeutics Research Pvt Ltd, Akshay Tech Park, No. 72 & 73, 2nd Floor, EPIP Zone, Phase I-Area, Whitefield, Bangalore 560066, India
Manipal University, Manipal, India

Naresh Shetty
M.S Ramaiah Medical College & Hospitals, MSR Nagar, MSRIT Post, Bangalore 560054, India

Vivek Pandey
Kasturba Medical College and Hospital, Madhav Nagar, Manipal 576104, India

Vikas Agarwal
Sanjay Gandhi Post Graduate Institute of Medical Sciences, Raebareli Road, Lucknow 226014, India

Shrikant Yeshwant Wagh
Jehangir Clinical Development Center, Jehangir Hospital, 33, Sasoon Road, Pune 411001, India

Tomasz Cudejko and Marike van der Leeden
Department of Rehabilitation Medicine, VU University Medical Center, Amsterdam, The Netherlands
Amsterdam Rehabilitation Research Centre Reade, Dr. J. van Breemenstraat 2, 1056 AB Amsterdam, 1040 HG Amsterdam, The Netherlands

Josien C. van den Noort
Department of Rehabilitation Medicine, VU University Medical Center, Amsterdam, The Netherlands
Department of Radiology and Nuclear Medicine, Musculoskeletal Imaging Quantification Center (MIQC), Academic Medical Center, Amsterdam, The Netherlands

Jaap Harlaar
Department of Rehabilitation Medicine, VU University Medical Center, Amsterdam, The Netherlands
Delft University of Technology, Delft, The Netherlands

Joost Dekker
Department of Rehabilitation Medicine, VU University Medical Center, Amsterdam, The Netherlands
Department of Psychiatry, VU University Medical Center, Amsterdam, The Netherlands

Martin van der Esch and Leo D. Roorda
Amsterdam Rehabilitation Research Centre Reade, Dr. J. van Breemenstraat 2, 1056 AB Amsterdam, 1040 HG Amsterdam, The Netherlands

Willem Lems
Amsterdam Rheumatology & Immunology Center, Amsterdam Medical Center, Reade, VU University Medical Center, Amsterdam, The Netherlands
Jan van Breemen ResearchInstitute, Reade, Amsterdam, The Netherlands

Jos Twisk
Department of Health Sciences, VU University Amsterdam, Amsterdam, The Netherlands
Department of Epidemiology and Biostatistics, VU University Medical Center, Amsterdam, The Netherlands

Martijn Steultjens and James Woodburn
School of Health and Life Sciences, Glasgow Caledonian University, Glasgow, United Kingdom

Matthew J. Parkes
Arthritis Research UK Centre for Epidemiology, Division of Musculoskeletal and Dermatological Sciences, Faculty of Biology, Medicine and Health, Manchester Academic Health Science Centre, University of Manchester, Manchester, UK
NIHR Manchester Musculoskeletal Biomedical Research Unit, Central Manchester University Hospitals NHS Foundation Trust, Manchester Academic Health Sciences Centre, Manchester, UK

Nasimah Maricar
Arthritis Research UK Centre for Epidemiology, Division of Musculoskeletal and Dermatological Sciences, Faculty of Biology, Medicine and Health, Manchester Academic Health Science Centre, University of Manchester, Manchester, UK
NIHR Manchester Musculoskeletal Biomedical Research Unit, Central Manchester University Hospitals NHS Foundation Trust, Manchester Academic Health Sciences Centre, Manchester, UK
Department of Physiotherapy, Salford Royal Hospital NHS Foundation Trust, Manchester, UK

Michael J. Callaghan
Arthritis Research UK Centre for Epidemiology, Division of Musculoskeletal and Dermatological Sciences, Faculty of Biology, Medicine and Health, Manchester Academic Health Science Centre, University of Manchester, Manchester, UK
NIHR Manchester Musculoskeletal Biomedical Research Unit, Central Manchester University Hospitals NHS Foundation Trust, Manchester Academic Health Sciences Centre, Manchester, UK
Department of Health Professions, Manchester Metropolitan University, Manchester, UK

David T. Felson
Arthritis Research UK Centre for Epidemiology, Division of Musculoskeletal and Dermatological Sciences, Faculty of Biology, Medicine and Health, Manchester Academic Health Science Centre, University of Manchester, Manchester, UK
NIHR Manchester Musculoskeletal Biomedical Research Unit, Central Manchester University Hospitals NHS Foundation Trust, Manchester Academic Health Sciences Centre, Manchester, UK
Clinical Epidemiology Unit, Boston University School of Medicine, Boston, MA, USA

Terence W. O'Neill
Arthritis Research UK Centre for Epidemiology, Division of Musculoskeletal and Dermatological Sciences, Faculty of Biology, Medicine and Health, Manchester Academic Health Science Centre, University of Manchester, Manchester, UK
NIHR Manchester Musculoskeletal Biomedical Research Unit, Central Manchester University Hospitals NHS Foundation Trust, Manchester Academic Health Sciences Centre, Manchester, UK
Department of Rheumatology, Salford Royal Hospital NHS Foundation Trust, Manchester, UK

Charles E. Hutchinson, Andrew D. Gait and Richard Hodgson
Imaging Sciences, University of Warwick, Warwick Medical School, Coventry, UK
Centre for Imaging Sciences, Institute of Population Health, The University of Manchester, Manchester, UK

Usman Ahmed and Attia Anwar
Warwick Medical School, Clinical Sciences Research Laboratories, University of Warwick, University Hospital, Coventry CV2 2DX, UK

Paul J. Thornalley and Naila Rabbani
Warwick Medical School, Clinical Sciences Research Laboratories, University of Warwick, University Hospital, Coventry CV2 2DX, UK
Warwick Systems Biology Centre, Senate House, University of Warwick, Coventry CV4 7AL, UK

Richard S. Savage
Warwick Systems Biology Centre, Senate House, University of Warwick, Coventry CV4 7AL, UK

Jianhua Xu, Jingyu Cai and Shuang Zheng
Department of Rheumatology and Immunology, Arthritis Research Institute, the First Affiliated Hospital of Anhui Medical University, 218 Jixi Street, Hefei, China

Kang Wang and Changhai Ding
Department of Rheumatology and Immunology, Arthritis Research Institute, the First Affiliated Hospital of Anhui Medical University, 218 Jixi Street, Hefei, China
Menzies Institute for Medical Research, University of Tasmania, Hobart, Tasmania 7000, Australia

Weiyu Han and Benny Antony
Menzies Institute for Medical Research, University of Tasmania, Hobart, Tasmania 7000, Australia

Eiichi Tsuda, Shugo Maeda, Eiji Sasaki and Yasuyuki Ishibashi
Department of Orthopaedic Surgery, Hirosaki University Graduate School of Medicine, Hirosaki, Japan

Daisuke Chiba
Department of Orthopaedic Surgery, Hirosaki University Graduate School of Medicine, Hirosaki, Japan
Department of Social Medicine, Hirosaki University Graduate School of Medicine, Hirosaki, Japan

Ippei Takahashi and Shigeyuki Nakaji
Department of Social Medicine, Hirosaki University Graduate School of Medicine, Hirosaki, Japan

Yalong Di
Department of Medical Imaging, Hebei General Hospital, Shijiazhuang 050051, China

Changxu Han, Liang Zhao and Yizhong Ren
Department of Sports Medicine, Second Affiliated Hospital of Inner Mongolia Medical University, Huhehaote 010030, China

Charles B. Eaton
Alpert Medical School of Brown University, Providence, USA
School of Public Health of Brown University, Providence, USA
Center of Primary Care and Prevention, Memorial Hospital of Rhode Island, 111 Brewster Street, Pawtucket, RI 02860, USA

Syeda Ameernaz and Mary B. Roberts
Center of Primary Care and Prevention, Memorial Hospital of Rhode Island, 111 Brewster Street, Pawtucket, RI 02860, USA

Maria Sayeed
Department of Medicine, Memorial Hospital of Rhode Island, 111 Brewster Street, Pawtucket, RI, USA

John D. Maynard
Vera Light Inc., 800 Bradbury Dr SE # 217, Albuquerque, NM, USA

Jeffrey B. Driban and Timothy E. McAlindon
Division of Rheumatology, Tufts Medical Center, 800 Washington Street, Boston, MA, USA

Cristóbal Orellana, Juan María García-Manrique, Noemí Navarro and Marta Larrosa
Rheumatology Department, Parc Tauli Sabadell University Hospital, Institute for Research and Innovation Parc Tauli (I3PT), Universitat Autónoma de Barcelona (UAB), 08208 Sabadell, Spain

Joan Calvet and Jordi Gratacós
Rheumatology Department, Parc Tauli Sabadell University Hospital, Institute for Research and Innovation Parc Tauli (I3PT), Universitat Autónoma de Barcelona (UAB), 08208 Sabadell, Spain
Departament de Medicina, Universitat Autónoma de Barcelona (UAB), 08003 Barcelona, Spain

José Chillarón and Juan Pedro-Botet
Departament de Medicina, Universitat Autónoma de Barcelona (UAB), 08003 Barcelona, Spain
Endocrinology and Nutrition Department, Hospital del Mar, 08003 Barcelona, Spain

Antoni Berenguer-Llergo
Biostatistics and Bioinformatics Unit, Institute for Research in Biomedicine Barcelona (IRB Barcelona), 08028 Barcelona, Spain

Assumpta Caixàs
Endocrinology and Nutrition Department, Parc Tauli Sabadell University Hospital, Institute for Research and Innovation Parc Tauli (I3PT), Universitat Autónoma de Barcelona (UAB), 08208 Sabadell, Spain

Index

O

P

R

S

T

V

www.ingramcontent.com/pod-product-compliance
Lightning Source LLC
LaVergne TN
LVHW080650210926
848485LV00003B/358